W9-BNL-543

Lipids and Vascular Disease

Current Issues

LIPIDS AND VASCULAR DISEASE

CURRENT ISSUES

Edited by

D John Betteridge BSc, PhD, MD, FRCP
Consultant Physician UCL Hospitals Trust, and
Professor of Endocrinology and Metabolism
University College London
Department of Medicine
Royal Free and University College Medical School
London W1N 8AA
UK

MARTIN DUNITZ

© Martin Dunitz Ltd 2000

First published in the United Kingdom in 2000 by
Martin Dunitz Ltd
The Livery House
7–9 Pratt Street
London NW1 0AE

Tel: +44 (0)20 7482 2202
Fax: +44 (0)20 7267 0159
E-mail: info.dunitz@tandf.co.uk
Website: http://www.dunitz.co.uk

Reprinted 2001

All rights reserved. No part of this publication may be
reproduced, stored in a retrieval system, or transmitted,
in any form or by any means, electronic, mechanical,
photocopying, recording or otherwise, without the
prior permission of the publisher or in accordance with
the provisions of the Copyright Act 1988.

A CIP catalogue record for this book is available from
the British Library

ISBN 1-85317-627-3

Composition by Wearset, Boldon, Tyne and Wear
Printed and bound in Great Britain by Biddles Ltd,
Guildford and King's Lynn

Contents

CONTENTS

Contributors

Mahmud Barbir
Consultant Cardiologist, Department of
Cardiology, Royal Brompton and Harefield
NHS Trust, Harefield Hospital, Harefield,
Middlesex UB9 6JH, UK

Ulrike Beisiegel
Professor, Medizinische Klinik,
Universitätkrankenhaus Eppendorf,
D-20246 Hamburg, Germany

Jean Davignon
Professor and Director, Hyperlipidemia and
Atherosclerosis Research Group, Clinical
Research Institute of Montréal (IRCM),
Montréal, QC H2W 1R7, Canada

Joep C Defesche
Department of Vascular Medicine, Academic
Medical Centre, University of Amsterdam,
PO Box 22660, 1100 DD Amsterdam, The
Netherlands

Robert Dufour
Hyperlipidemia and Atherosclerosis Research
Group, Clinical Research Institute of Montréal
(IRCM), Montréal, QC H2W 1R7, Canada

Patrick Duriez
Professor, U325 INSERM, Département
d'Athérosclerose, Institut Pasteur de Lille,
Université de Lille II, 59019 Lille, Cedex,
France

Ole Faergeman
Professor of Preventive Cardiology,
Department of Medicine and Cardiology,
Århus Amtssygehus University Hospital, 8000
Århus, Denmark

Bernhard Föger
Professor, Department of Internal Medicine,
Clinic of Internal Medicine, University of
Innsbruck, A-6020 Innsbruck, Austria

Jean-Charles Fruchart
Professor, Département de Recherche sur les
Lipoprotéines et l'Athérosclérose, INSERM
U325, Institut Pasteur de Lille, Université de
Lille II, 59019 Lille, France

Ian M Graham
Consultant Cardiologist, Adelaide-Meath
Hospital, incorporating the National
Children's Hospital, Dublin 24, Ireland

Sandeep Gupta
Consultant Cardiologist, Whipps Cross
Hospital, London E11, and St Bartholomew's
and The Royal London School of Medicine
and Dentistry, London E1 2AD, UK

Juan Carlos Kaski
Department of Cardiological Sciences, St
George's Hospital Medical School, Tooting,
London SW17 0RE, UK

Stefanie Koch
Medizinische Klinik, Universitätkrankenhaus
Eppendorf, D-20246 Hamburg, Germany

Malcolm Law
Wolfson Institute of Preventive Medicine,
Department of Environmental and Preventive
Medicine, St Bartholomew's and The Royal
London School of Medicine and Dentistry,
London EC1M 6BQ

Fawzi Lazem
Department of Cardiothoracic Surgery, Royal
Brompton and Harefield NHS Trust, Harefield
Hospital, Harefield, Middlesex UB9 6JH, UK

Gordon DO Lowe
Professor of Vascular Medicine and Honorary
Consultant Physician, University Department
of Medicine, Royal Infirmary, Glasgow G31
2ER, UK

Bharti Mackness
Research Associate, Department of Medicine,
Manchester Royal Infirmary,
Manchester M13 9WL, UK

Michael I Mackness
Lecturer in Medicine, Department of
Medicine, Manchester Royal Infirmary,
Manchester M13 9WL, UK

Raymond Meleady
Cardiologist, James Connolly Memorial
Hospital, Blanchardstown,
Dublin 15, Ireland

Josef R Patsch
Professor of Medicine and Chairman,
Department of Internal Medicine, Clinic of
Internal Medicine, University of Innsbruck, A-
6020 Innsbruck, Austria

Jacques E Rossouw
Deputy Director, Women's Health Initiative,
National Heart, Lung and Blood Institute,
Bethesda, MD 20892, USA

Bart Staels
Professor, U325 INSERM, Département
d'Athérosclerose, Institut Pasteur de Lille,
59019 Lille, Cedex, France

George Steiner
Professor of Medicine and Physiology,
Toronto General Hospital, University of
Toronto, Toronto, Ontario, M5G 2C4, Canada

Brian Tomlinson
Professor and Honorary Consultant Physician,
Division of Clinical Pharmacology,
Department of Medicine and Therapeutics,
The Chinese University of Hong Kong, Prince
of Wales Hospital, Shatin, NT, Hong Kong

Anthony F Winder
Professor, Department of Molecular Pathology
and Clinical Biochemistry, Royal Free and
University College London Medical School
(Royal Free Campus), and the Cardiovascular
Lipid Clinics, Royal Free NHS Hospital Trust,
London NW3 2QG, UK

David A Wood
Professor of Cardiology, National Heart and
Lung Institute, Imperial College School of
Medicine, London SW3 6LY, and Consultant
Cardiologist, Charing Cross Hospital,
Hammersmith Hospitals NHS Trust, London
W6 8RF, UK

Sir Magdi Yacoub
Professor of Cardiothoracic Surgery,
Department of Cardiothoracic Surgery, Royal
Brompton and Harefield NHS Trust, Harefield
Hospital, Harefield, Middlesex UB9 6JH, UK

Foreword

This book is not meant to be a comprehensive text on lipids and vascular disease. Rather, I have tried to identify important areas of current interest or controversy.

Much is now understood at the basic science and clinical level concerning low-density lipoprotein (LDL) cholesterol and vascular disease. Indeed there is probably no other area of medicine with such a comprehensive evidence base as that pointing to the benefits of LDL-lowering therapy for the primary and secondary prevention of vascular events. However, it is clear that patients still develop vascular events despite LDL lowering and attention is now focusing on other components of dyslipidaemia. For these reasons I have included chapters on postprandial lipaemia, high-density lipoprotein (HDL) and genetic determinants of lipid and lipoprotein concentrations. There is considerable excitement in the peroxisome proliferator activated receptor (PPAR) system; its impact on lipoprotein metabolism and as a target for pharmacological intervention makes it important to include. Lipoproteins are traditionally regarded as important in vascular terms so lipoproteins and the brain form a truly new frontier and a topic of great potential importance.

LDL cholesterol is regarded as the one essential risk factor for atherogenesis but other factors play an important role and there are chapters devoted to fibrinogen, homocysteine and chronic infection as emerging risk factors.

Important high-risk populations where lipids and lipoproteins are likely to enhance risk further and are open to therapeutic manipulation include those with hypertension, diabetes, heart transplantation and non-coronary vascular disease. Chapters are devoted to these areas together with a specific chapter devoted to women and coronary heart disease.

There is no doubt that the clinical availablity of the statin drugs has transformed the care of hypercholesterolaemic patients and has enabled large scale, randomised and double-blind trials with definitive vascular end-points to be performed. Chapters are devoted to the lipid-lowering trials and to an update on statins. Given the recent results of HDL Intervention Trial (VAHIT) fibrates still appear to have a place in management and this is discussed.

Finally, advances in clinical science are futile if they are not implemented in clinical practice and patients do not benefit. In the last couple of years new national and international guidelines on management have been published to help the practising physician. These are comprehensively reviewed in the final chapter.

My heartfelt thanks go to the contributors who have shown immense enthusiasm and timeliness towards this project and produced excellent chapters. My thanks also go to Martin Dunitz, and particularly to Alan Burgess and Mike Meakin for their expert help and encouragement.

1

Postprandial lipaemia

Bernhard Föger and Josef R Patsch

Why study postprandial lipaemia?

Triglyceride-rich lipoproteins (TRLs) transport both dietary fat from the intestine and endogenously synthesised fat from the liver to peripheral tissues for storage and utilization. Physiologically, triglyceride (TG) levels are increased in plasma for approximately 8 hours after a fatty meal,[1] indicating that healthy humans spend the major part of their lifetime in the postprandial state. Interestingly, the levels of fasting and postprandial TRLs in normolipidaemic, healthy, young to middle-aged subjects were found to be associated rather loosely ($r = 0.45$),[1] raising the question which of the two measures would be more informative pathophysiologically. In a seminal study addressing this issue, Patsch *et al.* quantified the triglyceridaemic response to a standardized fat meal in normolipidaemic subjects.[1] The authors observed that, when compared to fasting TG, the magnitude of postprandial lipaemia showed a much tighter inverse relationship to high density lipoprotein-2 (HDL_2) levels[1] and a much closer direct relationship to TG-enrichment of cholesterol-rich lipoproteins, particularly HDL_2.[2,3] The mechanism underlying this relationship relates to the exchange of neutral lipid core components between lipoprotein particles catalysed by cholesteryl ester transfer protein (CETP).[4] In animals that lack CETP, such as the mouse[4] and CETP-deficient humans,[4] cholesteryl esters generated in plasma by lecithin:cholesterol acyltransferase (LCAT) remain with their parent lipoprotein particle (HDL or low density lipoprotein LDL) until extracted from the circulation either by selective cholesteryl ester uptake via scavenger receptor class B, type I (SR-BI)[5] — as is the case with HDL — or by whole particle uptake via cellular receptors such as the LDL receptor, as is the case with LDL. By the same token, TG in chylomicrons and very low density lipoprotein (VLDL), again in the absence of CETP, remain with their respective parent lipoprotein particles leading to a very strict separation between lipoproteins carrying mainly cholesteryl esters (HDL, LDL) and lipoproteins carrying mainly TG (chylomicrons, VLDL) in their core. However in humans, circulating CETP catalyses homo- and hetero-exchange of apolar core lipids — TG and cholesteryl esters (CE) — between all lipoprotein classes, effecting the diversion of CE originally transported with HDL to TRLs on one hand and TG-enrichment of HDL (and LDL) at the expense of TRLs on the other.

CETP action has far-reaching metabolic consequences. Unlike TG, CE transported with TRLs cannot be degraded in the plasma compartment because cholesteryl ester hydrolase activity is absent in plasma, such that

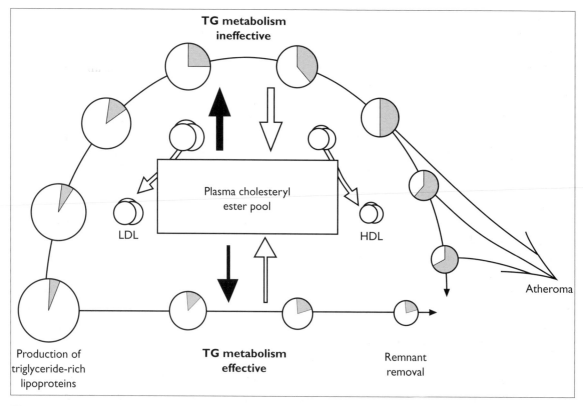

Fig. 1.1

Triglyceride (TG) metabolism: contribution to atherogenesis. In individuals with effective triglyceride metabolism, triglyceride-rich lipoproteins do not accumulate and therefore do not become significantly enriched in cholesteryl esters (CE) (areas with grey tint) through core lipid exchange with the plasma CE pool (arrows with grey tint). In individuals with ineffective triglyceride metabolism, on the contrary, triglyceride-rich lipoproteins are present in high concentrations for a prolonged time, permitting their extensive enrichment with CE derived from the plasma CE pool. CE-enriched remnants are diverted from their physiological removal pathway and deposited at sites where they cause atheromata. The CE withdrawn from the CE pool are replaced by triglycerides (white arrows), the hydrolysis of which leads to a reduction in the size of LDL and HDL. Detectable signs of the atherogenic sequence of events are thus retained on the lipoproteins carrying the plasma CE pool, i.e. LDL and HDL. Reproduced with permission.[6]

particle size is not reduced properly and, eventually, receptor-mediated catabolism of TG-rich remnant particles is impaired. On the other hand, TG transferred to HDL and LDL may subsequently be hydrolysed by lipases such as hepatic lipase, resulting in a reduction of particle core size, and the generation of smaller, denser HDL and LDL species. Thus, CETP action leads to the rerouting of 'good' cholesterol transported with HDL to apoB-containing lipoproteins, which eventually may contribute to atheroma formation (Figure 1.1).

Studies in the postprandial phase by Patsch *et al.*[1-3] illustrated that these adverse consequences of triglyceridaemia were not confined to frank hypertriglyceridaemia (TG = 222–2500 mg/dl),[7] but were also operative in normolipidaemia, attesting to the central role of TG in lipoprotein metabolism in apparently healthy individuals. Two different views of the role of TG in atherogenesis have been advanced. According to one school of thought chylomicron remnants, the TG-depleted end-products of chylomicron catabolism, are particularly atherogenic, at least in part because of their high content of dietary cholesterol. This point of view has been referred to as the 'Zilversmit hypothesis'.[8] The second school of thought was advanced by Patsch and Miesenböck who proposed that any kind of TRL can be atherogenic by virtue of its potential to extract CE from HDL and LDL.[6,9] Schneemann *et al.*[10] and Karpe *et al.*[11] observed that the postprandial increase in TRL-cholesterol is mainly accounted for by apoB-100-carrying VLDL, rather than by apoB-48-carrying chylomicron remnants. The reason for VLDL accumulation in the postprandial phase is both competition with chylomicrons for TG hydrolysis, in other words delayed VLDL catabolism,[10] and increased hepatic VLDL synthesis triggered by increased delivery of dietary free fatty acids to the liver. Based on this observation the authors have challenged the Zilversmit hypothesis and proposed a crucial atherogenic role for postprandial VLDL.[12,13] A third hypothesis proposes that small, dense LDL (LDL pattern B) is a crucial and possibly independent cause of atherogenesis.[14]

While each of these views is biologically plausible and backed up by substantial experimental data, it appears that they are not mutually exclusive. In fact, one wonders whether any of the above tenets is more than a facet of disordered TG metabolism. If so, a broader view of hypertriglyceridaemia can be taken, encompassing the above hypotheses, where

raised TRLs first extract cholesterol from LDL and HDL and in this way become atherogenic and deposit this cholesterol in the vessel wall. The LDL which become small and dense after loss of CE to TRL, then display decreased affinity for the LDL receptor[15] and increased susceptibility for oxidation[16] and subsequent uptake into macrophages via scavenger receptors.[17] Adverse effects on HDL include decreased HDL-cholesterol and a predominance of the HDL$_3$ subfraction.[1–3,8,9] This more comprehensive view of hypertriglyceridaemia has been labelled the 'triglyceride intolerance hypothesis'.[6,9] It proposes that impaired overall TG metabolic capacity imparts CHD risk and that both intestinal and hepatic TRLs may prove to be atherogenic. Thus, the idea behind measuring postprandial lipaemia is to use it not as a surrogate measure for atherogenic lipoproteins confined to the postprandial state, but rather as a challenge test that characterises TG metabolic capacity much more precisely than simple fasting TG levels when the TG clearing machinery is unchallenged and relaxed.

One of the core differences between the above concepts relates to the search for the atherogenic lipoprotein in the postprandial phase, a project which appears to be nowhere near comparison. While most people would agree that all atherogenic lipoproteins contain apoB-48 or apoB-100, few data are available to allow compensation of the atherogenicity of apoB-48 versus apoB-100 containing lipoproteins in humans. In the presence of several heparin-binding sites in the carboxy-terminal 52% of the apoB-100 molecule might be expected to lead to binding to the intimal matrix and retention of the respective lipoprotein particle in the vessel wall, thus adding to the atherogenicity of apoB-100 particles. ApoB-48, on the other hand, lacks the LDL receptor-binding site which also resides in the carboxy-terminal half of apoB-100, a fact that renders apoB-48-containing lipoprotein particles critically dependent on the presence of functional apoE for receptor-mediated clearance from the circulation. Thus, delayed clearance of apoB-48 may promote atherogenicity of these particles. To address this issue, Farese et al.[18] have used targeted mutagenesis of the mouse apoB gene to generate mice that synthesise exclusively either apoB-48 or apoB-100. After crossbreeding both mutant mice to the apoE −/− background, they observed higher VLDL-IDL-LDL cholesterol levels in apoB-48-only mice when compared with both the wild type and, even more so, with apoB-100-only mice.[18] Not surprisingly for a CETP-deficient animal species, both groups showed similar HDL levels. The extent of aortic atherosclerosis correlated strongly with plasma cholesterol levels. The authors concluded that in this mouse model, there are probably no major differences in the intrinsic atherogenicity of apoB-48 and apoB-100 particles, when corrected for plasma cholesterol concentrations.[19] Coming back to the question of postprandial lipaemia and atherogenesis in humans, the study by Farese et al. offers no support for a particular atherogenicity of either intestinal or hepatic lipoproteins. Therefore, the search for a particularly atherogenic lipoprotein may well become more or less moot.

Determinants of postprandial lipaemia

The magnitude of postprandial lipaemia is controlled by numerous genes involved in the transport of both dietary and endogenously synthesised lipids. So far, such a role has been demonstrated for lipoprotein lipase (LPL),[8,20,21] the major enzyme involved in catabolism of TRLs. In addition apoC-II, the activator of LPL, apoC-III, which interferes with receptor-mediated remnant removal, and apoE as a ligand for LDL receptor-related protein (LRP) hold major roles as determinants of the magnitude of postprandial lipaemia. Potentially important are apoB, microsomal triglyceride transfer protein (MTP) and hepatic lipase (HL). Proteins such as CETP,[22,23] phospholipid transfer protein (PLTP),[24,25] and lecithin:cholesterol acyltransferase (LCAT) modulate the response of HDL to postprandial lipaemia.

Fasting and postprandial triglyceride-rich lipoproteins and atherosclerosis

In the following section, a brief review is presented of epidemiological studies, clinical trials, dyslipidaemic settings in humans and in animals, and cell biological studies of the association of TG and postprandial lipaemia with atherosclerosis.

Epidemiological studies

Clinical interest in plasma triglycerides was triggered by epidemiological studies which indicated a role for TRLs in atherogenesis. In numerous cross-sectional studies dating back to the 1950s, elevated plasma TG levels in the fasting[26] and in the postprandial[27] state were found to be more prevalent in patients with coronary heart disease (CHD) than in healthy controls. The univariate association of TG with CHD was corroborated in numerous prospective studies.[28–32] In multivariate data analysis, however, TG was often eliminated by HDL and thus did not constitute an independent risk factor for CHD.[33,34] This fact cannot discount elevated TG levels as cause for CHD, because elevated TG levels are well known to lower HDL-cholesterol.[1–3,7] Thus, elimination of TG in multivariate analysis by HDL-cholesterol would likely imply that elevated TG levels cause CHD by lowering levels of protective HDL. However, many authorities in the field feel strongly that this view does not fully reflect the crucial role of TG in atherogenesis and this notion has gained increasing support in recent studies. Why may the effect of TRLs have been underestimated in these multivariate analyses? One reason could be that lipid analyses have most often been performed in a postabsorptive state, when lipoprotein concentrations in plasma have reached a steady state. However, several lines of thought indicate that TG should not be measured in the fasting state but rather in the postprandial state, when influx of dietary chylomicrons disturbs the steady state equilibrium for hours.[1] Secondly, the area under the incremental TG concentrations in plasma measured after a standardised fatty meal, that is, postprandial lipaemia, shows a much tighter inverse relationship with HDL-cholesterol than fasting TG.[1] Thus, assessment of postprandial lipaemia characterises the TG metabolic capacity considerably better than simple fasting TG levels. Thirdly, whereas postprandial lipaemia is highly reproducible, the biological variability of fasting TG values is in the order of 20%, much higher than the biological variability of HDL-determinations, which is less than 10%.[35] Accordingly, Patsch *et al.* hypothesised that an independent contribution of TRLs to atherogenesis might be more easily discernible using postprandial TG values.[36] In a large cross-sectional study examining 61 men with severe coronary artery disease (CAD) and 40 healthy men without CAD (verified by angiography) the investigators measured cholesterol, TG, HDL-cholesterol, HDL$_2$-cholesterol, and apolipoproteins A-I, A-II, and B in fasting plasma and TG before and 2, 4, 6 and 8 hours after a standardised test meal. Both the maximal TG increase and the magnitude of post-

prandial lipaemia (area under the TG curve for 8 hours after the test meal) were higher in patients than in controls. Single postprandial TG values taken 6 and 8 hours after the meal were highly discriminatory ($P < 0.001$) and, by logistic regression analysis, displayed an accuracy of 68% in predicting the presence or absence of CAD. In this regard, the accuracy of TG levels was higher than that of HDL$_2$-cholesterol levels (64%) and equal to that of apoB levels (68%), the most discriminatory fasting parameter. Multivariate logistic regression analysis selected postprandial but not fasting TG into the most accurate model that also contained the accepted risk factors HDL$_2$-cholesterol, apoB, and age. This model classified disease status of 82% of the subjects correctly. The authors concluded that TG levels are independent predictors of CAD in multivariate analyses that include HDL-cholesterol, provided that a challenge test of TG metabolism (such as postprandial lipaemia) is used. By its multivariate design, this study corroborated and extended previous investigations linking deranged postprandial lipoprotein metabolism to CAD.

Simons *et al.*[37] reported an increased postprandial apoB-48:apoB-100 ratio in TRL in 82 patients with CHD. Simpson *et al.*[38] noted exaggerated and prolonged postprandial lipaemia in 34 cases when compared with 18 controls. In addition, they observed increased retinyl palmitate concentrations in the plasma fraction d < 1.006 g/ml measured at 24 hours in patients with CHD.[38] Retinyl palmitate is secreted from the intestine with chylomicrons and stays with the particle until chylomicron remnants are taken up by the liver. As retinyl esters are not re-secreted from the liver with VLDL they serve as a marker of intestinal lipoproteins.[39] Based on these findings, the authors implicated TRLs and, in particular, chylomicron remnants in atherogenesis. Groot *et al.*[40] confirmed these results in strictly normotriglyceridaemic men (TG < 200 mg/dl), again illustrating the fact that postprandial TG values are much more informative and more closely linked with disease than fasting TG. In a carefully conducted study, Syvänne *et al.*[41] determined TG, retinyl palmitate, and cholesterol in plasma and in six TRL fractions separated by density in four groups of men (each $n = 15$): type 2 diabetic men with and without CAD and non-diabetic men with and without CAD. Postprandial TG and retinyl palmitate responses were higher in both diabetic groups than in healthy controls and higher in non-diabetic CAD patients than in healthy controls. The most marked differences were found in large VLDL (Svedberg flotation rate (Sf) = 60–400). Somewhat unexpectedly, however, no differences were observed between type 2 diabetic men with CAD (verified by angiography) and those without CAD (verified by thallium-exercise scan). The authors cautioned that a relatively small sample size, cross-sectional design and lack of angiographic assessment of disease status in type 2 diabetic men without CAD may have contributed to the negative result of the study regarding postprandial TRLs and atherosclerosis in diabetic patients.

In a large, community based study of postprandial lipaemia, Ginsberg *et al.* measured plasma TG, TG in plasma fraction d < 1.006, and plasma retinyl palmitate in 92 men and 113 women either with or without newly diagnosed exercise-induced angina pectoris.[42] In men with a body mass index (BMI) of less than 30 kg/m^2, postprandial TG (odds ratio 1.83, $P < 0.05$) and postprandial retinyl palmitate (odds ratio 2.77, $P < 0.05$) were included separately in multivariate models explaining disease status. In addition to postprandial lipids, these models included fasting TG, LDL-cholesterol and hypertension. In contrast, the investigators found no correlation between postprandial TG, retinyl palmitate and disease status in men with BMI > 30 kg/m^2 or in women. The authors suggest that postprandial hyperlipidaemia in obese subjects may be less closely linked with CHD than in non-obese subjects, possibly because of a preponderance of large-sized, less atherogenic TRLs in obesity. This view has received support from the Atherosclerosis Risk in Communities (ARIC) study which examined the postprandial TG response in subjects with and without asymptomatic carotid artery atherosclerosis determined by ultrasonography.[43] Again, postprandial lipaemia in obese white men and women was similar in cases and controls. In contrast, non-obese white men and women had significantly increased postprandial lipaemia compared with controls. Importantly, this study failed to observe a sex difference in this relationship. In a smaller previous study, Ryu *et al.*[44] related the results of a fat tolerance test to carotid artery wall thickness in 47 asymptomatic middle-aged individuals, as measured by B-mode ultrasound. Peak TG response was significantly and directly associated with carotid wall thickness in univariate and multivariate analysis, thereby providing the first link between postprandial hyperlipidaemia and carotid atherosclerosis. To assess the importance of postprandial lipaemia as a predisposing factor for atherosclerosis, Slyper *et al.*[45] studied postprandial lipaemia and chylomicron clearance (using a vitamin A–fat load test) in children of parents with early CHD. No difference was observed between the two study groups, a finding that is at variance with a previous study employing a similar design performed by Uiterwaal and coworkers.[46] Taken together, studies in the postprandial state provide strong support for an important role of TG in the development of atherosclerosis.

In the meantime, subsequent studies have been able to conclusively establish the connection between TG levels and CHD using the more usual but less powerful marker of TG metabolism, in other words postabsorptive TG levels. A recent meta-analysis of 17 prospective, population-based studies conducted between 1965 and 1997 showed that plasma TG is indeed a risk factor for cardiovascular disease independent of HDL-cholesterol.[47] This study attributes a relative risk for CHD of 1.32 for men and of 1.76 for women for each 1 mmol/l (88 mg/dl) increase in plasma TG.[47] Also, the 8-year follow-up data from the prospective Copenhagen Male Study have identified fasting TG as an independent risk factor for CHD in middle-aged and elderly white men.[48] After adjustment for confounding variables such as HDL-cholesterol, the authors attributed a relative risk for CHD of 1.5 and 2.2 to men with TG in the middle and highest tertile when compared with men in the lowest tertile. Complementing the data in men, a previous report from Framingham has already established TG as an independent risk factor in women between the ages of 50 and 69 years.[28] In the Paris Prospective Study, Fontbonne *et al.* identified hypertriglyceridaemia as the sole independent risk factor for CHD mortality among middle-aged men with impaired glucose tolerance or type 2 diabetes.[30] However, HDL-cholesterol levels were not available in these subjects.

Taken together, epidemiological studies suggest that triglycerides cause atherosclerosis by effects both dependent and independent of HDL lowering. They indicate that TG levels are a substantially stronger independent risk factor in women than in men[28,47] and, perhaps (although to date this remains to be proven) a stronger independent risk factor in diabetic patients than in the general population.[30,49] Triglycerides interact synergistically with other lipoproteins. In other words, elevated TG levels impart risk preferentially to subjects concomitantly displaying high LDL and low HDL levels,[31,50] which also explains the finding that, among populations, hypertriglyceridaemia is less closely related to CHD incidence than plasma cholesterol.[51] This concept of interaction between risk factors, referred to as the 'lipid triad', that is high TG levels, small, dense LDL particles, and low HDL levels, is plausible physiologically and has been gaining widespread acceptance lately.

Clinical trials

The most crucial test for a risk factor is reversibility. Does lowering TG levels decrease CHD? As interventions that lower solely TG are not available now and most likely will not be in the future, the closest answer to the above question comes from clinical trial data from studies of drugs that lower primarily TG levels. In primary prevention, treatment with clofibrate led to a 20% reduction in CHD incidence in the WHO Co-operative Study.[52] Treatment with gemfibrozil, another fibric-acid derivative, resulted in a 34% reduction in CHD incidence in the Helsinki Heart Study.[53] However, a concomitant decrease in LDL-cholesterol of approximately 10% precludes one from assigning the beneficial effects of gemfibrozil solely to TG lowering. One of two recent fibrate trials in the secondary prevention of CHD avoids this ambiguity.[54,55] The Department of Veterans Affairs High-Density Lipoprotein Cholesterol Intervention Trial (HIT) studied the effects of gemfibrozil versus placebo in 2500 men with CHD and TG < 300 mg/dl, LDL-cholesterol < 140 mg/dl, and HDL-cholesterol < 40 mg/dl.[54] The study thus recruited subjects with two common lipoprotein phenotypes, namely HTG with low HDL and isolated low HDL. These phenotypes are found in 14.7% and 4%, respectively, of kindreds with premature CHD.[56] In HIT, gemfibrozil lowered TG by 24% and increased HDL-cholesterol by 7.5%, whereas LDL remained virtually unchanged. Thus, the decrease of 22% in CHD incidence definitely reflects a beneficial effect of gemfibrozil other than LDL lowering. The above trials clearly establish that fibrates prevent CHD events, specifically nonfatal myocardial infarction. This could be due to retardation of atherosclerosis progression *per se*, or it could be caused by an improved haemostatic balance as fibrates have been shown to decrease fibrinogen[57] and plasminogen-activator inhibitor-1 (PAI-1) levels.[58]

Unequivocal support for a direct antiatherogenic role of fibrates has come from two recent angiographic trials. The Bezafibrate Coronary Atherosclerosis Intervention Trial (BCAIT) evaluated whether treatment with bezafibrate for 5 years could retard angiographic progression in dyslipidaemic survivors of a premature myocardial infarction.[59] Bezafibrate lowered TG levels by 31% and increased HDL-cholesterol by 9%, whereas LDL-cholesterol did not change. Bezafibrate significantly reduced atherosclerosis progression and the quantity of the favourable effect was similar to that achieved in trials using HMG-CoA reductase inhibitors. In addition, bezafibrate significantly reduced the clinical endpoints, that is coronary events. The positive results of BCAIT are corroborated by the results of the Lopid Coronary Angiography Trial (LOCAT) which randomly assigned 395 men with low HDL-cholesterol after coronary artery bypass grafting to either placebo or gemfibrozil.[60,61] Gemfibrozil reduced lesion progression in native vessels and virtually abolished development of new lesions in grafted vessels. Interestingly, VLDL was the lipoprotein most predictive of the development of new lesions in vein grafts.[61] These exciting findings are in line with previous angiography trials linking fasting and postprandial TRLs to CHD progression. In the drug-treatment groups of both the Cholesterol Lowering Atherosclerosis Study (CLAS) and the Monitored Atherosclerosis Regression Study (MARS), the apoC-III concentration in the heparin precipitate (apoC-III HP) emerged as the major determinant of atherosclerosis progression in multivariate analyses.[62,63] ApoC-III, secreted by the liver as a component of VLDL, delays plasma clearance of TRLs primarily by interfering with hepatic uptake of TRL remnants. Thus, transfer of apoC-III from its storage pool in plasma (HDL) to VLDL delays TRL catabolism, indicating compromised TG metabolic capacity. The observation that subjects with high levels of apoC-III in the heparin precipitate, that is apoB-containing lipoproteins, were much more susceptible to disease progression provides clear evidence for an important role of TG in secondary prevention. This role was particularly evident when the accepted, strong risk factor of LDL-cholesterol was removed by aggressive lipid-lowering (with niacin plus colestipol in CLAS and lovastatin in MARS). In a subset of subjects in MARS, investigators tried to pin down the atherogenic lipoprotein, as defined by apolipoprotein composition, and attributed much of the atherogenicity of apoB-containing lipoproteins to lipoproteins containing both apoB and apoA-II, apoC, apoD, and apoE in various combinations (i.e. LpB:C, LpB:C:E, LpA-II:B:C:D:E).[64] Another interesting finding of these studies was the fact that TRLs appeared to be more important for the progression of mild and moderate lesions compared with severe lesions.[63] Currently, large clinical endpoint studies are underway to measure the effects of fenofibrate in primary and secondary prevention in the diabetic population.

The only study to investigate the relationship of postprandial lipoproteins to the angiographic progression of coronary atherosclerosis was performed by Karpe *et al.*[65] Measuring apoB-48 and apoB-100 levels in lipoprotein fractions corresponding to chylomicrons, large VLDL and small VLDL in 17 normotriglyceridaemic postinfarction patients, 15 hypertriglyceridaemic postinfarction patients, and 10 healthy controls they found a direct association with apoB-48 in small VLDL, in other words a surrogate marker of chylomicron remnants with CAD progression. The strength of this relationship was not altered after adjustment for possible confounders, like HDL-cholesterol or apoB concentration in dense LDL. However, apoB-48 concentration in small VLDL did not differ between the three study groups and was unrelated to the extent of CAD at baseline. The authors conclude that small chylomicron remnants probably contribute to the progression of coronary atherosclerosis.

Cell biological studies

The first cell biological studies to define more clearly the atherogenic potential of TRLs were performed by Gianturco *et al.*[66] They observed that hypertriglyceridaemic, but not normotriglyceridaemic VLDL particles were able to induce lipid accumulation in peritoneal macrophages. The authors emphasized that large VLDL and chylomicrons are the only native plasma lipoproteins that, without prior modification *in vitro*, can induce foam cell formation. In contrast to chylomicrons, which are too large to penetrate the endothelium, chylomicron remnants and small VLDL (Sf < 60, corresponding to a particle diameter of less than 35 nm) readily enter the intima.[67] In fact, isolation of TRLs from atherosclerotic plaques by anti-apoB immunosorption has established definitely that TRLs can directly contribute to atherogenesis in humans.[68] In studies with cholesterol-fed rabbits, chylomicron and VLDL remnants have previously been identified as major contributors to atheroma formation in the aorta.[69]

Studies of human and animal models

Analysis of human monogenic dyslipidaemias has highlighted the non-linearity of the relationship between TG levels and CHD. Some dissenting voices notwithstanding,[70] most researchers believe that type I-hyperlipoproteinaemia due to homozygous LPL deficiency does not constitute a pro-atherogenic state despite plasma TG levels of several thousands on an unrestricted diet and very low HDL levels.[71] This is readily explainable considering that unlipolysed chylomicrons are unable to enter the vessel wall and that LDL levels in this condition are also very low. A similar situation has been noted in the rabbit, where chylomicronaemia induced by alloxan-diabetes actually has an anti-atherosclerotic effect.[72] In contrast, accumulation of smaller, partially lipolysed remnant particles of intestinal and hepatic TRLs in type III-hyperlipoproteinaemia leads to a high incidence of premature vascular disease.[73] Accumulation of remnants in type III results from a combination of homozygosity for a mutant form of apoE (apoE-2), which binds poorly to lipoprotein receptors, and VLDL overproduction. Type III-hyperlipoproteinaemia illustrates the critical role of lipoprotein remnants in the pathogenesis of atherosclerosis. In keeping with this view is the observation from PROCAM in which there was a positive, virtually linear association between TG levels and CHD up to TG ~500 mg/dl, beyond which the relationship is less strong.

Animal models of atherosclerosis generated by transgenic and gene-targeting approaches have advanced significantly our understanding of dyslipidaemia and atherogenesis. Although beyond the direct scope of this review, we feel that three major findings are very valuable in complementing the concepts outlined above. First, increased plasma HDL levels achieved by overexpression of human apoA-I in different animal models[74–76] protect against the development of atherosclerosis, clearly indicating a direct anti-atherogenic role of HDL. Second, overexpression of LPL protects against[77] and deficiency of apoE predisposes towards[78] the development of atherosclerosis, demonstrating that delays in both the first and the second step of chylomicron catabolism are potentially pro-atherogenic. Third, isolated hypertriglyceridaemia without major changes in HDL in mice overexpressing human apoC-III is moderately pro-atherogenic.[79] Interpretation of these studies is facilitated by the deficiency in mice of CETP, the major link between TG and HDL. Thus, perturbations in TG metabolism can be studied in isolation, without major concomitant changes in HDL.

Conclusion

Studies in the postprandial state have proven to be particularly informative regarding TG metabolic capacity and have been extremely helpful in establishing hypertriglyceridaemia as an important risk factor for the development and progression of coronary heart disease. Interventions that lower triglycerides and raise HDL constitute a promising complementary approach to LDL lowering in the primary and secondary prevention of coronary heart disease.

References

1. Patsch JR, Karlin JB, Scott LW, *et al.* Inverse relationship between blood levels of high density lipoprotein subfraction 2 and magnitude of postprandial lipemia. *Proc Natl Acad Sci USA* 1983; 80:1449–53.

2. Patsch JR, Prasad S, Gotto AM Jr, Bengtsson-Olivecrona G. Postprandial lipemia: A key for the conversion of high density lipoprotein$_2$ into high density lipoprotein$_3$ by hepatic lipase. *J Clin Invest* 1984; 74:2017–23.

3. Patsch JR, Prasad S, Gotto AM Jr, Patsch W. High density lipoprotein$_2$: Relationship of the plasma levels of this lipoprotein species to its composition, to the magnitude of postprandial lipemia, and to the activities of lipoprotein lipase and hepatic lipase. *J Clin Invest* 1987; 80:341–7.

4. Tall AR. Plasma cholesteryl ester transfer protein. *J Lipid Res* 1993; 34:1255–74.

5. Acton S, Rigotti A, Landschulz K, *et al.* Identification of scavenger receptor SR-BI as a high-density lipoprotein receptor. *Science* 1996; 271:518–20.

6. Miesenböck G, Patsch JR. Postprandial hyperlipidemia: the search for the atherogenic lipoprotein. *Curr Opin Lipidol* 1992; **3**: 196–201.

7. Eisenberg S, Gavish D, Oschry Y, *et al.* Abnormalities in very low, low, and high density lipoproteins in hypertriglyceridemia. *J Clin Invest* 1984; 74:470–82.

8. Zilversmit DB. Atherogenesis: A postprandial phenomenon. *Circulation* 1979; **60**:473–85.

9. Miesenböck G, Hölzl B, Föger B, *et al.* Heterozygous lipoprotein lipase deficiency due to a missense mutation as the cause of impaired triglyceride tolerance with multiple lipoprotein abnormalities. *J Clin Invest* 1993; 91:448–55.

10. Schneemann BO, Kotite L, Todd KM, Havel RJ. Relationships between the responses of triglyceride-rich lipoproteins in blood plasma containing apolipoproteins B-48 and B-100 to a fat-containing meal in normolipidemic humans. *Procl Natl Acad Sci USA* 1993; **90**: 2069–73.

11. Karpe F, Steiner G, Olivecrona T, *et al.* Metabolism of triglyceride-rich lipoproteins during alimentary lipemia. *J Clin Invest* 1993; 91:748–58.

12. Björkegren J, Karpe F, Milne RW, Hamsten A. Differences in apolipoprotein and lipid composition between human chylomicron remnants and very low density lipoproteins isolated from fasting and postprandial plasma. *J Lipid Res* 1998; **39**:1412–20.

13. Karpe F, Hellenius ML, Hamsten A. Differences in the postprandial concentrations of very-low-density lipoprotein and chylomicron remnants between normotriglyceridemic and hypertriglyceridemic men with and without coronary heart disease. *Metabolism* 1999; **48**:301–7.

14. Austin MA, Breslow JL, Hennekes CH, *et al.* Low density lipoprotein subclass patterns and risk of myocardial infarction. *JAMA* 1988; **260**: 1917–21.

15. McKeone BJ, Patsch JR, Pownall HJ. Plasma triglycerides determine low density lipoprotein composition, physical properties, and cell-specific binding in cultured cells. *J Clin Invest* 1993; **91**:1926–33.

16. De Graaf J, Hendriks JCM, Demacker PNM, Stalenhoef AFH. Identification of multiple dense LDL subfractions with enhanced susceptibility to in vitro oxidation among hypertriglyceridemic subjects. *Arteriosclerosis Thromb* 1993; **13**:712–19.

17. Lechleitner M, Hoppichler F, Föger B, Patsch JR. Low density lipoproteins of the postprandial state induce increased cellular cholesteryl ester accumulation in macrophages. *Arteriosclerosis Thromb* 1994; **14**:1799–807.

18. Farese RV Jr, Veniant MM, Cham CM, *et al.* Phenotypic analysis of mice expressing exclusively apolipoprotein B48 or apolipoprotein B100. *Proc Natl Acad Sci USA* 1996; **93**: 6393–8.

19. Veniant MM, Pierotti V, Newland D, *et al.* Susceptibility to atherosclerosis in mice expressing exclusively apolipoprotein B48 or apolipoprotein B100. *J Clin Invest* 1997; **100**:180–8.

20. Föger B, Königsrainer A, Palos G, *et al.* Effect of pancreas transplantation on lipoprotein lipase, postprandial lipaemia, and HDL cholesterol. *Transplantation* 1994; **58**:899–904.

21. Föger B, Königsrainer A, Palos G, *et al.* Effects of pancreas transplantation on distribution and composition of plasma lipoproteins. *Metabolism* 1996; **45**:856–61.

22. Föger B, Ritsch A, Doblinger A, *et al.* Relationship of plasma cholesteryl ester transfer protein to HDL cholesterol. Studies in normotriglyceridemia and moderate hypertriglyceridemia. *Arteriosclerosis Thromb Vasc Biol* 1996; **16**:1430–6.

23. Ritsch A, Drexel H, Amann FW, *et al.* Deficiency of cholesteryl ester transfer protein. Description of the molecular defect and the dissociation of cholesteryl ester and triglyceride transport in plasma. *Arteriosclerosis Thromb Vasc Biol* 1997; **17**:3433–41.

24. Föger B, Santamarina-Fojo S, Shamburek RD, *et al.* Plasma phospholipid transfer protein: adenovirus mediated overexpression in mice leads to decreased plasma HDL and enhanced hepatic uptake of phospholipids and cholesteryl esters from HDL. *J Biol Chem* 1997; **272**: 27393–400.

25. Jiang X, Bruce C, Mar J, *et al.* Targeted mutation of phospholipid transfer protein gene markedly reduces high-density lipoprotein levels. *J Clin Invest* 1999; **103**:907–14.

26. Gofman JW, deLalla O, Glazier F, *et al.* The serum lipoprotein transport system in health, metabolic disorders, atherosclerosis and coronary artery disease. *Plasma* 1954; **2**:413–84.

27. Albrink MJ, Man EB. Serum triglycerides in coronary artery disease. *Arch Intern Med* 1959; **103**:4–8.

28. Castelli WP. Epidemiology of triglycerides: a view from Framingham. *Am J Cardiol* 1992; **70(suppl.)**:3H–9H.

29. Carlson LA, Böttiger LE, Ahfeldt PE. Risk factors for myocardial infarction in the Stockholm prospective study. *Acta Med Scand* 1979; **206**:351–60.

30. Fontbonne A, Eschwege E, Cambien F, *et al.* Hypertriglyceridemia as a risk factor of coronary heart disease mortality in subjects with impaired glucose tolerance or diabetes. *Diabetologia* 1989; **32**:300–4.

31. Assmann G, Schulte H. Relation of high-density lipoprotein cholesterol and triglycerides to incidence of atherosclerotic coronary artery disease (the PROCAM experience). *Am J Cardiol* 1992; **70**:733–7.

32. Bainton D, Miller NE, Bolton CH, *et al.* Plasma triglyceride and high-density lipoprotein cholesterol as predictors of ischemic heart disease in British men: the Caerphilly and Speedwell Collaborative Heart Disease Studies. *Br Heart J* 1992; **68**:60–6.

33. Hulley SB, Roseman RH, Bawol RD, Brand RJ. Epidemiology as a guide to clinical deci-

sions. The association between triglyceride and coronary heart disease. *N Engl J Med* 1980; **302**:1383–9.

34. Criqui MH, Heiss G, Cohn R, *et al*. Plasma triglyceride level and mortality from coronary heart disease. *N Engl J Med* 1993; **328**: 1220–5.

35. Durrington PN. Triglycerides are more important in atherosclerosis than epidemiology has suggested. *Atherosclerosis* 1998; **141**(suppl.):S57–S62.

36. Patsch JR, Miesenböck G, Hopferwieser T, *et al*. The relationship of triglyceride metabolism and coronary artery disease: Studies in the postprandial state. *Arteriosclerosis Thromb* 1992; **12**:1336–45.

37. Simons LA, Dwyer T, Simons J, *et al*. Chylomicrons and chylomicron remnants in coronary artery disease: A case-control study. *Atherosclerosis* 1987; **65**:181–9.

38. Simpson HS, Williamson CM, Olivecrona T, *et al*. Postprandial lipemia, fenofibrate and coronary artery disease. *Atherosclerosis* 1990, **85**:193–202.

39. Goodman WS, Blomstrand R, Werner B, *et al*. The intestinal absorption and metabolism of vitamin A and β-Carotene in man. *J Clin Invest* 1966; **45**:1615–23.

40. Groot PHE, van Stiphuit WAHJ, Krauss XH, *et al*. Postprandial lipoprotein metabolism in normolipidemic men with and without coronary artery disease. *Arteriosclerosis Thromb* 1991; **11**:653–62.

41. Syvänne M, Hilden H, Taskinen MR. Abnormal metabolism of postprandial lipoproteins in patients with non-insulin-dependent diabetes mellitus is not related to coronary artery disease. *J Lipid Res* 1994; **35**:15–26.

42. Ginsberg HN, Jones J, Blaner WS, *et al*. Association of postprandial triglyceride and retinly palmitate responses with newly diagnosed exercise-induced myocardial ischemia in middle-aged men and women. *Arteriosclerosis Thromb Vasc Biol* 1995; **15**:1829–38.

43. Sharrett AR, Chambless LE, Heiss G, *et al*., for the ARIC investigators. Association of postprandial triglyceride and retinly palmitate responses with asymptomatic carotid artery atherosclerosis in middle aged men and women. *Arteriosclerosis Thromb Vasc Biol* 1995; **15**:2122–9.

44. Ryu JE, Howard G, Craven TE, *et al*. Postprandial triglyceridemia and carotid atherosclerosis in middle-aged subjects. *Stroke* 1992; **23**:823–8.

45. Slyper AH, Zereva S, Schectman G, *et al*. Normal postprandial lipemia and chylomicron clearance in offspring of parents with early coronary artery disease. *J Clin Endocrinol Metab* 1998; **83**:1106–13.

46. Uiterwaal CSPM, Grobbee DE, Witteman JCM, *et al*. Postprandial triglyceride response in young adult men and familial risk for coronary atherosclerosis. *Ann Intern Med* 1994; **121**:576–83.

47. Hokanson JE, Austin MA. Plasma triglyceride level is a risk factor for cardiovascular disease independent of high-density lipoprotein cholesterol level: a meta-analysis of population-based prospective studies. *J Cardiovasc Res* 1996; **3**:213–19.

48. Jeppesen J, Hein HO, Suadicani P, Gyntelberg F. Triglyceride concentration and ischemic heart disease. *Circulation* 1998; **97**:1029–36.

49. Laakso M, Lehto S, Penttilä I, Pyörälä K. Lipids and lipoproteins predicting coronary heart disease mortality and morbidity in patients with non-insulin-dependent diabetes. *Circulation* 1993; **88**:4121–30.

50. Manninen V, Tenkanen L, Koskinen P, *et al*. Joint effects of serum triglyceride and LDL cholesterol concentrations on coronary heart disease risk in the Helsinki Heart Study. *Circulation* 1992; **85**:37–45.

51. Simons LA. Interrelations of lipids and lipoproteins with coronary artery disease mortality in 19 countries. *Am J Cardiol* 1986; **57**:5G–10G.

52. Oliver MF, Heady JA, Morris JN, Cooper J. A co-operative trial in the primary prevention of ischemic heart disease using clofibrate. *Br Heart J* 1978; **40**:1069–118.

53. Frick MH, Elo O, Haapa K, *et al*. Helsinki Heart Study: primary prevention trial with gemfibrozil in middle-aged men with dyslipidemia. *N Engl J Med* 1987; **317**:1237–45.

54. Rubins HB, Robins SJ, Iwane MK, *et al*. Rationale and design of the Department of Veterans Affairs high-density lipoprotein cholesterol intervention trial (HIT) for secondary preven-

tion of coronary artery disease in men with low high-density lipoprotein cholesterol and desirable low-density lipoprotein cholesterol. *Am J Cardiol* 1993; **71**:45–52.

55. Goldbourt U, Brunner D, Behar S, Reicher-Reiss H. Baseline characteristics of patients participating in the Bezafibrate Infarction Prevention (BIP) study. *Eur Heart J* 1998; **19(suppl.)**:H42–H47.

56. Genest Jr JJ, Martin-Munley SS, McNamara JR, *et al.* Familial lipoprotein disorders in patients with premature coronary artery disease. *Circulation* 1992; **85**:2025–33.

57. Föger B, Tröbinger G, Ritsch A, *et al.* Treatment of primary mixed hyperlipidemia with etophylline clofibrate: effects on lipoprotein composition, lipoprotein-modifying enzymes, and postprandial lipoprotein metabolism. *Atherosclerosis* 1995; **117**:253–61.

58. Eriksson P, Nilsson L, Karpe F, Hamsten A. Very-low-density lipoprotein response element in the promoter region of the human plasminogen activator inhibitor-1 gene implicated in the impaired fibrinolysis of hypertriglyceridemia. *Arteriosclerosis Thromb Vasc Biol* 1998; **18**:20–6.

59. Ericsson CG, Hamsten A, Nilsson J, *et al.* Angiographic assessment of effects of bezafibrate on progression of coronary artery disease in young male postinfarction patients. *Lancet* 1996; **347**:849–53.

60. Frick MH, Syvänne M, Nieminen MS, *et al.*, for the Lopid Coronary Angiography Trial (LOCAT) Study Group. Prevention of the angiographic progression of coronary and vein-graft atherosclerosis by gemfibrozil after coronary bypass surgery in men with low levels of HDL cholesterol. *Circulation* 1997; **96**:2137–43.

61. Syvänne M, Nieminen MS, Frick MH, *et al.* Associations between lipoproteins and the progression of coronary and vein-graft atherosclerosis in a controlled trial with gemfibrozil in men with low baseline levels of HDL cholesterol. *Circulation* 1998; **98**:1993–9.

62. Blankenhorn DH, Alaupovic P, Wickham E, *et al.* Prediction of angiographic change in native human coronary arteries and aortocoronary bypass grafts: lipid and nonlipid factors. *Circulation* 1990; **81**:470–6.

63. Hodis HN, Mack WJ, Azen SP, *et al.* Triglyceride- and cholesterol-rich lipoproteins have a differential effect on mild/moderate and severe lesion progression as assessed by quantitative coronary angiography in a controlled trial of lovastatin. *Circulation* 1994; **90**:42–9.

64. Alaupovic P, Mack WJ, Knight-Ginson C, Hodis HN. The role of triglyceride-rich lipoprotein families in the progression of atherosclerotic lesions as determined by sequential coronary angiography from a controlled clinical trial. *Arteriosclerosis Thromb Vasc Biol* 1997; **17**:715–22.

65. Karpe F, Steiner G, Uffelman K, *et al.* Postprandial lipoproteins and progression of coronary atherosclerosis. *Atherosclerosis* 1994; **106**:83–97.

66. Gianturco SH, Bradley WA, Gotto AM Jr. Hypertriglyceridemic very low density lipoproteins induce triglyceride synthesis and accumulation in mouse peritoneal macrophages. *J Clin Invest* 1982; **70**:168–76.

67. Shaikh M, Wootton R, Nordestgaard BG. Quantitative studies of transfer in vivo of low density, Sf 12-60, and Sf 60-400 lipoproteins between plasma and arterial intima in humans. *Arteriosclerosis Thromb* 1991; **11**:569–77.

68. Rapp JH, Lespine A, Hamilton RL, *et al.* Triglyceride-rich lipoproteins isolated by selected-affinity anti-apolipoprotein B immunosorption from human atherosclerotic plaque. *Arteriosclerosis Thromb* 1994; **14**: 1767–74.

69. Daugherty A, Lange LG, Sobel BE, Schonfeld G. Aortic accumulation and plasma clearance of beta-VLDL and HDL: effects of diet-induced hypercholesterolemia in rabbits. *J Lipid Res* 1985; **26**:955–63.

70. Benlian P, de Gennes JL, Foubert L, *et al.* Premature atherosclerosis in patients with familial chylomicronemia caused by mutations in the lipoprotein lipase gene. *N Engl J Med* 1996; **335**:848–54.

71. Brunzell JD. Familial lipoprotein lipase deficiency and other causes of the chylomicronemia syndrome. In: Scriver CR, Beaudet AL, Sly WS, Valle D, eds. *The metabolic and molecular basis of inherited disease*, 7th edn. New York: McGraw-Hill; 1995: 1913–32.

72. Nordestgaard BG, Stender S, Kjeldsen K. Reduced atherogenesis in cholesterol fed dia-

betic rabbits. Giant lipoproteins do not enter the arterial wall. *Arteriosclerosis* 1988; 8:421–8.

73. Mahley WH, Rall SC Jr. Type III hyper-lipoproteinemia (dysbetalipoproteinemia): The role of apolipoprotein E in normal and abnormal lipoprotein metabolism. In: Scriver CR, Beaudet AL, Sly WS, Valle D, eds. *The metabolic and molecular basis of inherited disease*, 7th edn. New York: McGraw-Hill; 1995: 1953–80.

74. Rubin EM, Krauss RM, Spangler EA, *et al.* Inhibition of early atherogenesis in transgenic mice by human apolipoprotein AI. *Nature* 1991; 353:265–7.

75. Plump AS, Scott CJ, Breslow JA. Human apolipoprotein A-I gene expression increases high density lipoprotein and suppresses atherosclerosis in the apolipoprotein E-deficient mouse. *Proc Natl Acad Sci USA* 1994; 91:9607–11.

76. Duverger N, Kruth H, Emmanuel F, *et al.* Inhibition of atherosclerosis development in cholesterol-fed human apolipoprotein A-I-transgenic rabbits. *Circulation* 1996; 94:713–17.

77. Yagyu H, Ishibashi S, Zhong C, *et al.* Over-expressed lipoprotein lipase protects against atherosclerosis in apolipoprotein E knockout mice. *Circulation* 1998; 98:I–2.

78. Zhang SH, Reddick RL, Burkey B, Maeda N. Diet induced atherosclerosis in mice heterozygous and homozygous for apolipoprotein E gene disruption. *J Clin Invest* 1994; **94**: 937–45.

79. Hayek T, Masucci-Magoulas L, Jiang XC, *et al.* Decreased early atherosclerotic lesions in hypertriglyceridemic mice expressing cholesteryl ester transfer protein gene. *J Clin Invest* 1995; **96**:2071–4.

2

HDL: are there any benefits in raising it?

Michael I Mackness and Bharti Mackness

Introduction

Among the many independent risk factors for coronary heart disease (CHD) identified by epidemiological studies, low plasma concentrations of high density lipoprotein (HDL) is one of the strongest.[1] The Framingham Heart Study demonstrated that for any given low density lipoprotein (LDL) concentration, HDL-cholesterol concentration is inversely correlated with CHD risk.[2] A review of 19 prospective risk factor studies for CHD by an NIH consensus panel in 1992 indicated that 15 of the studies reported a significant association between low HDL levels and CHD while three of the other studies showed a non-significant trend towards this association.[3] Prospective studies conducted since this time have continued to show a strong association between low HDL levels and CHD.[4,5] The protective role of HDL against the development or progression of CHD has also been shown in interventional trials, particularly those using fibrates such as the Helsinki Heart Study and the Bezafibrate Coronary Atherosclerosis Intervention Trial.[6,7]

It is now beyond dispute that HDL protects against the development of CHD. The questions arise as to how this protection is achieved, what is the mechanism involved and can this be modulated to achieve greater protection against the development of CHD or even cause the regression of pre-existing disease?

Mechanisms of the anti-atherosclerotic action of HDL

Reverse cholesterol transport (RCT)

Traditionally the central role of HDL in RCT has been invoked to explain its anti-atherosclerotic action.[8] However, despite many years of research, grave doubts remain that this is the case, as it remains unproven that RCT occurs *in vivo* and many animal species use HDL rather than LDL to transport cholesterol to peripheral tissues. The transport of excess cholesterol from the peripheral tissues to the liver for disposal would be essential to cholesterol homeostasis to prevent cholesterol build-up in the peripheral tissues, particularly the arteries. Briefly, small HDL precursors, known as pre-β HDL,[9] in the tissue fluid take free cholesterol from cell membranes [the competing mechanistic theories of how this occurs have been the subject of several excellent recent reviews[10] and will not be dealt with here]. Once on the pre-β particle, the free cholesterol is esterified by the action of lecithin-cholesterol-acyl transferase (LCAT) which renders it more hydrophobic. The cholesteryl ester moves to the centre of the particle and a gradi-

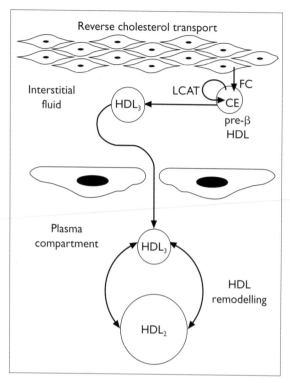

Reverse cholesterol transport

Interstitial fluid

LCAT   FC

HDL₃   CE

pre-β
HDL

Plasma
compartment

HDL₃

HDL
remodelling

HDL₂

Fig. 2.1
Simplified representation of reverse cholesterol transport.

ent for the movement of free cholesterol from the cell membrane to the pre-β HDL particle is established (Figure 2.1). Continued uptake of cholesterol results in the formation of larger, α migrating HDL₃ which diffuses from the tissue fluid into the plasma. Once in the circulation, HDL 'remodelling' occurs through the action of cholesteryl ester transfer protein (CETP), phospholipid transfer protein (PLTP), hepatic and lipoprotein lipase and the transfer of apolipoproteins from other lipoproteins,[11,12] resulting in a mixture of HDL₂ and HDL₃ species which fall into two main categories: those containing apoA-I but no apoA-II, and

those containing both of these apolipoproteins. The fate of the cholesterol within the HDL pool has not been fully elucidated but it can be taken up by the liver for reuse or excretion as bile acids, or it can be used by tissues such as the adrenals and reproductive organs for synthesis of steroid hormones. Alternatively, it can be transferred back to VLDL or LDL by CETP.

Prevention of oxidation

The oxidation of LDL polyunsaturated fatty acids resulting in a pro-atherosclerotic, pro-inflammatory particle is central to current theories on the initiation and progression of atherosclerosis (see Chapter 1). Several laboratories have reported results consistent with HDL being able to retard directly the oxidation of LDL *in vitro* or to prevent the pro-inflammatory and cytotoxic properties of oxidised LDL in a variety of arterial cells in culture (Table 2.1).

Although the mechanism of the anti-oxidative action of HDL remained obscure for a long time, there are now two overlapping theories which could explain this action. These can be broadly termed the 'direct metabolism' and 'transfer' theories (Figure 2.2).

Direct metabolism theory

In this model, HDL comes into contact with LDL, probably in the subintimal space, and acts to prevent LDL oxidation by metabolising LDL lipid hydroperoxides. Ours was the first laboratory to show that the ability of HDL to retard LDL oxidation was by a mechanism that was largely enzymatic and which acted at a specific point in the lipid peroxidation cascade.[13] We went on to show that the HDL-associated enzyme paraoxonase (PON1) could prevent LDL lipid peroxidation *in vitro*.[14,15] These initial studies have been confirmed and extended in other laboratories. PON1 has

HDL prevents		Reference(s)
LDL oxidation	*in vitro*	13–17, 18, 19, 20
	in vivo	21–23
Macrophage uptake of oxidised LDL		24, 25
Oxidised LDL cytotoxicity to endothelial and smooth muscle cells		26–28
TGRL cytotoxicity to macrophages and endothelial cells		29, 30
Oxidised LDL inhibition of intracellular communications		31
Oxidised LDL inhibition of guanyl cyclase		32
Oxidised LDL induction of MCP-1		33, 34
Lyso-PC-induced cytotoxicity to smooth muscle cells		35
Oxidised LDL induced endothelial cell death		36
Oxidised LDL dysregulation of arterial tone		37

Table 2.1
Prevention of LDL oxidation and the effects of oxidised LDL by HDL.

been shown to act by hydrolysing phospholipid and cholesteryl ester hydroperoxides derived from arachidonic and linoleic acid.[16,17]

PON1 displays a substrate activity polymorphism. The molecular basis of the PON1 activity polymorphism has been shown to be an amino acid substitution at position 192 (or position 191 when alanine is defined as the N-terminal residue). The Q (low activity towards paraoxon) isoenzyme has glutamine at position 192 and the R (high activity towards paraoxon) isoenzyme has arginine at position 192.[38]

Recent studies by Davies *et al.*[39] have further explored PON1 substrate activity polymorphism. While the R alloenzyme is more active towards some substrates such as paraoxon, other substrates such as phenylacetate do not discriminate between the alloenzymes. It now emerges that yet other substrates such as diazoxon and the nerve gases sarin and soman are hydrolysed faster by the Q alloenzyme. Another polymorphism at amino acid 55, a leucine (L) to methionine (M) substitution, was not believed to effect PON1 activity.[38] However, Blatter-Garin *et al.*[40] reported that the 55 polymorphism modulated activity in type 2 diabetes mellitus through an effect on PON1 concentration. In a study of 300 healthy people we have shown that the 55 polymorphism modulates PON1 activity independently of the 192 polymorphism.[41] Thus serum from individuals homozyous for the QQ/MM polymorphisms has the lowest hydrolytic activity towards paraoxon and that from RR/LL homozygotes has the highest activity.

In the last few years, several laboratories have reported the results of case–control studies investigating the relationship between the PON1 192 genetic polymorphism and the presence of CHD. Although it is possible to criticise the experimental method of these

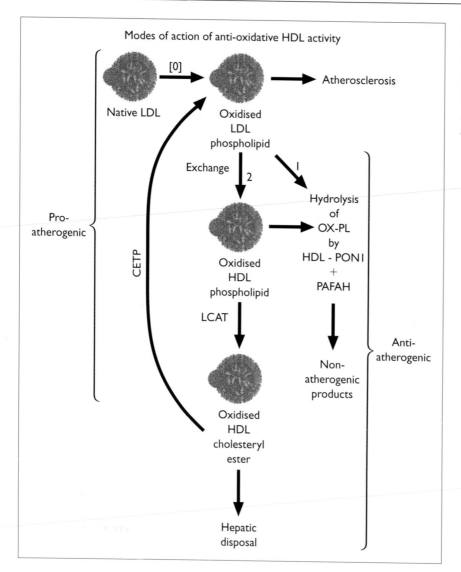

Modes of action of anti-oxidative HDL activity

Fig. 2.2
Possible modes of action to explain the anti-oxidative activity of high-density lipoprotein. 1, Direct metabolism; 2, transfer.

studies, six have reported no relationship between the polymorphism and CHD while four have reported a positive result.[42] Yet another study reported a positive relationship in Singapore Indians but no relationship in Singapore Chinese. However, it is important to note that there have been no negative stud- ies. Surprisingly, it was the R allele (high activ- ity towards paraoxon) that was positively associated with the presence of CHD. These findings were the opposite of those expected, especially as PON1 prevented LDL-lipid per- oxidation, but later it was realised that the Q allele was associated with the highest PON1 activity towards certain substrates. Thus, the QR and RR PON1 genotype may have a much more marked difference in activity compared with the QQ genotype with respect to a naturally occurring substrate crucial to the development of atheroma. However, detailed genetic analysis of an Asian Indian population has indicated that a Cys → Ser polymorphism of codon 310 (310S) of PON2 must be present with the PON1 R allele for there to be an association with the risk of development of CHD.[23]

Relatively few studies have reported on investigations of the PON1-55 polymorphism and CHD. In a study of 408 Caucasian type 2 diabetic patients, homozygosity for the L allele was an independent risk factor for CHD.[40] However, a second study could find no association of the PON1-55 polymorphism with CHD in Asian Indians and Chinese.[44]

In an attempt to answer the questions posed by epidemiological studies, we investigated the ability of HDL containing the different PON1 isoenzymes to protect LDL against oxidative modification. HDL protected LDL from oxidative modification, whatever the combination of alloenzymes present in it. However, HDL from QQ/MM homozygotes was most effective at protecting LDL, while HDL from RR/LL homozygotes was least effective. Thus after 6 hours of co-incubation of HDL and LDL with Cu^{2+}, PON1-QQ HDL retained 57% ($\pm 6.3\%$) of its original ability to protect LDL from oxidative modification, while PON1-QR HDL retained less at 25.1% ($\pm 4.5\%$) ($P < 0.01$) and PON1-RR HDL retained only 0.75% ($\pm 0.40\%$). In similar experiments HDL from LL and LM genotypes retained 21.8% ($\pm 7.5\%$) and 29.5% ($\pm 6.6\%$) ($P = NS$), respectively, of their protective ability, whereas PON1-MM HDL maintained 49.5% ($\pm 5.3\%$) ($P < 0.01$). Thus the reactivity of the PON1 alloenzymes reflects diazoxon

hydrolysis more than paraoxon hydrolysis and the relationship between R and L alleles and CHD could be explained by the differential hydrolysis of lipid hydroperoxides by the PON1 alloenzymes.[45-47]

PON1 activity and/or mass are low in several disease states associated with increased susceptibility to CHD[48,49] and also in CHD-prone animal models,[50-52] it is possible that perturbation of PON1 activity leads to increased susceptibility to disease.

Immunohistochemical localisation studies have shown PON1 to be present in the normal artery.[53] The concentration of PON1 in the artery wall increases massively as atherosclerosis progresses, possibly a response to increased oxidative stress. It is also worth noting that active PON1 is present in human interstitial fluid[54] and is therefore perfectly positioned to prevent LDL lipid peroxidation. HDL isolated from the serum of chicken, ostrich and turkey completely lacks PON1 protein and activity and is unable to prevent LDL oxidation,[55] providing further evidence for a central role of PON1 as an anti-inflammatory enzyme.

Two other HDL-associated enzymes, LCAT and platelet-activating factor acetylhydrolase (PAF-AH) have also been shown to directly inhibit LDL lipid peroxidation *in vitro*.[18,56,57] Compared to PON1, relatively little work has been done to characterise the role of LCAT. The activity of PAF-AH is the subject of some controversy, with some workers claiming that the hydrolysis of phospholipid hydroperoxides by PAF-AH is anti-inflammatory.[56,57] Yet other workers claim that this is a pro-inflammatory process because of the products of the reaction.[58]

There is some evidence that the anti-oxidant activity of HDL occurs *in vivo*. Rabbits made hypercholesterolaemic by cholesterol feeding were injected with 200 mg of human HDL3. Total conjugated dienes and trienes were reduced by 20–30% and phospholipid hydroperoxides by 50% after 6 hours and remained at this level for up to 24 hours after the HDL3 injection.[21] The same authors have also reported a negative correlation between the plasma concentration of HDL-cholesterol and that of plasma conjugated dienes.[21] Over-expressing human apoA-1 in mice also results in the inhibition of LDL oxidation, further strengthening the concept of a function for HDL in limiting the accumulation of lipid per-oxides in the circulation.[22]

To study the *in vivo* role of PON1, Shih *et al.*[23] created PON1-knockout mice through gene targeting. HDL isolated from PON1-deficient mice were unable to prevent LDL oxidation in a cell co-culture model of the artery wall, and both the HDL and LDL isolated from PON1-knockout mice were more susceptible to oxidation by co-culture cells compared with the lipoproteins of wild-type littermates. These results are consistent with human epidemiological and tissue culture studies suggesting that PON1 has the capacity to destroy certain pro-inflammatory lipids contributing to atherosclerosis. Interestingly, PAF-AH activity was not reduced in null mice, yet HDL was ineffective in destroying biologically active oxidised lipids. This indicates either that, when present on HDL, PAF-AH alone is unable to destroy biologically active lipids in mildly oxidised LDL, and/or there is a delicate balance of oxidised species and the enzymes capable of destroying them. Therefore, in the absence of PON1 and in the absence of a compensatory increase in PAF-AH, HDL is unable to destroy the biologically active lipids in mildly oxidised LDL.

Transfer theory

Parthasarathy *et al.*[24] were the first to suggest that HDL acted to protect LDL against lipid peroxidation by acting as a reservoir for lipid peroxides generated on LDL and therefore breaking the chain of lipid peroxide propagation in LDL. Consistent with this, other work-ers have reported that HDL is the principal carrier of lipid hydroperoxides in plasma[59] and that oxidised cholesteryl esters in HDL are taken up to a greater extent and more rapidly catabolised by hepatic cells and perfused rat liver than unoxidised cholesteryl ester. Oxi-dised cholesteryl esters of LDL, on the other hand, were neither taken up nor catabolised by the perfused liver.[60,61]

This theory has been extended by Klimov and colleagues.[62] In essence this theory requires the transfer of LDL phospholipid hydroperoxides (PLHP) to HDL. In experi-ments designed to test the validity of this the-ory, LDL bound to sepharose was oxidised and then incubated with HDL. There was an increase in total lipid hydroperoxide content of re-isolated HDL which was not seen in the absence of oxidised LDL.[62] Once attached to HDL, there could then be two fates for the PLHP. Either they could be hydrolysed by the action of PON1, PAF-AH and LCAT, either singly or in combination, to give non-athero-genic products, or they could be transferred by the action of LCAT to cholesterol to form oxi-dised cholesteryl esters in HDL (see Figure 2.2). Evidence for this theory is provided by the work of Nagata *et al.*[63] Phospholipid con-taining linoleic acid hydroperoxide in the Sn-2 position was added to human plasma at 37°C. Following incubation, the main products were lysophospholipid and cholesteryl ester con-taining oxidised linoleic acid. The formation of oxidised cholesteryl ester was stimulated by the addition of HDL, but not LDL, and inhib-ited by DTNB suggesting transfer of oxidised fatty acid was catalysed by LCAT. HDL then transports the oxidised cholesteryl esters to the liver for disposal, which again represents an anti-atherogenic pathway.

HDL effect	Reference(s)
Reduces blood viscosity	64
Downregulates thrombin generation	65
Inhibits endothelial cell cytokine induced VCAM-1 expression	66, 67
Modulation of endothelial cell prostaglandin/thromboxane synthesis ratio	68, 69
Modulation of platelet activity	70, 71
Activation of fibrinolysis	72
Stimulation of endothelin-1 secretion by endothelial cells	73

Table 2.2
Miscellaneous, possible anti-atherogenic properties of HDL.

It is possible, however, that oxidised cholesteryl esters could be returned to LDL through the action of CETP. This may be a pro-atherogenic pathway, particularly in situations where CETP activity is increased, for example in diabetes mellitus.

Miscellaneous beneficial effects

As can be seen from Table 2.2, HDL has been shown to have a number of effects which may be regarded as beneficial. These effects appear to be mainly anti-thrombotic. The findings presented in Table 2.2 require confirmation and it is not yet known if HDL exhibits any of these functions *in vivo*.

Are there benefits to raising HDL?

Overexpressing various components of human HDL, for example apoA-1 and LCAT in animal models, leads to increased concentrations of HDL-cholesterol and an increased resistance to the development of atherosclerosis.[74–76] In transgenic rabbits overexpressing human apoA-1, the increase in HDL is dependent on the number of copies of the human gene that are expressed. However, only those animals expressing the highest copy numbers appear to be very resistant to developing atherosclerosis when fed a high cholesterol diet. Plasma from these animals is more efficient at promoting cellular cholesterol efflux than plasma from wild-type littermates, presumably because of the high concentration of HDL.[76]

Interventional studies in humans have shown that several drugs such as fibrates and niacin can raise HDL-cholesterol concentrations. Drugs that lower primarily LDL-cholesterol concentrations, such as the HMG-CoA reductase inhibitors (vastatins), also marginally raise HDL levels and have been associated with a lack of progression of pre-existing coronary atherosclerosis. However, niacin combined with bile acid sequestrants raises HDL levels significantly and is associated with significant regression of pre-existing coronary atherosclerosis. These studies argue strongly that disease regression is caused by the increase in HDL levels.[77]

A case can be made that raising HDL levels would result in significant clinical benefit and, presumably, the lower the HDL concentration at the outset, the larger the benefit that would result. Doubts, however, remain. HDL is a very heterogeneous mixture of particles and certain specific protective functions may reside in specific particles, so that raising HDL by current methods may not increase specific sub-fractions. Another problem is how we measure HDL. Most clinical trials (and indeed most routine laboratories) measure HDL-cholesterol and report an increase in levels as an increase in HDL concentration. The two are not necessarily the same. For an increase in HDL to be effective, an increase in particle number will be required.

The potentially important anti-oxidative enzymes PON1 and PAFAH have a very selective distribution amongst the HDL subfractions. PON1 is associated with a specific HDL subspecies also containing apoA-1 and clusterin.[78] PAFAH is associated with denser HDL subspecies. To increase the anti-oxidative activity of HDL, a different pharmaceutical approach will be required, in other words the selective targeting of specific HDL components. This would require the discovery of components that can upregulate selectively, for example PON1.

One approach which may prove beneficial is to increase the concentration of selective HDL components by somatic gene transfer. Adenovirus-mediated transfer of human apoA-1 to mice has resulted in a clear anti-atherogenic effect. Such an approach with other HDL components may prove equally or even more successful. However, several problems which affect gene expression after viral transfer will have to be solved before this approach can be applied to humans.

Conclusion

The anti-atherosclerotic functions of HDL are well documented and clinical benefit should accrue from raising it. However, this may best be achieved by selective targeting of the anti-atherosclerotic components of HDL rather than attempting to raise the total HDL concentration.

Acknowledgements

The authors would like to thank Professors PN Durrington and AN Klimov for helpful discussions and Ms C Price for excellent assistance in typing the manuscript.

References

1. Miller GJ, Miller NE. Plasma high-density lipoprotein concentration and the development of ischaemic heart disease. *Lancet* 1975; i:16–19.
2. Castelli WP, Garrison RJ, Wilson PW, *et al.* Incidence of coronary heart disease and lipoprotein cholesterol levels. The Framingham Study. *JAMA* 1986; **256**:2835–8.
3. Consensus Statement. Triglyceride, high-density lipoprotein and coronary heart disease. 1992; **10**:1–28.
4. Assmann G, Schulte H, von Eckardstein A, Huang Y. High density lipoprotein cholesterol as a predictor of coronary heart disease risk. The PROCAM experience and pathophysiological implications for reverse cholesterol transport. *Atherosclerosis* 1996; **124**:S11–S20.
5. Tanne D, Yaari S, Goldbourt U. High-density lipoprotein cholesterol and risk of ischaemic stroke mortality. A 21 year follow-up of 8586 men from the Israeli Ischaemic Heart Disease Study. *Stroke* 1997; **21**:83–7.
6. Frick MH, Elo O, Haapa K, *et al.* Helsinki Heart Study: primary prevention trial of gemfibrozil in middle aged men with dyslipidaemia. Safety of treatment, changes in risk factors, and incidence of coronary heart disease. *N Engl J Med* 1987; **12**:1237–45.
7. de Faire U, Ericsson CG, Grip L, *et al.* Secondary preventive potential of lipid-lowering drugs. The Bezafibrate Coronary Atherosclerosis Intervention Trial (BECAIT). *Eur Heart J* 1996; **17F**:37–42.
8. Barter PJ, Rye R-A. High density lipoproteins

and coronary heart disease. *Atherosclerosis* 1996; **121**:1–12.

9. Castro GR, Fielding CJ. Early incorporation of cell-derived cholesterol into pre-β migrating high-density lipoprotein. *Biochemistry* 1988; **27**:25–9.

10. Rothblat GH, de la Llera-Moya M, Atger V, *et al.* Cell cholesterol efflux: integration of old and new observations provides new insights. *J Lipid Res* 1999; **40**:781–96.

11. Navab M, Hama SY, Hough GP, *et al.* High density lipoprotein associated enzymes: their role in vascular biology. *Curr Opin Lipidol* 1998; **9**:449–56.

12. Bisgaier CL, Pape ME. High density lipoprotein: are elevated levels desirable and achievable? *Curr Pharmaceut Design* 1998; **4**:53–70.

13. Mackness MI, Abbott CA, Arrol S, Durrington PN. The role of high density lipoprotein and lipid-soluble antioxidant vitamins in inhibiting low-density lipoprotein oxidation. *Biochem J* 1993; **294**:829–35.

14. Mackness MI, Arrol S, Durrington PN. Paraoxonase prevents accumulation of lipoperoxides in low-density lipoprotein. *FEBS Letts* 1991; **286**:152–4.

15. Mackness MI, Arrol S, Abbott CA, Durrington PN. Protection of low-density lipoprotein against oxidative modification by high-density lipoprotein associated paraoxonase. *Atherosclerosis* 1993; **104**:129–35.

16. Watson AD, Berliner JA, Hama SY, *et al.* Protective effect of high density lipoprotein associated paraoxonase — Inhibition of the biological activity of minimally oxidised low-density lipoprotein. *J Clin Invest* 1995; **96**:2882–91.

17. Aviram M, Billecke S, Sorenson R, *et al.* Paraoxonase active site required for protection against LDL oxidation involves its free sulphydryl group and is different from that required for its arylesterase/paraoxonase activities: selective active of human paraoxonase alloenzymes Q and R. *Arteriosclerosis Thromb Vasc Biol* 1998; **10**:1617–24.

18. Klimov AN, Nikiforova AA, Pleskov VM, *et al.* The protective action of high-density lipoproteins, their subfractions and lecithin-cholesterol acyltransferase in the peroxide modification of low-density lipoproteins. *Biokkimiya* 1989; **54**:118–23.

19. Ohta T, Takata S, Morino Y, Matsuda I. The protective effects of lipoproteins containing apoprotein A-I on Cu^{2+}-catalysed oxidation of human low-density lipoprotein. *FEBS Letts* 1989; **257**:435–8.

20. Kunitake ST, Jarvis MR, Hamilton RL, Kane JP. Binding of transition metals by apolipoprotein A-I-containing plasma lipoproteins: inhibition of oxidation of low density lipoproteins. *Proc Natl Acad Sci USA* 1992; **89**:6993–7.

21. Klimov AN, Gurevich VS, Nikiforova AA, *et al.* Antioxidative activity of high-density lipoproteins *in vivo*. *Atherosclerosis* 1993; **100**:13–19.

22. Hayek T, Oikuiue J, Danker G, *et al.* HDL apolipoprotein A-I attenuates oxidative modification of low density lipoprotein: studies in transgenic mice. *Eur J Clin Chem Clin Biochem* 1995; **33**:721–5.

23. Shih DM, Gu L, Xia Y-R, *et al.* Mice lacking serum paraoxonase are susceptible to organophosphate toxicity and atherosclerosis. *Nature* 1998; **394**:284–7.

24. Parthasarathy S, Barnett J, Fong LG. High-density lipoprotein inhibits the oxidative modification of low-density lipoprotein. *Biochim Biophys Acta* 1990; **1044**:275–83.

25. Miyazaki A, Sakai M, Suginohara Y, *et al.* Acetylated low density lipoprotein reduces its ligand activity for the scavenger receptor after interaction with reconstituted high-density lipoprotein. *J Biol Chem* 1994; **269**:5264–9.

26. Hessler JR, Robertson AL, Chisholm GM. LDL-induced cytotoxicity and its inhibition by HDL in human vascular smooth muscle and endothelial cells in culture. *Atherosclerosis* 1979; **32**:213–29.

27. Hessler JR, Morel DW, Lewis LJ, Chisholm GM. Lipoprotein oxidation and lipoprotein induced cytotoxicity. *Arteriosclerosis* 1983; **3**:215–22.

28. Morel DW, Hessler JR, Chisholm GM. Low density lipoprotein cytotoxicity induced by free radical peroxidation of lipid. *J Lipid Res* 1983; **24**:1070.

29. Chung BH, Segrest JP, Smith K, *et al.* Lipolytic surface remnants of triglyceride-rich lipoproteins are cytotoxic to macrophages but not in the presence of high density lipoprotein. *J Clin Invest* 1989; **83**:1363–74.

30. Speidel MT, Booyse FM, Abrams A, *et al.* Lipolyzed hypertriglyceridaemic serum and triglyceride-rich lipoprotein cause lipid accumulation in and are cytotoxic to cultured human endothelial cells. High density lipoproteins inhibit this cytotoxicity. *Thrombosis Res* 1990; **58**:251–64.

31. Zwijsen RM, de Haan LH, Kuivenhoven JA, Nusselder IC. Modulation of low-density lipoprotein-induced inhibition of intercellular communication by antioxidants and high-density lipoproteins. *Food Chem Toxicol* 1991; **29**:615.

32. Schmidt K, Klatt P, Graier WF, *et al.* High density lipoprotein antagonizes the inhibitory effects of oxidised low density lipoprotein and lysolecithin on soluble gyanyl cyclase. *Biochem Biophys Res Commun* 1992; **182**:302.

33. Navab M, Imes SS, Hama SY, *et al.* Monocyte transmigration induced by modification of low density lipoprotein in cocultures of human aortic wall cells is due to induction of monocyte chemotactic protein 1 synthesis and is abolished by high density lipoprotein. *J Clin Invest* 1991; **88**:2039–46.

34. Maier JAM, Barenghi L, Pagani F, *et al.* The protective role of high-density lipoprotein on oxidised-low-density-lipoprotein-induced U937/endothelial cell interactions. *Eur J Biochem* 1994; **221**:35–41.

35. Nilsson J, Dahlgren B, Ares M, *et al.* Lipoprotein-like phospholipid particles inhibit the smooth muscle cell cytotoxicity of lysophosphatidylcholine and platelet activating factor. *Arteriosclerosis Thromb Vasc Biol* 1998; **18**:13–19.

36. Suc I, Blanc IE, Troly M, *et al.* HDL and apo A prevent cell death of endothelial cells induced by oxidised LDL. *Arteriosclerosis Thromb Vasc Biol* 1997; **17**:2158–66.

37. Ota Y, Kugiyama K, Sugiyama S, *et al.* Complexes of apo A-I with phosphatidylcholine suppress dysregulation of arterial tone by oxidised LDL. *Am J Physiol* 1997; **273**:H1215–H1222.

38. La Du BN. Human serum paraoxonase/arylesterase. In: Kalow W, ed. *Pharmacogenetics of Drug Metabolism.* New York: Pergamon Press; 1992: 51–91.

39. Davies HG, Richter RJ, Keifer M, *et al.* The effect of the human serum paraoxonase polymorphism is reversed with diazoxon, soman and sarin. *Nature Genetics* 1996; **14**:334–6.

40. Blatter-Garin MC, James RW, Dussoix P, *et al.* Paraoxonase Polymorphism Met-Leu 54 is associated with modified serum concentrations of the enzyme. *J Clin Invest* 1997; **99**:62–6.

41. Mackness B, Mackness MI, Arrol S, *et al.* Effect of the molecular polymorphisms of human paraoxonase (PON1) on the rate of hydrolysis of paraoxon. *Br J Pharmacol* 1997; **112**:265–8.

42. Mackness MI, Mackness B, Durrington PN, *et al.* Paraoxonase and coronary heart disease. *Curr Opin Lipidol* 1998; **9**:319–24.

43. Sanghera DK, Aston CE, Saha N, Kamboh MI. DNA polymorphisms in two paraoxonase genes (PON1 and PON2) are associated with the risk of coronary heart disease. *Am J Hum Genet* 1998; **62**:36–44.

44. Sanghera DK, Saha N, Kamboh MI. The codon 55 polymorphism of the paraoxonase 1 gene is not associated with risk of coronary heart disease in Asian Indians and Chinese. *Atherosclerosis* 1998; **136**:217–23.

45. Mackness MI, Arrol S, Mackness B, Durrington PN. The alloenzymes of paraoxonase determine the effectiveness of high-density lipoprotein in protecting low density lipoprotein against lipid-peroxidation. *Lancet* 1997; **349**:851–2.

46. Mackness B, Mackness MI, Arrol S, *et al.* Effect of the human serum paraoxonase 55 and 192 genetic polymorphisms on the protection by high density lipoprotein against low density lipoprotein oxidative modification. *FEBS Letts* 1998; **423**:57–60.

47. Mackness B, Durrington PN, Mackness MI. Polymorphisms of paraoxonase genes and low-density lipoprotein lipid peroxidation. *Lancet* 1999; **353**:468–9.

48. Ayub A, Mackness MI, Arrol S, *et al.* Serum paraoxonase after myocardial infarction. *Arteriosclerosis Thromb Vasc Biol* 1999; **19**:330–5.

49. Mackness B, Mackness MI, Arrol S, *et al.* Serum paraoxonase (PON1) 55 and 192 polymorphism and paraoxonase activity and concentration in non-insulin dependent diabetes mellitus. *Atherosclerosis* 1998; **139**:341–9.

50. Hayek T, Fuhrman B, Vaya J, *et al*. Reduced progression of atherosclerosis in apolipoprotein E deficient mice following consumption of red wine, or its polyphenols quercetin or catechin, is associated with reduced susceptibility of LDL to oxidation and aggregation. *Arteriosclerosis Thromb Vasc Biol* 1997; **17**: 2744–52.

51. Navab M, Hama-Levy S, van Lenten BJ, *et al*. Mildly oxidised LDL induces an increased apolipoprotein J/paraoxonase ratio. *J Clin Invest* 1997; **99**:2005–19.

52. Shih DM, Gu L, Hama S, *et al*. Genetic-dietary regulation of serum paraoxonase expression and its role in atherogenesis in a mouse model. *J Clin Invest* 1996; **97**:1630–9.

53. Mackness B, Hunt R, Durrington PN, Mackness MI. Increased immunolocalisation of paraoxonase, clusterin and apolipoprotein AI in the human artery wall with progression of atherosclerosis. *Arteriosclerosis Thromb Vasc Biol* 1997; **17**:1233–8.

54. Mackness MI, Mackness B, Arrol S, *et al*. Presence of paraoxonase in human interstitial fluid. *FEBS Lett* 1997; **416**:377–80.

55. Mackness B, Durrington PN, Mackness MI. Lack of protection against oxidative modification of LDL by avian HDL. *Biochem Biophys Res Comm* 1998; **247**:443–6.

56. Stafforini DM, Prescott SM, McIntyre TM. Human plasma platelet-activating factor acetylhydrolase. *J Biol Chem* 1987; **262**: 4223–30.

57. Watson AD, Navab M, Hama SY, *et al*. Effect of platelet-activating factor-acetylhydrolase on the formation and action of minimally oxidised low-density lipoprotein. *J Clin Invest* 1995; **95**:774–82.

58. Macphee C, Moores KE, Boyd HF, *et al*. Lipoprotein-associated phospholipase A2, platelet-activating factor acetylhydrolase, generates two bioactive products during the oxidation of low-density lipoprotein: use of a novel inhibitor. *Biochem J* 1999; **338**:479–87.

59. Bowry VW, Stanley KK, Stocker R. High density lipoprotein is the major carrier of lipid hydroperoxides in human blood plasma from fasting donors. *Proc Natl Acad Sci USA* 1992; **89**:10316–20.

60. Sattler W, Stacker R. Greater selective uptake by Hep G2 cells of high density lipoprotein cholesterylester hydroperoxides than anoxidised cholesterylesters. *Biochem J* 1993; **294**:771–6.

61. Christison J, Karjalaineu A, Brauman J, *et al*. Rapid reduction and removal of HDL but not LDL-associated cholesterylester hydroperoxides by rat liver perfused in situ. *Biochem J* 1996; **314**:737–42.

62. Klimov AN, Nikiforova AA, Kuzmin AA, *et al*. Is high density lipoprotein a scavenger for oxidised phospholipids of low density lipoprotein? In: *Advances in Lipoprotein and Atherosclerosis Research, Diagnostics and Treatment*. Jena: Gustav Fischer Verlag; 1998: 78–82.

63. Nagata Y, Yamamoto Y, Niki E. Reaction of phosphatidylcholine hydroperoxide in human plasma: the role of peroxidase and lecithin: cholesterol acyltransferase. *Arch Biochem Biophys* 1996; **329**:24–36.

64. Sloop GD, Mercante DE. Opposite effects of low-density and high-density lipoprotein on blood viscosity in fasting subjects. *Clin Hemoriheal Microcirc* 1998; **19**:197–203.

65. Griffin JH, Kojima K, Kanka CL, *et al*. High-density lipoprotein enhancement of anticoagulant activities of plasma proteins and activated protein C *J Clin Invest* 1999; **103**:219–27.

66. Baker PW, Rye K-E, Gamble JR, *et al*. Ability of reconstituted high-density lipoproteins to inhibit cytokine-induced expression of vascular cell adhesion molecule-1 in human umbilical vein endothelial cells. *J Lipid Res* 1999; **40**:345–53.

67. Calabresi L, Franceschini G, Sirtori CR, *et al*. Inhibition of VCAM-1 expression in endothelial cells by reconstituted high density lipoproteins. *Biochem Biophys Res Comm* 1997; **238**:61–5.

68. Oravec S, Demuth K, Myara I, Hornych A. The effect of high-density lipoprotein subfractions on endothelial eicosanoid secretion. *Thromb Res* 1998; **92**:65–71.

69. Beitz A, Beitz J. Antiatherosclerotic potency of high density lipoprotein of different origins: a review and some new findings. *Prostaglandins Leukotrienes Essential Fatty Acids* 1998; **58**: 221–30.

70. Lerch PG, Spycher DO, Doran JE. Reconstituted high density lipoprotein (rHDL)

modulates platelet activity *in vitro* and *ex vivo*. *Thromb Haemost* 1998; **80**:316–20.

71. Nofer JR, Walter M, Kehrel B, *et al.* HDL3-mediated inhibition of thrombin-induced platelet aggregation and fibrinogen binding occurs via decreased production of phospho-inositide-derived second messengers 1,2-diacyl-glycerol and inositol 1,4,5-tri-phosphate. *Arteriosclerosis Thromb Vasc Biol* 1998; **18**:861–9.

72. Saku K, Ahmad M, Glas-Greewalt P, Kashyap ML. Activation of fibrinolysis by apolipoproteins of high density lipoproteins in man. *Thromb Res* 1985; **39**:1–8.

73. Hu RM, Chuang MY, Prins B, *et al.* High density lipoprotein stimulate the production and secretion of endothelin-1 from cultured bovine aortic endothelial cells. *J Clin Invest* 1994; **93**:1056–62.

74. Badimon JJ, Badimon L, Fuster V. Regression of atherosclerotic lesions by high-density lipoprotein fraction in cholesterol-fed rabbit. *J Clin Invest* 1990; **85**:1234–41.

75. Rubin EM, Krauss RM, Spungier EA, *et al.* Inhibition of early atheorgenesis in transgenic mice by human apolipoprotein A-I. *Nature* 1991; **353**:265–7.

76. Duverger N, Kruth H, Emmanuel F, *et al.* Inhibition of atherosclerosis development in cholesterol-fed human apolipoprotein A-I transgenic rabbits. *Circulation* 1996; **94**:713–17.

77. Kashyab ML. Mechanistic studies of high-density lipoproteins. *Am J Cardiol* 1998; **82**:42U-48U.

78. Blatter M-C, James RW, Messmer S, *et al.* Identification of a distinct human high-density lipoprotein subspecies defined by a lipoprotein-associated protein, K-85: Identity of K-85 with paraoxonase. *Eur J Biochem* 1993; **211**:871–9.

79. Benoit P, Emmanuel F, Caillund JM, *et al.* Somatic gene transfer of human apo A1 inhibits atherosclerosis progression in mouse models. *Circulation* 1999; **99**:105–10.

80. Van Vlijmen BJM, Herz J. Gene targets and approaches for raising HDL. *Circulation* 1999; **99**:12–14.

3

The PPAR system and regulation of lipoprotein metabolism

Bart Staels

Introduction

Epidemiological and interventional studies have established dyslipidaemia as a major risk factor for atherosclerosis and coronary artery disease (CAD). Primary[1] and secondary[2] interventional trials with HMG-CoA reductase inhibitors have provided evidence that a drastic reduction in LDL-cholesterol levels reduces the cardiovascular risk in hypercholesterolaemic patients and even in patients considered to have normal LDL-cholesterol levels.[3] In addition, other dyslipidaemias, such as hypoalphalipoproteinaemia (low plasma HDL concentrations) with or without concomitant hypertriglyceridaemia, may be the cause of a substantial number of cases of CAD.[4]

Whereas HMG-CoA reductase inhibitors are currently first-line drugs for the treatment of hypercholesterolaemia, fibrates are useful for the treatment of hypoalphalipoproteinaemia with or without hypertriglyceridaemia. Fibrates are a group of lipid modifying agents, chemically related to clofibrate, which was the first fibrate in clinical use. Second generation fibrates that are widely used include beclofibrate, bezafibrate, ciprofibrate, etofibrate, fenofibrate, and gemfibrozil. The recommendation for the use of fibrates in certain types of dyslipidaemia has gained support from a subgroup analysis of the Helsinki Heart Study[5] which showed a greater than 70% reduction in CHD risk in overweight patients with a baseline LDL:HDL-cholesterol ratio of greater than 5 and a triglyceride level of 200 mg/dl treated with gemfibrozil.[6,7] Results from two secondary prevention angiographic studies using bezafibrate and gemfibrozil revealed that fibrate treatment retards the progression of coronary atherosclerosis and decreases the number of coronary events.[8,9] Recently, results from the VA-HIT (Veterans Affairs-High Density Lipoprotein Cholesterol Intervention Trial) study with gemfibrozil[10] demonstrated that raising HDL-cholesterol and lowering triglycerides, even in the absence of a significant lowering of LDL-cholesterol, reduced both CAD mortality and non-fatal myocardial infarction in men with documented CAD and low HDL-cholesterol ($\leq$40 mg/dl), low LDL-cholesterol ($\leq$140 mg/dl) and low triglyceride levels ($\leq$300 mg/dl).

Although fibrates have been used in clinical practice for over three decades, knowledge of the molecular mechanisms of their normolipidaemic effects was lacking until recently. It was known for several years that fibrates induce peroxisome proliferation in rodents due to the induction of the transcription of genes involved in peroxisomal β-oxidation, a process mediated by transcription factors belonging to the peroxisome proliferator activated receptor (PPAR) family.[11] Recently, it became clear that fibrates exert their effects on lipoprotein metabolism principally via activation of the PPARα form. Importantly, fibrates exert their effects on lipoprotein metabolism in humans, without inducing any peroxisome proliferation response. In this chapter, we will present a brief overview of the characteristics of the PPAR family of nuclear receptors, followed by a review of current knowledge on how PPARs regulate lipoprotein metabolism.

Peroxisome proliferator activated receptors: the molecular mediators of fibrate action

Peroxisome proliferator activated receptors (PPARs) constitute a subfamily of the nuclear receptors.[11] Nuclear receptors are ligand-activated transcription factors. Three distinct PPARs, termed α, δ(β) and γ, each encoded by a separate gene and showing a distinct tissue distribution pattern, have been cloned so far. Natural and synthetic ligands that induce the transcriptional activity of PPARs have been subsequently identified. Whereas all PPARs are activated by fatty acids, a number of eicosanoids appear to be more selective natural activators of certain PPARs, such as leukotriene B4 (LTB4), 8(S)hydroxyeicosatetraenoic acid and 8(S)hydroxyeicosapentaenoic acid for PPARα[12–14] and prostaglandin J2 derivatives, 9-hydroxyoctadecadienoic acid and 13-hydroxyoctadecadienoic acid for PPARγ.[15–17] In addition, fibrates bind to and activate PPARα, albeit with low affinity.[13,14] However, selectivity for the PPARα form differs between the currently used fibrates. Whereas fenofibrate and ciprofibrate are more selective PPARα activators, gemfibrozil and bezafibrate are much less selective, the latter

being similarly active on all three PPAR forms.

Activated PPARs heterodimerise with another nuclear receptor, the 9-cis retinoic acid receptor RXR, and alter the transcription of target genes after binding to specific peroxisome proliferator response elements (PPREs). PPREs consist of a direct repeat of the nuclear receptor hexameric AGGTCA DNA core recognition motif separated by one or two nucleotides (DR1 and DR2) (Figure 3.1). This mechanism of transcriptional regulation explains the majority of the actions of PPARα on lipid and lipoprotein metabolism. In addition, PPARα has been shown to repress gene transcription by interfering with the NFκB, Stat and AP-1 signalling pathways in a DNA-binding-independent fashion (see Figure 3.1). These actions of PPARα are probably at the basis of the recently discovered anti-inflammatory actions of fibrates, as described by Pineda Torra et al.[18]

Clinical actions of fibrates

Fibrates are first-line drugs in the treatment of primary hypertriglyceridaemia and are very useful in the treatment of hypoalphalipoproteinaemia, combined hyperlipidaemia, type III dyslipoproteinaemia and secondary lipid abnormalities observed in type 2 diabetic and obese individuals.

The most pronounced effect of fibrates is a decrease in plasma triglyceride-rich lipoproteins. Levels of LDL-cholesterol generally decrease in individuals with elevated baseline plasma concentrations and HDL-cholesterol levels are usually increased when baseline plasma concentrations are low.[19] LDL particles display significant size heterogeneity, existing in three major subclasses: large light, intermediate and small dense LDL. The small dense LDL fraction exhibits a diminished resistance to oxidation and an enhanced

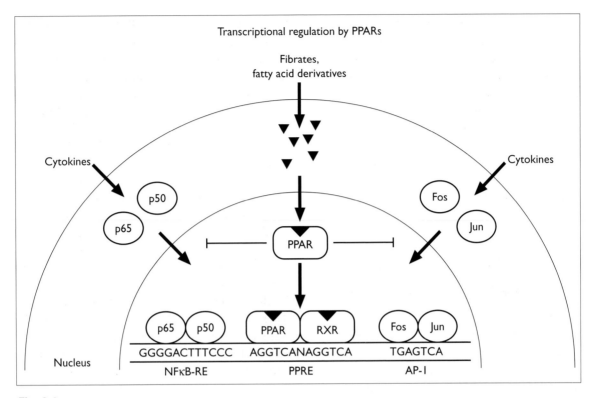

Fig. 3.1
Mechanisms of transcriptional regulation by peroxisome proliferator activated receptors (PPARs).

atherogenic potential. Fibrate treatment of patients with an atherogenic LDL profile results in a reduction of these dense LDL particles with an equivalent increase in the intermediate subfraction.

The increased HDL concentrations found after fibrate treatment are generally reflected by increased plasma levels of apoA-I and apoA-II. Human HDL also consists of particles of different size and apolipoprotein composition, and can be separated into large light HDL_2 and small dense HDL_3. Based on its apoA-I and apoA-II content, HDL may also be separated into particles containing only apoA-I (LpA-I) or both apoA-I and apoA-II (LpAI:AII). Fibrates increase HDL levels, a change that is associated with an increase in LpA-I:A-II, and a decrease in LpA-I concentrations.[19]

In the following sections we will review our current knowledge of the molecular mechanisms underlying the actions of fibrates via PPARα on lipid and lipoprotein metabolism.

Effect of fibrates on triglyceride metabolism

One of the major effects of PPARα activators is to reduce triglyceride levels. The decrease in plasma levels of triglyceride-rich lipoproteins

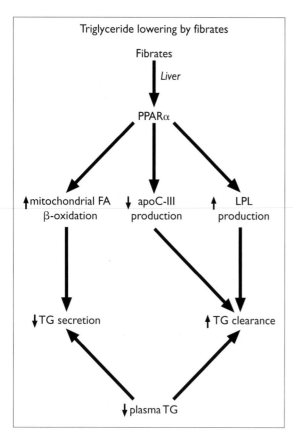

Fig. 3.2
Mechanism of triglyceride lowering activity of fibrates.

is due to a decrease in their synthesis rates combined with an acceleration of their intravascular catabolism (Figure 3.2).

Effects on intracellular fatty acid metabolism

Recent studies have shown that fibrates increase cellular fatty acid (FA) catabolism resulting in inhibition of hepatic VLDL triglyceride synthesis and secretion.

PPARα is highly expressed in tissues with elevated rates of FA catabolism, where it regulates genes involved in FA uptake, activation

into acyl-CoA esters, degradation via the peroxisomal and mitochondrial β-oxidation pathways and ketone body synthesis.[11] Intracellular FA concentrations are partly determined by a regulated import system that is controlled by FA transport proteins, such as FATP and FAT/CD36. Coupling of FA uptake to their activation in acyl-CoA esters by the activity of acyl-CoA synthetase (ACS) results in a positive import gradient. Fibrates, via activation of PPARα, induce FATP, FAT and ACS mRNA levels in rat liver.[20,21] This regulation of FATP and ACS expression by PPARα activators occurs at the transcriptional level and is also observed *in vitro* in hepatocyte cell culture systems.

Once activated, fatty acids are transported into the mitochondria. Expression of muscle- and liver-type carnitine palmitoyltransferase (CPT)-I, a pivotal enzyme in the mitochondrial FA uptake in these tissues, is induced by fibrates via PPARα binding to a PPRE localised in their promoter regions.[22,23] Moreover, the expression of the muscle CPT-I gene is decreased in PPARα-deficient mice and PPARα activators do not induce its expression in hearts of PPARα-deficient mice. These results show that PPARα regulates the entry of FAs into the mitochondria, which is a crucial step in their metabolism, especially in tissues like heart, skeletal muscle and brown adipose tissue, in which FAs are a major source of energy. Finally, PPARα activators regulate the expression of mitochondrial enzymes of the FA β-oxidation pathway. The recent observation that PPARα activators may also regulate the expression of uncoupling proteins (UCP),[24] raises the intriguing possibility that these drugs induce, under certain conditions, FA catabolism without ATP generation, an action which may be beneficial in obese patients.

Altogether, these data show that PPARα activators stimulate different steps in FA oxidative metabolism in different organs, particularly in the liver where they reduce the quantity of FA available for VLDL synthesis and secretion, as has been observed with gemfibrozil and fenofibrate in liver cells.[25,26]

Effect of fibrates on intravascular triglyceride metabolism

Fibrates also increase VLDL- and chylomicron-triglyceride hydrolysis. Two distinct mechanisms appear to be involved in the induction of intravascular lipolytic activity by fibrates. The first is induction of LPL gene expression leading to a higher hydrolytic activity of the enzyme. The second involves alterations in the composition of triglyceride-rich lipoproteins secreted by the liver following treatment with fibrates, producing particles with a higher susceptibility for lipolysis.

A PPRE in the human LPL promoter which mediates a positive responsiveness of the LPL gene to PPARα activators in rat liver has been identified.[27] Furthermore, fibrates repress the expression of the triglyceride metabolism antagonist, apoC-III, in liver. ApoC-III may delay the catabolism of triglyceride-rich particles through different mechanisms. ApoC-III appears to inhibit the binding of triglyceride-rich lipoproteins to the endothelial surface and lipolysis by LPL, to interfere with apoE-mediated receptor clearance of remnant particles as well as to decrease VLDL glycosaminoglycan binding in an apoE-independent manner.[28–33] In humans a common genetic variant of the apoC-III promoter has been identified, which results in impaired downregulation of apoC-III expression by insulin and which may therefore represent a major contributing factor to the development of hypertriglyceridaemia.[34] Elevated apoC-III synthetic rates have been observed in hypertriglyceridaemic patients.[35] In contrast, subjects deficient in apoC-III exhibit an increased catabolic rate of VLDL.[36]

In severe primary hypercholesterolaemia, fenofibrate therapy decreases apoC-III and lipoprotein particles containing both apoC-III and apoB.[37] Fibrates lower apoC-III mRNA levels in a dose- and time-dependent manner both *in vivo* in rat livers as well as *in vitro* in primary cultures of human and rat hepatocytes.[38,39] Using PPARα-deficient mice, an obligatory role for PPARα in the repression of apoC-III gene expression by fibrates was demonstrated.[40] The regulation of apoC-III gene transcription is complex, being governed by an ensemble of transcription factor binding sites within 1Kb upstream of the transcription initiation site. Among these sites is the C3P (also called CIIIB) site, to which a number of nuclear receptors such as HNF-4, ARP-1, Ear/COUP-TF,[41] RXR and PPARα bind.[41,42] Whereas HNF-4, RXR and PPARα[42,43] can activate apoC-III gene transcription via this site, ARP-1 and Ear3/COUP-TF act as repressors.[41] The transcriptional suppression of apoC-III gene expression by fibrates can be due to one or more of the following mechanisms. First, the suppression of apoC-III by PPARα activators may be due to a displacement of the strong transcriptional activator HNF-4 by the less active PPARα/RXR complex, resulting in lower apoC-III promoter activity.[43] Second, PPARα activators such as MEDICA 16 may decrease the expression of HNF-4, although this effect has not been observed with clinically used fibrates such as fenofibrate or ciprofibrate.[44] Third, PPARα activators may induce the expression of repressor proteins, such as ARP-1, Ear3/COUP-TF or Rev-erbα. Interestingly, fibrates induce Rev-erbα expression both in rat and human liver cells via PPARα interacting with a PPRE in the Rev-erbα gene promoter.[44,45] Furthermore, Rev-erbα-deficient mice exhibit increased plasma triglycerides and apoC-III concentrations and liver apoC-III mRNA levels are elevated.[46] Finally, activated PPARα has been shown to interfere with certain transcription factor pathways, such as AP-1,[47] NF-κB[48,49] and STAT,[50] which are all operative in liver cells and the participation of such a mechanism in the repression of apoC-III expression is a possibility.

Effects of fibrates on HDL metabolism

Fenofibrate increases the apoA-I synthetic rate and to a lesser extent its catabolic rate in hypercholesterolaemic patients.[51] However, unlike their effects on plasma triglycerides, fibrates influence HDL-cholesterol and apoA-I differently in humans and rodents. In rats, fibrate treatment results in a considerable lowering of plasma HDL concentrations.[52,53] Recent studies have demonstrated that in humans, fibrates increase plasma HDL concentrations, at least in part, through the induction of the expression of the human apoA-I and apoA-II genes,[54–56] while in rodents they decrease plasma HDL concentrations because of a marked decrease of the expression of these genes in liver.[53,56] Whereas fibrates repress apoA-I gene transcription in rat hepatocytes, they enhance its expression and production *in vivo* in humans and *in vitro* in both human hepatocytes and hepatoma cells[44,54] and cynomolgus monkey hepatocytes.[57]

Although fibrates have opposite effects on HDL metabolism in rodents and humans, a large body of evidence indicates that these drugs act via activation of PPARα in both species. Studies in PPARα-deficient mice[40,58] have demonstrated that fibrates regulate apoA-I expression via PPARα in this species. In PPARα-deficient mice both HDL-cholesterol and plasma apoA-I levels are elevated. Furthermore, hepatic apoA-I mRNA levels are elevated in PPARα-deficient mice. A significant

decrease in both hepatic apoA-I mRNA and plasma apoA-I levels is seen after treatment with PPARα ligands only in PPARα wild-type, but not in PPARα-deficient animals. Thus, fibrates alter HDL-cholesterol levels in mice through PPARα regulating apoA-I gene expression.

Using human apoA-I transgenic mice, in which the expression of the transgene is driven by its own human promoter, it was demonstrated that the opposing regulation of human versus mouse apoA-I by fibrates is due to differences in cis-acting sequence elements.[56] Furthermore, treatment of those human apoA-I transgenic mice with fibrates increased HDL-cholesterol and human apoA-I plasma concentrations concomitantly with an increase in hepatic human apoA-I mRNA levels. Unpublished data from our laboratory show that fenofibrate acts by both increasing human apoA-I synthesis and decreasing the fractional catabolic rates of plasma HDL cholesteryl esters and apoA-I. Furthermore, a significant induction of hepatic SR-BI receptor protein levels is observed, resulting in a net mass flux of HDL cholesteryl esters to the liver of fenofibrate treated animals.

Fibrates induce the transcription rate of the human apoA-I gene via PPARα, interacting with a positive PPRE located in the A site of the human apoA-I gene promoter liver specific enhancer (Figure 3.3).[54] The absence of induction of rat apoA-I gene expression by fibrates is due to three nucleotide differences between the rat and the human apoA-I promoter A site, rendering the PPRE in the human apoA-I promoter non-functional in rats.[44] In contrast, rat but not human apoA-I transcription is repressed by the nuclear receptor Rev-erbα, which binds to a negative response element adjacent to the TATA box of the rat, but not the human apoA-I promoter. Interestingly, both in humans and rats, fibrates increase liver

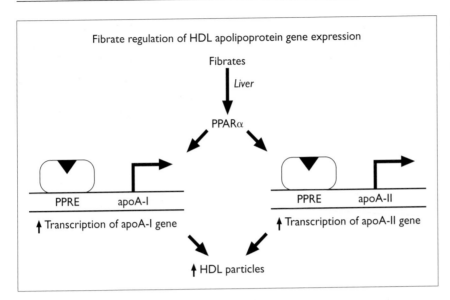

Fibrate regulation of HDL apolipoprotein gene expression

Fibrates

Liver

PPARα

PPRE   apoA-I

↑ Transcription of apoA-I gene

PPRE   apoA-II

↑ Transcription of apoA-II gene

↑ HDL particles

Fig. 3.3
Regulation of HDL apolipoprotein gene expression by fibrates via PPARα.

Rev-erbα gene expression. Therefore, it appears that the opposite regulation of apoA-I expression in humans versus rodents is linked to differences in cis-elements in their respective promoters leading to repression by Rev-erbα of rat apoA-I and activation by PPARα of human apoA-I (Figure 3.4).

Fibrates also induce the expression of the second most abundant HDL apolipoprotein, apoA-II, in primary cultures of human hepatocytes and in human hepatoblastoma Hep G2 cells.[55] A DR1-type PPRE in the J-site of the human apoA-II promoter was furthermore identified, which binds PPARα with high affinity (see Figure 3.3). Thus, fibrates increase apoA-II plasma levels by stimulating transcription of its gene through the interaction of activated PPARα with the apoAII-PPRE.

Using a transgenic rabbit model, which expresses the human apoA-I gene under control of its homologous regulatory regions,

including the fibrate-response elements previously shown to be active in mice,[56] it was demonstrated that fibrate actions on apoA-I metabolism occur independently of peroxisome proliferation.[59] In these human apoA-I transgenic rabbits, administration of fenofibrate increased plasma human apoA-I concentrations via an increased expression of the human apoA-I gene in the liver without increasing liver weight or ACO activity. These data provide *in vivo* evidence that the beneficial increase in apoA-I levels can occur mechanistically dissociated from any deleterious activity on peroxisome proliferation and possibly hepato-carcinogenesis.

Conclusion

Our knowledge on the physiological role of the PPAR family of transcription factors in the regulation of lipid and lipoprotein metabolism

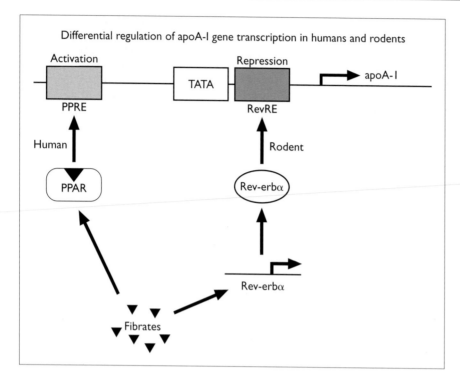

Differential regulation of apoA-I gene transcription in humans and rodents

Fig. 3.4
Mechanism of the differential regulation between human and rodents of apoA-I gene transcription by fibrates.

has evolved enormously over the last 5 years. It is now clear that PPARα activators, such as fibrates, may exert beneficial effects on atherosclerosis development through their normolipidaemic activities. In addition, recent studies, not discussed in the present article, indicate that PPARα activators also exert direct effects on the vascular wall, resulting in the inhibition of vascular inflammation and thrombogenesis. Such actions are undoubtedly beneficial in the treatment of atherosclerosis. Further studies using new molecules that are more potent and more specific PPARα activators than the presently available drugs will certainly provide additional information on the role of PPARα in lipoprotein metabolism and atherogenesis and should offer new therapeutic perspectives.

References

1. Shepherd J, Cobbe SM, Ford I, *et al.* Prevention of coronary heart disease with pravastatin in men with hypercholesterolemia. *N Engl J Med* 1995; **333**:1301–7.

2. Pedersen TR, Kjekshus J, Berg K, *et al.* Randomised trial of cholesterol lowering in 4444 patients with coronary heart disease: The Scandinavian Simvastatin Survival Study (4S). *Lancet* 1994; **344**:1383–9.

3. Sacks FM, Moye LA, Davis BR, *et al.* Relationship between plasma LDL concentrations during treatment with pravastatin and recurrent coronary events in the Cholesterol and Recurrent Events trial. *Circulation* 1998; **97**: 1446–52.

4. Saku K, Zhang B, Ohta T, Arakawa K. Quantity and function of high density lipoprotein as an indicator of coronary atherosclerosis. *J Am Coll Cardiol* 1999; **33**:436–43.

5. Frick MH, Elo O, Haapa K, *et al*. Helsinki Heart Study: primary prevention trial with gemfibrozil in middle-aged men with dyslipidemia. Safety of treatment, changes in risk factors, and incidence of coronary heart disease. *N Engl J Med* 1987; **317**:1237–45.

6. Huttunen J, Manninen V, Manttari M, *et al*. The Helsinki Heart Study: central findings and clinical implications. *Ann Med* 1991; **23**: 155–9.

7. Tenkanen L, Manttari M, Manninen V. Some coronary risk factors related to the insulin resistance syndrome and treatment with gemfibrozil. Experience of the Helsinki Heart Study. *Circulation* 1995; **92**:1779–85.

8. Ericsson CG, Hamsten A, Nilsson J, *et al*. Angiographic assessment of effects of bezafibrate on progression of coronary artery disease in young male postinfarction patients. *Lancet* 1996; **347**:849–53.

9. Frick MH, Syvanne M, Nieminen MS, *et al*. Prevention of the angiographic progression of coronary and vein-graft atherosclerosis by gemfibrozil after coronary bypass surgery in men with low levels of HDL cholesterol. *Circulation* 1997; **96**:2137–43.

10. Rubins HB. Veterans Affairs-High Density Lipoprotein Cholesterol Intervention Trial (VA-HIT). Plenary Session XII 'Late Breaking Clinical Trials' Scientific Sessions American Heart Association, Dallas; 1998.

11. Schoonjans K, Staels B, Auwerx J. The peroxisome proliferator activated receptors (PPARs) and their effects on lipid metabolism and adipocyte differentiation. *Biochim Biophys Acta* 1996; **1302**:93–109.

12. Kliewer SA, Sundseth SS, Jones SA, *et al*. Fatty acids and eicosanoids regulate gene expression through direct interactions with peroxisome proliferator-activated receptors α and γ. *Proc Natl Acad Sci USA* 1997; **94**:4318–23.

13. Forman BM, Chen J, Evans RM. Hypolipidemic drugs, polyunsaturated fatty acids, and eicosanoids are ligands for peroxisome proliferator-activated receptors α and δ. *Proc Natl Acad Sci USA* 1997; **94**:4312–17.

14. Devchand PR, Keller H, Peters JM, *et al*. The PPARα-leukotriene B4 pathway to inflammation control. *Nature* 1996; **384**:39–43.

15. Kliewer SA, Lenhard JM, Willson TM, *et al*. A prostaglandin J2 metabolite binds peroxisome proliferator-activated receptor γ and promotes adipocyte differentiation. *Cell* 1995; **83**:813–19.

16. Forman BM, Tontonoz P, Chen J, *et al*. 15-Deoxy-Δ12,14 prostaglandin J2 is a ligand for the adipocyte determination factor PPARγ. *Cell* 1995; **83**: 803–12.

17. Nagy L, Tontonoz P, Alvarez JGA, *et al*. Oxidized LDL regulates macrophage gene expression through ligand activation of PPARγ. *Cell* 1998; **93**:229–40.

18. Pineda Torra I, Gervois P, Staels B. PPARα in metabolic disease, inflammation, atherosclerosis and aging. *Curr Opin Lipidol* 1999; **10**: 151–9.

19. Staels B, Dallongeville J, Auwerx J, *et al*. The mechanism of action of fibrates on lipid and lipoprotein metabolism. *Circulation* 1998; **98**:2088–93.

20. Martin G, Schoonjans K, Lefebvre A-M, *et al*. Coordinate regulation of the expression of the fatty acid transporter protein (FATP) and acyl CoA synthetase (ACS) genes by PPARα and PPARγ activators. *J Biol Chem* 1997; **272**:28210–17.

21. Motojima K, Passilly P, Peters JM, *et al*. Expression of putative fatty acid transporter genes are regulated by peroxisome proliferator-activated receptor alpha and gamma activators in a tissue- and inducer-specific manner. *J Biol Chem* 1998; **273**: 16710–14.

22. Mascaro C, Acosta E, Ortiz JA, *et al*. Control of human muscle-type carnitine palmitoyltransferase I gene transcription by peroxisome proliferator-activated receptor. *J Biol Chem* 1998; **273**: 8560–3.

23. Brandt JM, Djouadi F, Kelly DP. Fatty acids activate transcription of the muscle carnitine palmitoyltransferase I gene in cardiac myocytes via the peroxisome proliferator-activated receptor alpha. *J Biol Chem* 1998; **273**: 23786–92.

24. Kelly LJ, Vicario PP, Thompson GM, *et al*. Peroxisome proliferator-activated receptors gamma and alpha mediate in vivo regulation of uncoupling protein (UCP-1, UCP-2, UCP-3) gene expression. *Endocrinology* 1998; **139**: 4920–7.

25. Kesaniemi YA, Grundy SM. Influence of

gemfibrozil and clofibrate on metabolism of cholesterol and plasma triglycerides in man. *J Am Med Assoc* 1984; 251:2241–6.

26. Hahn SE, Goldberg DM. Modulation of lipoprotein production in Hep G2 cells by fenofibrate and clofibrate. *Biochem Pharmacol* 1992; 43:625–33.

27. Schoonjans K, Peinado-Onsurbe J, Lefebvre A-M, *et al*. PPARα and PPARγ activators direct a distinct tissue-specific transcriptional response via a PPRE in the lipoprotein lipase gene. *EMBO J* 1996; 15:5336–48.

28. Quarfordt SH, Michalopoulos G, Schirmer B. The effect of human C apolipoproteins on the in vitro hepatic metabolism of triglyceride emulsions in the rat. *J Biol Chem* 1982; 257:14642–7.

29. Windler E, Chao Y, Havel RJ. Regulation of the hepatic uptake of triglyceride-rich lipoproteins in the rat. *J Biol Chem* 1980; 255:8303–7.

30. Clavey V, Lestavel-Delattre S, Copin C, *et al*. Modulation of lipoprotein B binding to the LDL receptor by exogenous lipids and apolipoproteins CI, CII, CIII, and E. *Arteriosclerosis Throm Vasc Biol* 1995; 15:963–71.

31. Aalto-Setälä K, Fisher EA, Chen X, *et al*. Mechanism of hypertriglyceridemia in human apolipoprotein (apo) CIII transgenic mice. Diminished very low density lipoprotein fractional catabolic rate associated with increased apo CIII and reduced apo E on the particles. *J Clin Invest* 1992; 90:1889–900.

32. Aalto-Setälä K, Weinstock PH, Bisgaier CL, *et al*. Further characterization of the metabolic properties of triglyceride-rich lipoproteins from human and mouse apo C-III transgenic mice. *J Lipid Res* 1996; 37:1802–11.

33. Ebara T, Ramakrishnan R, Steiner G, Schachter NS. Chylomicronemia due to apolipoprotein CIII overexpression in apolipoprotein E-null mice. Apolipoprotein CIII-induced hypertriglyceridemia is not mediated by effects on apolipoprotein E. *J Clin Invest* 1997; 99: 2672–81.

34. Li WW, Dammerman MM, Smith JD, *et al*. Common genetic variation in the promoter of the human apo CIII gene abolishes regulation by insulin and may contribute to hypertriglyceridemia. *J Clin Invest* 1995; 96:2601–5.

35. Malmendier CL, Lontie J-F, Delcroix C, *et al*. Apolipoproteins C-II and C-III metabolism in hypertriglyceridemic patients. Effect of a drastic triglyceride reduction by combined diet restriction and fenofibrate administration. *Atherosclerosis* 1989; 77:139–49.

36. Ginsberg HN, Le N-A, Goldberg IJ, *et al*. Apolipoprotein B metabolism in subjects with deficiency of apolipoproteins CIII and AI: evidence that apolipoprotein CIII inhibits catabolism of triglyceride-rich lipoproteins by lipoprotein lipase in vivo. *J Clin Invest* 1986; 78:1287–95.

37. Bard JM, Parra HJ, Camare R, *et al*. A multi-center comparison of the effects of simvastatin and fenofibrate therapy in severe primary hypercholesterolemia, with particular emphasis on lipoproteins defined by their apolipoprotein composition. *Metabolism* 1992; 41:498–503.

38. Staels B, Vu-Dac N, Kosykh VA, *et al*. Fibrates downregulate apolipoprotein C-III expression independent of induction of peroxisomal Acyl Coenzyme A Oxidase. *J Clin Invest* 1995; 95:705–12.

39. Haubenwallner S, Essenburg AD, Barnett BC, *et al*. Hypolipidemic activity of select fibrates correlates to changes in hepatic apolipoprotein C-III expression: a potential physiologic basis for their mode of action. *J Lipid Res* 1995; 36:2541–51.

40. Peters JM, Hennuyer N, Staels B, *et al*. Alterations in lipoprotein metabolism in PPARα-deficient mice. *J Biol Chem* 1997; 272: 27307–12.

41. Ladias JAA, Hadzopoulou-Cladaras M, Kardassis D, *et al*. Transcriptional regulation of human apolipoprotein genes apoB, apoCIII, and apoAII by members of the steroid hormone receptor superfamily HNF-4, ARP-1, EAR-2, and EAR-3. *J Biol Chem* 1992; 267:15849–60.

42. Vu-Dac N, Gervois P, Pineda-Torra I, *et al*. Retinoids increase human apo C-III expression at the transcriptional level via the retinoid X receptor. Contribution to the hypertriglyceridemic action of retinoids. *J Clin Invest* 1998; 102:625–32.

43. Hertz R, Bishara-Shieban J, Bar-Tana J. Mode of action of peroxisome proliferators as hypolipidemic drugs, suppression of

apolipoprotein C-III. *J Biol Chem* 1995; 270:13470–5.

44. Vu-Dac N, Chopin-Delannoy S, Gervois P, *et al*. The nuclear receptors PPARα and Reverbα mediate the species-specific regulation of apolipoprotein A-I expression by fibrates. *J Biol Chem* 1998; **273**:25713–18.

45. Gervois P, Chopin-Delannoy S, Fadel A, *et al*. Fibrates increase human Rev-erbα expression in liver via a novel PPAR response element. *Mol Endocrinol* 1998; **13**:400–9.

46. Duez H, Mansen A, Fiévet C, *et al*. Rev-erbα: an orphan nuclear receptor involved in lipoprotein metabolism. *Circulation* 1999; **17**:1–449.

47. Sakai M, Matsushima-Hibiya Y, Nishizawa M, Nishi S. Suppression of rat glutathione transferase P expression by peroxisome proliferators: interaction between Jun and peroxisome proliferator-activated receptor alpha. *Cancer Res* 1995; **55**:5370–6.

48. Staels B, Koenig W, Habib A, *et al*. Activation of human aortic smooth-muscle cells is inhibited by PPARα, but not by PPARγ activators. *Nature* 1998; **393**:790–3.

49. Poynter ME, Daynes DA. PPARα activation modulates cellular redox status, represses NFkB signalling and reduces inflammatory cytokine production in aging. *J Biol Chem* 1998; **273**:32833–41.

50. Zhou YC, Waxman DJ. Cross-talk between janus kinase-signal transducer and activator of transcription (JAK-STAT) and peroxisome proliferator-activated receptor-alpha (PPARα) signalling pathways. Growth hormone inhibition of PPARα transcriptional activity mediated by STAT5b. *J Biol Chem* 1999; **274**:2672–81.

51. Malmendier CL, Delcroix C. Effects of fenofibrate on high and low density lipoprotein metabolism in heterozygous familial hypercholesterolemia. *Atherosclerosis* 1985; **55**:161–9.

52. Staels B, van Tol A, Andreu T, Auwerx J. Fibrates influence the expression of genes involved in lipoprotein metabolism in a tissue-selective manner in the rat. *Arteriosclerosis Thromb* 1992; **12**:286–94.

53. Berthou L, Saladin R, Yaqoob P, *et al*. Regulation of rat liver apolipoprotein A-I, apolipoprotein A-II, and acyl-coenzyme A oxidase gene expression by fibrates and dietary fatty acids. *Eur J Biochem* 1995; **232**:179–87.

54. Vu-Dac N, Schoonjans K, Laine B, *et al*. Negative regulation of the human apolipoprotein A-I promoter by fibrates can be attenuated by the interaction of the peroxisome proliferator-activated receptor with its response element. *J Biol Chem* 1994; **269**:31012–18.

55. Vu-Dac N, Schoonjans K, Kosykh V, *et al*. Fibrates increase human apolipoprotein A-II expression through activation of the peroxisome proliferator-activated receptor. *J Clin Invest* 1995; **96**:741–50.

56. Berthou L, Duverger N, Emmanuel F, *et al*. Opposite regulation of human versus mouse apolipoprotein A-I by fibrates in human apo A-I transgenic mice. *J Clin Invest* 1996; **97**: 2408–16.

57. Kockx M, Princen HM, Kooistra T. Fibrate-modulated expression of fibrinogen, plasminogen activator inhibitor-1 and apolipoprotein A-I in cultured cynomolgus monkey hepatocytes: role of the peroxisome proliferator-activated receptor alpha. *Thromb Haemost* 1998; **80**:942–8.

58. Costet P, Legendre C, More J, *et al*. Peroxisome proliferator-activated receptor alpha-isoform deficiency leads to progressive dyslipidemia with sexually dimorphic obesity and steatosis. *J Biol Chem* 1998; **273**:2577–85.

59. Hennuyer N, Poulain P, Madsen L, *et al*. Beneficial effects of fibrates on apolipoprotein A-I metabolism occur independent of any peroxisome proliferative response. *Circulation* 1999; **99**:2445–51.

4

Genetics: determinants of lipid and lipoprotein concentrations

Ole Faergeman

Introduction

Biotechnology in the clinic is no longer a novelty. Laboratories inside and outside hospitals offer tests for mutations in various genes to physicians and sometimes to lay-persons. Some of this activity is appropriate, but some is predicated on simplistic notions about genes and disease. Using the metabolism of plasma lipoproteins as an example of a complex biological system, this chapter will indicate why genetic determinants of plasma concentrations of lipoproteins, and genetic diagnoses, are not always straightforward.

Metabolism of plasma lipoproteins

Before embarking on a discussion of genetic variation affecting lipoprotein concentrations, the reader should be acquainted with the salient features of the structure and function of the plasma lipoproteins. They consist of a lipid core of triglycerides (triacylglycerols) and esterified cholesterol surrounded by an amphiphilic monolayer of phospholipid, unesterified cholesterol and proteins called apolipoproteins. Their main function is transport of triglycerides, cholesterol and fat soluble vitamins in blood.

Most of the fuel for oxidative metabolism is transported in blood as fatty acids, either in non-esterified form or esterified to glycerol as triglyceride. Smaller amounts are transported as glucose, amino acids, ketone bodies and glycerol.[1] To be soluble in an aqueous solution such as blood, fatty acids and triglycerides are bound to proteins. Non-esterified fatty acids are attached to albumin by weak molecular bonds. They are released from adipose tissue by the action of hormone sensitive lipase, which hydrolyses triglycerides to glycerol and fatty acids. Although concentrations of non-esterified fatty acids in plasma are only about 5–15 mg/dl (0.13–0.39 mmol/l), the turnover rate is so high that more than 100 grams of fatty acid are transported in this manner every 24 hours, moving from adipose tissue to the liver and muscles, including the heart.

More complex lipids such as triglycerides and cholesteryl esters are packaged into the hydrophobic core of lipoproteins. The liver and especially the small intestine release up to 200 grams of fatty acid in the form of triglyceride every 24 hours. In the lumen of the small intestine, alimentary fat is partially hydrolysed to diglycerides and monoglycerides before absorption into epithelial cells. Here, fatty acids are re-esterified to glycerol and the resulting triglyceride is packaged into chylomicrons. These large lipoproteins are released into intestinal lymph (chyle) for transport through the lymphatic vessels to the left subclavian vein. In the liver, fatty acids are similarly esterified and packaged as triglyceride into very low density lipoproteins (VLDL).

Each lipoprotein macromolecule, be it a chylomicron or a VLDL, contains one molecule of apolipoprotein B (apoB). Intestinal apoB is termed apoB-48. It is approximately half the size of apoB-100, which is formed in the liver. In liver cells, apoB-100 is continuously synthesised but is degraded again if triglycerides and perhaps cholesteryl esters are not available for secretion. On the other hand, if these lipids are available, lipoproteins are secreted from the cell with amounts of triglyceride that vary according to rates of triglyceride synthesis.

Chylomicrons and VLDL are carried by blood to adipose tissue, where fatty acids are stored, or to muscles, where they are consumed in oxidative metabolism. Attached to endothelial cells of the capillaries of these tissues is an enzyme, lipoprotein lipase. With apolipoprotein C-II as a cofactor, this enzyme removes part of the core of chylomicrons and VLDL by hydrolysing triglycerides. Chylomicrons that are partially deprived of their core are called chylomicron 'remnants'. Similarly, VLDL 'remnants' are the progressively denser lipoproteins resulting from partial removal of triglyceride from VLDL. They are intermediate in density between VLDL and LDL and are called intermediate density lipoproteins (IDL). The liver removes chylomicron remnants and about half of VLDL remnants from plasma by several, partially interrelated mechanisms involving the LDL receptor, a multipurpose receptor called 'the LDL receptor related protein' and heparan sulphate proteoglycans. The other half of VLDL remnants are further catabolised to LDL. Remnant metabolism has recently been reviewed by Mahley and Ji.[2]

Concentrations of LDL in plasma, which

are closely related to atherogenesis are determined by the balance of rates of synthesis and removal. Although some LDL may be secreted directly from the liver, most are derived from the catabolism of VLDL. There are two mechanisms for the removal of LDL from plasma. Until recently it was thought that most LDL molecules are taken up by extrahepatic tissues, but it now seems clear that hepatic LDL receptors remove the bulk of these lipoproteins from blood plasma: only small amounts of LDL are taken up by LDL receptors in non-hepatic tissues to help satisfy requirements for cholesterol. There is also a receptor independent mechanism for removal of LDL from plasma, which occurs primarily in extrahepatic tissues. Whereas uptake of LDL by the LDL receptor is a saturable process, the non-receptor mediated uptake of LDL is linearly related to the concentration of LDL in plasma.

Cholesterol is derived from food and endogenous synthesis. A little less than half a gram of cholesterol is absorbed every 24 hours in the small intestine, and about twice as much is synthesised in various organs of the body. In many species, probably including man, substantially more than half of the endogenous cholesterol synthesis occurs in extrahepatic tissues. Only small amounts of cholesterol can be used for adrenal or gonadal steroid synthesis, and only small amounts are lost from the body by sloughing of epithelium from the gut and skin. The bulk of cholesterol is transported to the liver for conversion to bile acids or excretion into the bile as cholesterol. This transport process has been termed 'reverse cholesterol transport', but the term is inappropriate, because most cholesterol does not originate in the liver.[3]

The lipoproteins responsible for transport of most of the cholesterol to the liver are the high density lipoproteins (HDL). HDL are not formed in the same way as chylomicrons and VLDL. Precursors of HDL are bilayer discs of protein and phospholipids secreted from liver cells and possibly from intestinal cells. These discs are also called nascent HDL. They function as cholesterol acceptor proteins in extracellular fluids, where they take up cholesterol from cell membranes. In blood plasma, lecithin-cholesterol acyltransferase (LCAT) forms a lipid core of cholesteryl ester within the disc by catalysing the transfer of a fatty acid molecule from lecithin to cholesterol. The result is an HDL3 lipoprotein. As HDL particles enlarge by esterification of more cholesterol, HDL3 are converted into HDL2.

The esterified cholesterol of HDL is removed from the lipoprotein by an HDL receptor on liver cells (SR-B1). About half of cholesterol is transported to the liver in this manner. The rest is moved to the liver by a slightly different route. Cholesteryl esters in the core of HDL can exchange with triglycerides in the core of the apoB containing lipoproteins (VLDL, IDL and LDL). This exchange reaction requires a specific transfer protein called cholesteryl ester transfer protein. Once in the core of VLDL, IDL or LDL, cholesteryl esters are transported with these lipoproteins to the liver, where cholesterol is either excreted into the bile as cholesterol or converted to bile acids. We shall return to the conversion of cholesterol to bile acids at the end of this chapter.

This sketch of the intravascular metabolism of lipoproteins and barest outline of the intracellular metabolism of lipoprotein components serves to indicate that control must be exerted by many hundreds of proteins. As a corollary, the sketch also indicates that there must be myriad ways in which slight or not-so-slight variation in gene structure can affect concentrations of lipoproteins in plasma. Many of these genes are already known to have several and sometimes a very large number of such variations, each of which may or may not affect protein function. But with few exceptions, there is no straightforward or linear relationship between genetic variation and any biochemical or physiological variable, including concentrations of plasma lipoproteins.

Dyslipidaemia caused by variation in one gene

Genetic variations come in several shapes and sizes. The most easily understood are mutations that prevent a gene from encoding a truly key protein with normal function. Within the lipoprotein system, a good example of such a monogenic disease is familial hypercholesterolaemia, which is caused usually by a mutation in the gene for the LDL receptor. The mutation can prevent formation of any receptor protein at all, or it can cause the receptor to be so abnormal that it cannot perform its task of binding and ingesting LDL into the cell. This can result in severe hypercholesterolaemia and premature coronary heart disease. A special case of familial hypercholesterolaemia is discussed later in this chapter, and the disease is covered in full in Chapter 6.

Ligands for the LDL receptor are apolipoprotein B (apoB) and apolipoprotein E (apoE). Apart from its ligand function, apoB is also the main structural protein of chylomicrons, VLDL and LDL. In the case of VLDL, it shares the ligand function with apolipoprotein E. At least eight mutations in the apoB gene cause LDL concentrations to be very low (hypobetalipoproteinaemia) because of defects in synthesis of the protein, and at least two mutations do the reverse. The latter affect the part of the gene coding for the part of the protein that binds to the LDL receptor. One of them (Arg3500Gln) is fairly common, especially in central Europe, which is one of its places of origin. There the incidence is approximately

1 in 250, but further north in Europe it is about 1 in 1 000.[4] The mutation compromises ligand function sufficiently to cause hypercholesterolaemia that is only slightly less severe than that measured in patients with familial hypercholesterolaemia caused by defects in the receptor. The condition is called familial defective apolipoprotein B. The other mutation (Arg3531Cys) is rare, and ligand function is less affected.

ApoB-100 and apoB-48 seem to be apolipoproteins only. They have no known function apart from their structural and ligand functions in the metabolism of lipoproteins. Thus the apoB story and the LDL receptor story are fairly straightforward compared with that of the other ligand for the LDL receptor, namely apoE. We will discuss apoE later in this chapter.

Markers of pathogenetic genetic variation

More common than familial hypercholesterolaemia and familial defective apolipoprotein B are gene variations with modest effects on concentrations of lipoproteins and risk of atherosclerotic disease. To suggest that they are more common and less severe, such variations are termed polymorphisms rather than mutations, but there is no clear distinction between the two concepts.

Interesting polymorphisms do not necessarily have to be in exons, which are those parts of genes that code for proteins. They can occur in the intervening stretches of DNA, the introns, or they can be outside of the gene entirely. So long as they are not too far from the gene, they will almost always be transmitted with the gene from parent to child. As such, they will be good markers for any mutations in exons of the gene that do affect lipoprotein concentrations and risk of disease.

A large number of studies have exploited these marker relationships. As an example, let us consider the gene for lipoprotein lipase, situated on chromosome 8. It contains 10 exons and therefore nine introns. The enzyme protein itself has two functions: an enzyme function and a ligand function. One end of the protein (the N-terminal end) catalyses the hydrolysis of triglycerides in chylomicrons and VLDL as they pass through capillaries of muscle and fat tissue to produce chylomicron remnants or VLDL remnants. Having performed its enzymatic function, the enzyme then lets go of the capillary wall and travels with the remnant lipoproteins to the liver, where the C-terminal end of the enzyme, playing the role of ligand, can help the partially degraded lipoproteins to attach to receptors on liver cells. The cells engulf the lipoproteins and complete the degradation process.

About 30% of genes (alleles) for lipoprotein lipase contain one version of a polymorphic site in intron 8 that prevents a particular enzyme (HindIII), used in the laboratory, from cleaving the gene. The other version of this polymorphic site allows HindIII to cleave the gene. Plasma concentrations of HDL cholesterol are higher in people with two versions of the gene without the cleavage site than in persons with two versions of the gene with the cleavage site. People with both versions, for example a paternal gene without and a maternal gene with the cleavage site, have intermediate concentrations of HDL.[5]

The HindIII cleavage site, situated as it is in an intron, is very unlikely to affect gene function. However, the allele with resistance to cleavage by HindIII is almost always transmitted from generation to generation along with a quite different variation in another part of the gene. The latter is an exonic polymorphism. Genes with one version of this polymorphism encode lipoprotein lipase lacking two amino acids at the C-terminal end of the protein (Ser447Ter). This version of the protein occurs in about 20% of people, and it is associated with slightly higher concentrations of HDL cholesterol, slightly lower concentrations of triglycerides, and slightly lower risk of coronary artery disease.[6] Whether or not the Ser447Ter polymorphism increases the affinity of lipoprotein lipase for liver cell receptors is not known, but it is possible. If so, and if the ligand function of lipoprotein lipase really is important physiologically, it would suggest that lipoproteins, partially degraded by lipoprotein lipase and clearly atherogenic, are more effectively removed from plasma. Of course, it would also explain the relationship to the marker of Ser447Ter, namely the HindIII polymorphism in intron 8.

Studies of markers such as the HindIII polymorphism in the lipoprotein lipase gene have been very useful in demonstrating the degree to which variation in a particular gene can affect biochemical measurements and clinical disease. With the advent of machinery that can determine the sequence of base pairs in the long stretches of DNA that make up the exons and introns of a gene and its closest surroundings, such studies of markers are no longer so important.

The gene for lipoprotein lipase seems to be especially prone to mutation, and Ser447Ter is just one of 38 variations in the exons or the promoter of the lipoprotein lipase gene currently listed in OMIM (Online Mendelian Inheritance in Man), a regularly updated review of human genetic variation available on www.ncbi.nlm.nih.gov/Omim. Closer examination of the gene actually reveals even more variation.[7] Some of the other polymorphisms or mutations have much more profound effects on enzymatic function. For example, several different point mutations, deletions and duplications in the gene destroy its ability

to code for any functional enzyme at all. If both the paternal and the maternal genes are so affected (homozygosiity), triglyceride concentrations can exceed 100 mmol/l (about 10 000 mg/dl), and the patient may present with the chylomicronaemia syndrome (milky plasma, eruptive xanthomatosis and pancreatitis). Chylomicronaemia syndrome can be a result of homozygosity for several different mutations in the gene for apoC-II, the cofactor for lipoprotein lipase. Patients homozygous for severe deficiency of either lipoprotein lipase or apoC-II are victims of nature's knockout experiments with man.

Interactions

Although familial hypercholesterolaemia is one of the classical inborn errors of metabolism, the relationship between mutation, hypercholesterolaemia and coronary heart disease is not invariable. For example, the concentration of LDL cholesterol was on average 4.35 mmol/l (168 mg/dl) in Chinese patients with familial hypercholesterolaemia residing in China. In Chinese patients residing in Canada, on the other hand, the average level was 7.46 mmol/l (288 mg/dl), and age of onset of coronary heart disease was earlier than in China.[8] So environment (in this case probably diet), significantly modifies the effects of genetic variation. However, interactions come in many shapes and sizes, some of them unexpected.

The OMIM lists 58 allelic variants in the LDL receptor gene, and specialised registries of LDL receptor mutations now tally more than 350 such mutations, which have been reviewed recently.[9] While exploring the mutational spectrum in Danish families with familial hypercholesterolaemia, we found a mutation not in one but in two of the 18 exons of the same LDL receptor gene allele (either the paternal or the maternal one).[10] The mutation in exon 11 caused a single amino acid substitution in the protein, and the mutation in exon 17 deleted three amino acids from the part of the receptor that anchors it to the plasma membrane of cells. But which of the mutations was the culprit?

To try to answer that question, LDL receptor genes containing one or both of these mutations were incorporated (transfected) into cells in culture. Each of the mutations alone had little or no effect on the ability of the cells to take up LDL from the culture medium. However, receptor function was reduced by 75% when the transfected gene contained both mutations. Thus they acted in synergy to cause disease in that particular family. Had we stopped the study of the family when we found the first of these mutations, we might have declared it the culprit, when in fact it caused mischief only in the company of the other mutation. The study emphasises that it is important to ascertain the pathogenicity of any particular genetic variation before declaring to the patient (and the professional community) that it causes disease.

Other forms of interaction are much more common than this intragenic one. In fact, interactions of various kinds are probably the rule rather than the exception. Let us look at the gene for apolipoprotein E, the other ligand for the LDL receptor, which has interesting interactions with the environment and with other genes.

First, however, we should note that different variations in the gene promote quite different diseases. ApoE is much smaller than apoB-100 (299 versus 4535 amino acids), and it appears to have physiological functions apart from its role as a ligand for the interaction of chylomicrons and VLDL with receptors in the liver. Perhaps for these reasons, the pathophysiology associated with polymor-

phisms in the gene for apoE varies a lot. The most commonly occurring version (the 'wild type') of apoE is termed apoE-3. ApoE-2 is formed if arginine is replaced by cysteine at amino acid position 158. If cysteine is replaced by arginine at amino acid position 112, apoE-4 is formed. ApoE-3, apoE-4 and apoE-2 are the most common isoforms of apoE, but several other amino acid substitutions occur at other sites.

The common polymorphism is related to at least three disease entities. First, dysbeta-lipoproteinaemia can afflict people with two versions of the apoE-2 isoform. This rare form of hyperlipidaemia increases the risk of atherosclerotic disease. However, it is more severe when it is caused by mutations in the receptor binding domain of apoE (amino acids 136–150).

Second, people with one or especially two versions of apoE-4 (E-4/E-3, E-4/E-2 or E-4/E-4) are at slightly increased risk of developing Alzheimer's disease. ApoE serves to transport lipids in the nervous system and, in experimental settings, apoE-3 and apoE-4 affect neurite extension differently. Additional insights may be necessary to explain the relationship of variation in the apoE gene to Alzheimer's disease.

Third, the rate of coronary heart disease in people with apoE-4 is about 40% higher than that in people with apoE-3/E-3. This increase in risk may well be due to differences in the affinity of apoE-3 and apoE-4 for the various receptors involved in hepatic removal of remnants of VLDL and chylomicrons from plasma. ApoE-4 is not as good a ligand as apoE-3, and people with one or two versions of apoE-4 are slightly hyperlipidaemic.[2]

Quantitatively important gene–gene and gene–environment interactions are suggested by a recent study of the apoE polymorphism and risk of recurrence of coronary heart disease and

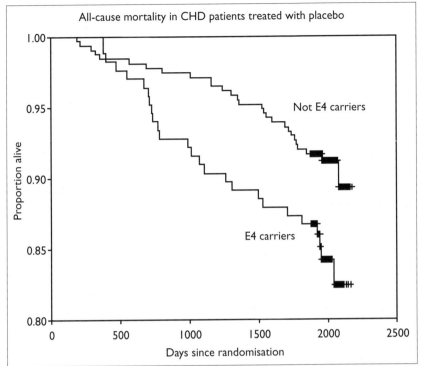

All-cause mortality in CHD patients treated with placebo

Not E4 carriers

E4 carriers

Proportion alive

Days since randomisation

Fig. 4.1
Kaplan–Meier curves for all-cause mortality in patients with coronary heart disease with and without the gene for apoE-4, when treated with placebo in the Scandinavian Simvastatin Survival Study. Reproduced with permission.[11]

death,[11] which formed a substudy of the Scandinavian Simvastatin Survival Study (4S). This latter study had shown that treatment of CHD patients with simvastatin increased survival by 30% in the course of 5.4 years.[12]

In the substudy, blood for apoE genotyping was available from 966 Danish and Finnish 4S patients. The relationship between the common apoE polymorphism and the risk of dying in placebo patients and in patients treated with simvastatin is depicted in Figures 4.1 and 4.2. In the placebo group, patients with apoE-4 had a 15.7% risk of dying during the course of the study. If they did not have the apoE-4 allele, risk was only 9.0%. Since simvastatin reduced those risks to 6.0 and 5.1%, respectively, reduction in risk was far greater in patients with the apoE-4 allele (9.7%) than in those without it (3.9%). This particular

genetic analysis identified patients who were both at greatest risk and most likely to benefit from preventive treatment. Since the drug is an environmental factor in this situation, these findings illustrate one kind of interaction between genes and environment.

The same substudy illustrated additive effects or interaction between genes. A small number of LDL molecules sometimes possess a protein in addition to apoB. This additional protein is called apolipoprotein(a) or apo(a). With apo(a) attached to LDL, the whole complex is called Lp(a) (pronounced 'LP little A'). This is a good illustration of the arcane language used by researchers in one field to keep everybody else at bay. Most population studies show that people with high concentrations of Lp(a) in plasma and, by extension, the risk of coronary artery disease attributable to Lp(a) in

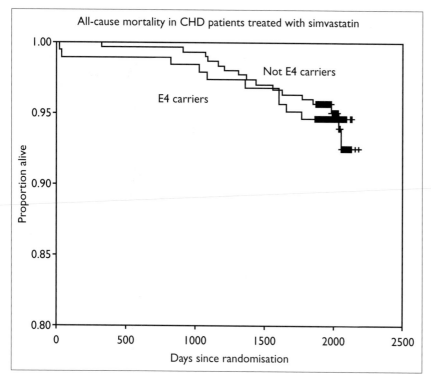

Fig. 4.2
Kaplan–Meier curves for all-cause mortality in patients with coronary artery disease with and without the gene for apoE-4, when treated with active drug in the Scandinavian Simvastatin Survival Study. Reproduced with permission.[11]

serum are at increased risk of coronary heart disease.[13] Conventionally, concentrations exceeding 30 mg/dl (0.78 mmol/l) are considered to be too high. We used this cut-off point in the study of the apoE polymorphism in 4S patients. A patient in the placebo group was fortunate if his Lp(a) level was below 30 mg/dl (0.78 mmol/l) and he had no apoE-4. In that case, risk of dying before the study ended was 6.5%. The risk was doubled if he or she had either the apoE-4 allele or Lp(a) concentrations over 30 mg/dl (0.78 mmol/l), and it was more than tripled if he or she had both risk factors. Again, treatment with simvastatin reduced risk of dying to the same low level (5–7%) in all of these groups. It was reduced by 13% in patients without apoE-4 and with low Lp(a) levels, by 50% in patients with either apoE-4 or high Lp(a) levels, and by 80% in patients with both risk factors.

The gene for apo(a) contains several variations. They will not be described in detail here, probably to the reader's relief. The important feature about them is that they largely determine concentrations of Lp(a) in plasma and, by extension, the risk of coronary artery disease attributed to Lp(a). Therefore the data from the 4S substudy illustrate not only that the genes for apoE and apo(a) interact or act additively to affect risk of death in patients with coronary artery disease, they also show that the drug cuts into the gene–gene interaction and creates a triple interactive process, the gene–gene–environment interaction. We abstained from looking for more interactions, but they were surely there.

There was one additional and remarkable finding in that study. LDL cholesterol concentrations in the placebo group and simvastatin group were the same, irrespective of the pres-

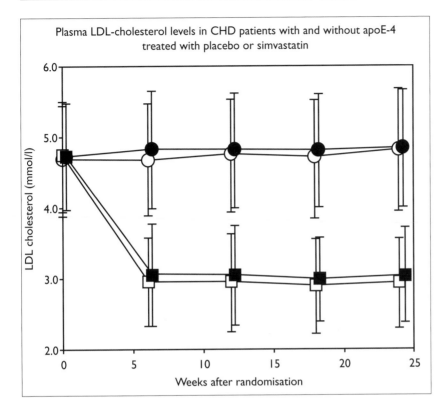

Plasma LDL-cholesterol levels in CHD patients with and without apoE-4 treated with placebo or simvastatin

Fig. 4.3
LDL-cholesterol concentrations in plasma of patients with coronary artery disease with (filled symbols) or without (empty symbols) the gene for apoE-4 during the first 24 weeks of treatment with placebo (upper curves) or simvastatin (lower curves) in the Scandinavian Simvastatin Survival Study. Reproduced with permission.[11]

ence of apoE-4 (Figure 4.3). We had no measurements of remnant lipoproteins in plasma, and the manner of drug interaction with the two kinds of genetic variation could therefore reside in drug effects on plasma lipid variables that were not measured. However, the complex interaction noted here could also have been produced by effects of the drug that were either unrelated or indirectly related to those on plasma lipoproteins.

Redundancy

The chylomicronaemia syndrome and familial hypercholesterolaemia are two of nature's several experiments with man, demonstrating how genetic variation can affect concentra-

tions of plasma lipoproteins and risk of disease. Analogous lessons emerge from many of man's experiments on animals genetically changed by breeding or genetic engineering. For example, inbreeding was used to develop the Watanabe Heritable Hyperlipidaemic (WHHL) rabbit, in which severe hyperlipidaemia is due to abnormal function of the LDL receptor. The animal develops atherosclerosis spontaneously. Mice without LDL receptors and mice without apoE have been produced by gene knockout.[14] The LDL receptor deficient mice have moderately severe hypercholesterolaemia similar to that in humans, but they do not develop atherosclerosis unless given fat and cholesterol to eat. In contrast, apoE deficient mice are severely hyperlipidaemic even on a normal diet, but the hyperlipidaemia differs from that in humans. When fed a diet resembling the average American human diet, cholesterol concentrations soar to 2000 mg/dl (51.8 mmol/l), and the mice develop severe atherosclerosis that is similar in several respects to atherosclerosis in humans. These experimental animals demonstrate how changes in one gene can affect dramatically the concentrations of plasma lipoproteins and propensity to develop atherosclerosis. However, if gene knockout produces no dramatic phenotypic change, it does not necessarily mean that the gene is unimportant. It might indicate that the gene and its product are the central or ancillary parts of a system of important back-up mechanisms. Redundancy is likely when vital functions are involved.

Let us consider again cholesterol transport to the liver. The body cannot break down the ring structure of cholesterol. Sterols obviously do not accumulate in tissues under normal circumstances: on the other hand, as we noted earlier, only small amounts of cholesterol are converted to steroid hormones or sloughed with skin and intestinal mucosa. Therefore there must be robust mechanisms for getting cholesterol out of the body. Most cholesterol is secreted as such into the bile or converted to bile acids and, as indicated in the introduction to this chapter, there are several mechanisms for getting cholesterol to the liver: it can be routed directly to an HDL receptor on liver cells, but it can also arrive there indirectly by way of VLDL and LDL, with the help of cholesterol ester transfer protein.

In the liver, there seems to be yet more redundancy in the systems for cholesterol removal.[15] Researchers knocked out the gene for 7α-hydroxylase in mice. This enzyme catalyses the attachment of a hydroxyl group to the seventh carbon atom of cholesterol, the initial step in the conversion of cholesterol to bile acid. The knockout mice, homozygous for 7α-hydroxylase deficiency, had malabsorption

of fat, skin abnormalities and general wasting. Given the physiological function of bile acids, the researchers had expected all of the mice to die, and that is what 90% of them did within 3 weeks of birth. However 10% of the mice recovered and survived normally, which was unexpected. These survivors had a back-up system, an additional 7α-hydroxylase, the gene for which had not been knocked out. This enzyme catalysed the 7α-hydroxylation, not of cholesterol, but of two oxysterols, to which cholesterol had been converted by hydroxylation of either the 25th or the 27th carbon atom. Therefore in a fortunate minority of the mice, there were at least two mechanisms for converting cholesterol to bile acids.

Hepatic removal of remnant lipoproteins from plasma[2] and intracellular esterification of cholesterol[16] provide still more examples of redundancy in the metabolism of lipids, but these should suffice to make the point that redundancy must be expected in vital biological processes. Evidence of redundancy can suggest exciting new biological pathways for analysis. However, it also deserves study in its own right. Like interactions between genes and between genes and environment, redundancy is likely to explain in part why genetic variations so often do not have the consequences we expect, if a gene in fact 'determined' concentrations of lipids or lipoproteins or so many other biochemical, physiological or clinical phenomena.

Conclusions

Our whole environment and all of our genes do, of course, determine almost everything in us, including plasma concentrations of lipids and lipoproteins. In this chapter we have emphasised that some genetic variations are only markers of the genetic variations that affect phenotypes, and we have looked at examples of various forms of interaction and redundancy in the metabolism of lipids and lipoproteins that demonstrably modify the relationships between genes and phenotypes.

Like other well used dualities, however, that of 'nurture and nature' is simplistic. Time is not implicit, for example, and time changes everything, almost always irreversibly. How we lived in the womb and soon after birth, whether or not we have been afflicted with disease, how we may have eaten earlier but not necessarily now, all are likely to modify the way genes and the immediate environment affect lipoprotein concentrations and risk of disease. Also not implicit in the duality, but emphasised in this chapter, is that the workings of nature and nurture are not simply additive: their mutual relationship is very unlikely to be neatly linear.

Irreversibility and non-linearity are said to characterise complex systems, of which the lipoprotein system is probably a good example. On the epistemological level, recognition of this complexity should encourage us to reduce it to component complexities like interaction and redundancy, if we do not belong to the increasing coterie of scientists that embraces holistic approaches such as neural networking.[17]

On a clinical level, recognition of complexity should temper enthusiasm for genetic testing as a way to advise patients about risks of genetic disease. At this stage of our understanding, it might be best to restrict non-research, clinical, genetic testing to looking for mutations in genes that almost always are pathogenetic. In the lipoprotein field, and in populations with a high intake of dietary fat, this means genes for the LDL receptor and apolipoprotein B when the concern is atherosclerotic disease, and the genes for lipoprotein lipase and apoC-II when the concern is chylomicronaemia syndrome.

Acknowledgement

This chapter was prepared during Ole Faergeman's tenure of grant 22511 from the Danish Heart Association.

References

1. Havel RJ. Caloric homeostasis and disorders of fuel transport. *N Engl J Med* 1972; **287**: 1186–92.
2. Mahley RW, Ji Z-S. Remnant lipoprotein metabolism: key pathways involving cell-surface heparan sulfate proteoglycans and apolipoprotein E. *J Lipid Res* 1999; **40**:1–16.
3. Dietschy JM. Theoretical considerations of what regulates low-density-lipoprotein and high-density-lipoprotein cholesterol. *Am J Clin Nutr* 1997; **65(suppl.)**:S1581–S1589.
4. Hansen PS, Nørgaard-Petersen B, Meinertz H, *et al.* Incidence of the apolipoprotein B-3500 mutation in Denmark. *Clin Chim Acta* 1994; **230**:101–4.
5. Gerdes C, Gerdes LU, Hansen PS, Faergeman O. Polymorphisms in the lipoprotein lipase gene and their associations with plasma lipid concentrations in 40-years old Danish men. *Circulation* 1995; **92**:1765–9.
6. Wittrup HH, Tybjærg-Hansen A, Nordestgaard BG. Lipoprotein lipase mutations, plasma lipids and lipoproteins, and risk of ischemic heart disease. A meta-analysis. *Circulation* 1999; **99**:2901–7.
7. Templeton AR, Clark AG, Weiss KM, *et al.* Recombinational and mutational hotspots with the human lipoprotein lipase gene. *Am J Hum Genet* 2000; **66**:69–83.
8. Pimstone SN, Sun X-M, du Souich C, *et al.* Phenotypic variation in heterozygous familial hypercholesterolemia: a comparison of Chinese patients with the same or similar mutations in the LDL-receptor gene living in China or Canada. *Arteriosclerosis Thromb Vasc Biol* 1995; **15**:1704–12.
9. Soutar A. Update on low density lipoprotein receptor mutations. *Curr Opin Lipidol* 1998; **9**:141–47.
10. Jensen HK, Jensen TG, Faergeman O, *et al.* Two mutations in the same low-density

lipoprotein receptor allele act in synergy to reduce receptor function in heterozygous familial hypercholesterolemia. *Hum Mutat* 1997; **9**:437–44.

11. Gerdes LU, Gerdes C, Kervinen K, *et al*. The apolipoprotein ε4 allele determines prognosis and the effect on prognosis of simvastatin in survivors of myocardial infarction. A substudy of the Scandinavian Simvastatin Survival Study (4S). *Circulation* (In press).

12. 4S Study Group. Randomised trial of cholesterol lowering in 4444 patients with coronary heart disease: the Scandinavian Simvastatin Survival Study (4S). *Lancet* 1994; **344**:1383–89.

13. Klausen IC, Sjøl A, Hansen PS, *et al*. Apolipoprotein(a) isoforms and coronary heart disease in men. A nested case-control study. *Atherosclerosis* 1997; **132**:77–84.

14. Smith JD. Mouse models of atherosclerosis. *Lab Anim Sci* 1998; **48**:573–79.

15. Schwartz M, Lund EG, Russell DW. Two 7α-hydroxylase enzymes in bile acid biosynthesis. *Curr Opin Lipidol* 1998; **9**:113–18.

16. Farese RV. Acyl CoA:cholesterol acyltransferase genes and knockout mice. *Curr Opin Lipidol* 1998; **9**:119–23.

17. Coveney P, Highfield R. *Frontiers of Complexity*. New York: Ballantine Books; 1995.

5

Lipoproteins in the brain: a new frontier?

Stefanie Koch and Ulrike Beisiegel

Introduction

Lipoproteins in plasma have been studied extensively and various diseases have been related to defects in lipoprotein metabolism. However, even though the percentage of lipids within the central nervous system (CNS) is higher than in any other organ[1] only comparatively few studies have been performed on lipoproteins in brain. Neurological symptoms have been observed in abetalipoproteinemia, a disease in which no chylomicrons are formed in the intestine and uptake of lipids and lipophilic vitamins is considerably decreased. These symptoms are thought to be caused by the reduced supply of lipophilic vitamins and possibly also essential fatty acids to the brain. This observation emphasizes the importance of the supply of lipophilic substances to the brain and indicates the necessity for a lipid transport system within the cerebrospinal fluid (CSF). However, until now the mechanism for the delivery of lipids to the CNS has not been thoroughly investigated and the question of how essential fatty acids and lipophilic vitamins enter the brain has not been answered. It is a fact that the brain, although not metabolically dependent on fatty acid oxidation, still needs to be supplied with essential fatty acids[2] and vitamins. In addition to cellular cholesterol synthesis, cholesterol uptake might also be important for neuronal growth and repair,

in particular during brain development. On the other hand, oxidized lipids, including oxysterols (which are formed during nerve cell degeneration and cell death), need to be removed to prevent accumulation of these toxic metabolites in the brain.[3] All these lipophilic substances must be associated with lipoproteins for transport. Therefore CSF-lipoproteins (CLP), together with their respective receptors, are essential for lipid homeostasis in the brain and consequently for brain function.

Plasma lipoproteins cannot pass the blood–brain barrier (BBB) and an independent lipid metabolism and distinct lipid transport system in the brain and CSF must be postulated. Until recently there was only very limited information available on the lipoprotein system of the brain and it is only now that more detailed data are beginning to appear in the literature, characterizing lipoproteins in the CSF and lipoprotein syntheses in astrocytes.[4]

Lipoproteins, which provide lipids for cellular metabolism, need to be taken up via receptor mediated processes. Several members of the LDL receptor family, important in the uptake of apolipoprotein (apo) E containing lipoproteins,[5] have been found to be expressed in the CNS.[6] The physiological role of these receptors in lipoprotein uptake in the brain has not yet been demonstrated. However, recent data have indicated a function for some

	Plasma	CSF
Apolipoproteins (mg/dl)		
apoE	4[10]	0.31
apoA-I	130[10]	0.04
Lipids (mg/dl)		
total	500	2.3[9]
cholesterol	190	0.8[9]
phospholipids	200	0.4[11]
triglycerides	100	0.4[11]
total fatty acids	340	1.0[9]

Table 5.1

Concentrations of apolipoproteins and lipids in human CSF compared to plasma

members of the LDL receptor family in the transduction of signals necessary for cell migration.[7]

Last but not least, the observation that apoE-4 is associated with late onset Alzheimer's disease (AD) has raised a great deal of interest in the role of lipoproteins in the human brain.[8] An important point raised by the current research in AD is lipid peroxidation, which is shown to be increased in people with AD in comparison to controls.[9] Unsaturated fatty acids are the substrate for lipid peroxidation and lipophilic vitamins are important inhibitors of oxidative processes. The balance in supply to the brain of unsaturated (essential) fatty acids and lipophilic antioxidants such as vitamin E might be important for the oxidation status in the CSF.

In this chapter we summarize the current knowledge of the lipoprotein system in the CSF and give an overview of the potential physiological role of lipoproteins, apolipoproteins and their receptors, as well as their potential pathophysiological relevance in neurological diseases.

CSF-lipoproteins, apolipoproteins, and enzymes

A comparison of the concentrations of some lipoprotein constituents in the CSF versus levels found in plasma is given in Table 5.1. The concentration of all lipids and apoA-I is more than 100-fold less in CSF compared to plasma. Thus the measurement of these parameters and consequently the investigation of lipoproteins in the CSF is quite sophisticated. Data on CSF composition are available mainly from human CSF (fresh or postmortem material from lumbar or ventricular punctures). In contrast, studies of localization and gene expression of proteins relevant in lipoprotein metabolism in the brain are performed mostly in animal models. Those results are reviewed elsewhere.[12]

CSF-lipoproteins (CLP) were first detected by Swahn et al. in 1961,[13] and the first qualitative and semi-quantitative analysis of some apolipoproteins (A-I, C-II, C-III and E) was performed in 1979 by Roheim et al.[14] Since that time, to our knowledge, only four other

Reference	Method	Particles described	Density (g/ml)	Size (nm)	Apolipoprotein content
Pitas et al. 1987[15]	density gradient, affinity-chromatography	apoE-fraction apo-A-I-fraction	1.09–1.15 1.09–1.15	14 14	E + CE, C, (PE), PC, Sph A-I + CE, C, (PC)
Borghini et al. 1995[16]	gelfiltration, affinity-chromatography (parallel and sequential)	CSF-LpE CSF-LpA-I third population		20 20 32	A-I, A-IV, D, E, J A-I, A-IV, D, E, J A-IV, D, J
Koudinov et al. 1996[17]	sequential flotation ultracentrifugation	CSF-VLDL/LDL CSF-HDL$_2$ CSF-HDL$_3$ CSF-VHDL	0.99–1.063 1.063–1.125 1.125–1.21 1.21–1.25		A-IV, E A-I, A-II, A-IV, C-II, D, E, J, Aβ A-I, A-II, A-IV, C-II, D, E, J, Aβ A-I, A-II, A-IV, J, Aβ
Guyton et al. 1998[18]	density gradient gelfiltration	HDL$_1$	1.006–1.060	18	E

There is no unified nomenclature yet for CSF-lipoproteins. C, cholesteryl; CE, cholesterol ester; PE, phosphatidyl-ethanolamine; PC, phosphatidylcholine; Sph, sphingomyelin.

Table 5.2
Subpopulations of CSF-lipoproteins

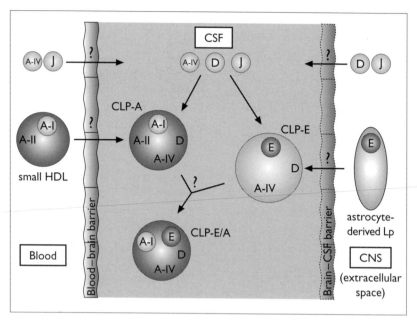

Fig. 5.1
ApoA-I lipoproteins are believed to be derived from the plasma (CLP-A). ApoE particles are synthesized as discoidal precursors from astrocytes and it is hypothesized that they are converted to spherical particles by acquiring cholesteryl esters within the parenchyma of the CNS before reaching the CSF as CLP-E.[4] Here CLP-E/A might be formed by interaction between these two particles. The apolipoproteins A-IV, D, and J might either be soluble or lipoprotein-associated in the CSF.

groups have tried to characterize CLP in terms of size, density, and/or apolipoprotein and lipid content[15–18] and their results are summarized in Table 5.2.

There is no final classification of CLP yet, but taking together all of the findings regarding distribution and origin of CSF apolipoproteins, we propose a scheme for the lipoprotein system in the CSF which is presented in Figure 5.1. ApoE and apoA-I are the main structural apolipoproteins in the CSF (in contrast to the merely lipoprotein associated apolipoproteins, such as apoA-IV, D, and Cs). The structural apolipoproteins are responsible for the formation of different classes of CLP. The size range of CLP is rather small (5–20 nm) and comparable to the 5–15 nm of apoA-I containing particles (HDL) in plasma. The apoB containing particles in plasma are much larger (20–1000 nm) and are not present in CSF. Therefore it can be assumed that the metabo-

lism and function of CLP is somewhat different from plasma lipoproteins.

It has been shown that apoE containing CLP are synthesized by astrocytes within the brain[4] in contrast to apoA-I lipoproteins which most probably originate from plasma. Therefore one can predict the existence of at least two distinct CLP classes. In accordance with this, Koudinov *et al.*[17] found less dense apoE containing particles (an observation that was later confirmed by Guyton *et al.*[18]), as well as very dense apoA-I containing CLP (see Table 5.2). In addition they found a large CLP population with the density of plasma-HDL (CSF-HDL$_2$ and CSF-HDL$_3$), containing various apolipoproteins. Separation of lipoproteins by density does not allow a statement of whether all those apolipoproteins are found in the same or distinct particles. In addition, loosely associated apolipoproteins can easily dissociate during ultracentrifugation. However in earlier studies, Borghini *et al.*[16] used affinity chromatography to show that apoE and apoA-I can be found in the same particle. Taking these results together, one could hypothesize that larger apoE-CLP interact with small apoA-I-CLP resulting in a medium-sized E/A-I particle produced by an exchange of apolipoproteins and presumably also lipids. In addition to these three CLP classes (CLP-E, CLP-A and CLP-E/A), Borghini *et al.* found a fourth group of CLP containing neither apoE nor apoA-I but apoA-IV, D and J. This observation is not unexpected, as in plasma these apolipoproteins are found both lipoprotein associated and free, or bound with only a few lipids. Our recent data on human CLP confirm the presence of a lipid-poor apolipoprotein fraction (Koch *et al.*, manuscript in preparation).

Two groups have already tried to shed some light on the function of CLP.[19,20] Fagan *et al.*[20] demonstrated the ability of apoE-3 enriched CLP to promote neurite outgrowth, a process that seems to be LRP mediated. On the other hand, Rebeck *et al.*[19] showed that CLP can decrease intracellular levels of cholesterol, a process that has been shown to be mediated in plasma by apoA-I containing HDL. Further studies are needed to clarify finally whether these different functions can be attributed to one or the other CLP of the above mentioned classes.

Most plasma apolipoproteins, with the exception of apoB, have been detected in the CSF and at least three (apoE, apoD and apoJ) are synthesized in the mammalian brain. Others, such as apoA-I, apoA-II and apoA-IV, most probably originate from plasma, crossing the blood–brain barrier conceivably by transcytosis or paracellular transport of small lipoproteins[21] (Table 5.3).

The complex morphology of the brain and variations in the localization between species mean that a detailed description of the expression pattern of apolipoproteins in different brain regions and cell types would be beyond the purpose of this review and what is known so far has already been described elsewhere.[12] Instead, we will summarize the current knowledge of the functions of apolipoproteins and enzymes in plasma and the brain.

ApoA-I

ApoA-I in plasma is found mainly on HDL particles participating in reverse cholesterol transport, a process known to be important for cholesterol removal from peripheral tissues. As already mentioned, apoA-I is not expressed in the brain, but porcine brain endothelial cells seem to be able to synthesize apoA-I.[27] It has been shown that CSF lipoproteins can decrease intracellular levels of cholesterol.[19] This effect could be the result of the presence of CLP-A, which resembles plasma HDL. Further studies are required to show whether it can be attributed to a certain CLP subpopulation which might provide a transport system in the CSF for the removal of excess cholesterol and/or modified lipids, comparable to the reverse cholesterol transport in the plasma.

ApoA-II

ApoA-II in plasma is associated with apoA-I containing HDL and seems to play a major role in maintaining HDL levels by interaction with hepatic lipase. ApoA-II has been detected in the CSF[15] and the formation of homo- and heterodimeric complexes has been studied under normal and pathological conditions.[19] Nevertheless the function of apoA-II in the brain remains obscure.

ApoA-IV

ApoA-IV is found both lipoprotein associated and in the lipoprotein free plasma fraction

Apolipoprotein	Plasma Function	Concentration (mg/dl)	Detection in CSF	Brain Function	References
apoA-I	structural protein of HDL, activation of LCAT, reverse cholesterol transport	120–140	+	nerve regeneration	Dawson et al.[22]
apoA-II	activation of HL, triglyceride metabolism	35–50	+	?	Tso et al.[23]
apoA-IV	activation of LCAT	<5	+	satiety signal, nerve regeneration	Boyles et al.[24]
apoB-100	structural protein of all Lp except HDL, cholesterol metabolism	70–90	–	–	
apoB-48	binding to LDL receptor	<5	–	–	
apoC-I	inhibition of Lp binding to liver receptors, activation of LCAT	5–8	–	–	
apoC-II	activation of LpL	3–7	+	activation of LpL?	
apoC-III	inhibition of LpL, inhibition of Lp binding to receptors	10–12	+	–	
apoD	activation and stabilization of LCAT, 'multiligand-multifunction' protein	8–10	+*	degenerative and regenerative processes	Boyles et al.[24]
apoE	ligand for lipoprotein receptors	3–5	+*	neuronal repair, neurite outgrowth, synaptic plasticity	Swartz et al.[25]
apoH	binding to phospholipids (PL)	15–30	+*	transport of PL across BBB?	Shayo et al.[26]
apoJ	distribution of cholesterol	7–20	+*	transport of β-amyloid across BBB?	

*, synthesized in the brain; Aβ, β-amyloid; Lp, lipoproteins.

Table 5.3
Human apolipoproteins in plasma and CSF

and affects mainly triglyceride metabolism. It has been proposed that apoA-IV is a circulating signal released in response to fat intake, regulating satiety and inhibiting gastric acid secretion. ApoA-IV seems to act centrally since its concentration in CSF is increased after a lipid rich meal.[23] However, the mechanism for this regulation has not yet been clarified. ApoA-IV has been detected in tanycytes and astrocytes,[28] and an accumulation of this apolipoprotein was described under pathological conditions, namely in regenerating and remyelinating mammalian peripheral nerves.[24]

ApoC

No expression of the various proteins of the apoC family has been found in the brain. Roheim *et al.*[14] detected reasonable amounts of apoC-II and apoC-III in the CSF by electroimmunoassay, but since then no other investigators have been able to show apoC proteins in CSF. Borghini *et al.*[16] found traces of these apolipoproteins, but did not present the data, and we and others[29] were unable to detect any apoC. In plasma, apoC-II is a necessary activator for LpL activity and, given the results of several studies of lipoprotein lipase (LpL) activity in brain tissues,[30] the presence of apoC-II as an cofactor for LpL in human CSF can be postulated.

ApoD

ApoD was originally described in plasma by McConathy and Alaupovic.[31] It was found to be structurally unrelated to other apolipoproteins; rather, it belongs to the lipocalin superfamily, whose members carry small lipophilic ligands.[32] It is expressed in many tissues, including the brain, where it is synthesized by a variety of cell types.[33] It is proposed to be important for cholesterol transport in compartments without direct contact with the blood. Several lines of evidence suggest a role

in the nervous system in degenerative and regenerative processes. ApoD was shown to be induced in regenerating nerves following crush injury.[24] In Niemann–Pick disease type C and in pharmacological (kainate) induced neurodegeneration in rats, apoD accumulates in cells destined for subsequent cell death.[34,35] In patients with AD or other neuropathologies, apoD levels are increased in the CSF.[36] These data suggest an important function for apoD beyond lipoprotein metabolism.

ApoE

ApoE is a well studied apolipoprotein in plasma, occurring in three major genetically determined isoforms (E-2, E-3 and E-4). It is a key regulator of plasma lipid levels and plays an active role in the catabolism of triglyceride rich lipoproteins. Via apoE, these lipoproteins can be recognized by all members of the LDL receptor family.[37] Studies from several laboratories have shown that apoE is synthesized in the brain and does not enter the brain from the plasma. The most convincing experiment demonstrated that, after liver transplantation from a donor with a different apoE genotype, the apoE isoforms in brain did not change.[38] Several lines of evidence indicate that apoE has important functions in the brain both within and beyond lipoprotein metabolism. It is the major apolipoprotein in the CSF[14] and, next to the liver, the brain is the organ with highest levels of apoE mRNA.[39] ApoE synthesis increases dramatically in response to nerve injury[24] and it has been implicated in neurite outgrowth[40] and synaptic plasticity.[41] On the other hand, it has been shown that apoE is not essential for delivery of cholesterol for axonal growth[42] and mice deficient in the apolipoprotein do not have an obvious neurological phenotype. Regeneration and reutilization of cholesterol after nerve injury occur in the absence of both apoE and apoA-I.[43] This suggests that considerable redundancy is built into the lipoprotein assisted process of cholesterol redistribution.

An association of the isoform E-4 with late onset AD was reported in 1993.[8] This observation was confirmed by many other laboratories and was recently summarized by Mahley and Huang.[44] ApoE has been localized in senile plaques in AD patients, but until now the biochemical basis for this association has not been revealed. Several experimental approaches examined isoform specific binding of apoE to β-amyloid (*ex vivo*), the main component of the senile plaques in AD,[45] as well as to tau (*in vitro*), a microtubule associated protein forming the paired helical filaments in AD brains.[46] Pathological hyperphosphorylation of the tau protein leads to the formation of tangles and apoE-3 and E-2 have been described as interacting with tau and protecting it from hyperphopshorylation, whereas apoE-4 does not have this effect. However, there is no evidence of apoE entering the cytosol, an action that would be needed for a direct interaction with tau.[47] An interaction between apoE and β-amyloid on lipoproteins seems to be reasonable and may be relevant in preventing plaque formation. Against the background of our preliminary data on lipid levels in the CSF of AD patients, and from the general understanding of lipoprotein metabolism, we propose that the association of apoE-4 with AD might be related to the different lipid levels and lipoprotein composition in apoE-4 carriers, rather than to the different structure of apoE-4 itself. In favor of this hypothesis is the finding of a reduction of cholesterol, phospholipids and fatty acids, suggesting an altered lipid homeostasis and lipoprotein pattern in the brain of AD patients.[48,49]

ApoH

ApoH (β_2-glycoprotein-I) is predominantly a plasma protein, but 30% is found associated with lipoproteins. The role of apoH in lipid metabolism has not been fully established. It has been shown to activate LpL and to stimulate the removal of triglycerides. It is also thought to have different physiological functions as well as pathological properties attributed to its binding to acidic phospholipids, that is regulation of platelet dependent thrombosis and antiphospholipid syndrome.[50] ApoH is expressed in the brain[51] and has been shown to be recognized by LRP2/megalin,[52] as is also described for apoJ. So far this finding has been discussed only with respect to implications in the kidney, but given the fact that LRP2/megalin is expressed in brain microvessels, one could also assume a function for apoH in the transport of phospholipids across the blood–brain barrier.

ApoJ

ApoJ (also called clusterin or SGP-2) was described in 1990 by de Silva *et al.*[53] and Illingworth and Glover[54] and is now recognized as a multifunctional glycoprotein with numerous proposed roles in complement mediated cytolysis, cell aggregation and chemotaxis, cell death and lipoprotein metabolism.[55] It was found to be synthesized throughout the CNS in various cell populations,[56] and has been implicated in the binding and scavenging of excess lipids from membrane debris in damaged tissues, for example the brain in neurodegenerating diseases and the aortic wall during atherosclerosis. It was also found to interact with β-amyloid[57] and this complex can be recognized by LRP2/megalin, an important member of the LDL receptor family.[58] This interaction may play a role in transport of β-amyloid across the blood–brain barrier.

β-*Amyloid*

Recently β-amyloid, known to accumulate in AD in the senile plaques, has been found to be associated with lipoproteins in human CSF[17] and is secreted as lipoprotein particles together with apoJ and transthyrethin from hepatoma cells.[59] It can therefore be considered as an apolipoprotein, although its physiological function remains to be elucidated.

Enzymes

Lipoprotein lipase (LpL) is an important hydrolytic enzyme in plasma, responsible for the catabolism of triglyceride rich lipoproteins. It is produced and is functionally active in rat brain.[30] LpL also seems to play a role in the transfer of vitamin E to tissues and may provide a lipid enriched and antioxidant supplemented milieu for neuronal survival.[60] However, functional studies dealing with these questions are still required. Recent data from Huey *et al.*[61] propose that LpL might be critical in myelin synthesis in the peripheral nervous system, especially in response to nerve injury.

Lecithin: cholesteryl-acyltransferase (LCAT) is an important enzyme for the esterification of cholesterol on HDL in plasma. The activity of this enzyme in CSF was described a number of years ago by Illingworth and Glover.[54] In plasma, most LCAT is found associated with lipoproteins containing apoD. Synthesis of both proteins has been detected in the brain in distinct cell populations.[62] The finding that patients with familial LCAT deficiency sometimes have CNS impairments implies an important role for this enzyme in the brain.[63]

Two other enzymes are also expressed in the human brain: cholesteryl ester transfer protein (CETP)[64] and phospholipid transfer protein (PLTP).[65] These might also be relevant in CSF-lipoprotein metabolism but there are not sufficient data to report on their functions at the present time.

Lipoprotein receptors in the brain

The LDL receptor is an endocytotic receptor responsible for the uptake and subsequent degradation of LDL. Its structure and function have been described fully by Brown and Goldstein,[66] in particular with regard to familial hypercholesterolemia, a severe disease in which this receptor is defective and which causes very early coronary heart disease. In the last 10 years several receptors with high homology to the LDL receptor have been detected; as well as binding lipoproteins, these multifunctional receptors have relevance far beyond lipoprotein metabolism. The most important are LRP, LRP2/megalin, the VLDL receptor and apoE-R2.[67] These receptors have distinct tissue distributions, but are all expressed in the brain.[12]

The current thinking in lipoprotein metabolism could easily include these receptors in the concept of lipoprotein uptake and reverse cholesterol transport in the brain. However, studies on the function of the receptor in lipoprotein metabolism in the brain are still missing. Instead a new frontier in lipoprotein receptor research has been opened. The VLDL receptor and the apoE-R2 have been found to interact directly with both extracellular (reelin) and cytosolic (mDab1) signaling proteins that are necessary for the correct positioning of migrating neurons during brain development.[7] Therefore these receptors seem to be directly responsible for the transduction of extracellular signals resulting in the activation of intracellular protein kinases. A function beyond lipoprotein metabolism has been described recently for LRP2/megalin. In binding and internalizing vitamin and

and mRNAs during optic nerve degeneration. *J Biol Chem* 1986; **261**:5681–84.

23. Tso P, Liu M, Kalogeris TJ. The role of apolipoprotein A-IV in food intake regulation. *J Nutr* 1999; **129**:1503–6.

24. Boyles JK, Notterpek LM, Anderson LJ. Accumulation of apolipoproteins in the regenerating and remyelinating mammalian peripheral nerve. Identification of apolipoprotein D, apolipoprotein A-IV, apolipoprotein E, and apolipoprotein A-I. *J Biol Chem* 1990; **265**:17805–15.

25. Swartz RH, Black SE, George-Hyslop P. Apolipoprotein E and Alzheimer's disease: a genetic, molecular and neuroimaging review. *Can J Neurol Sci* 1999; **26**:77–88.

26. Shayo M, McLay RN, Kastin AJ, Banks WA. The putative blood–brain barrier transporter for the beta-amyloid binding protein apolipoprotein j is saturated at physiological concentrations. *Life Sci* 1997; **60**:L115–L118.

27. Mockel B, Zinke H, Flach R, Weiss B, Weiler-Guttler H, Gassen HG. Expression of apolipoprotein A-I in porcine brain endothelium in vitro. *J Neurochem* 1994; **62**:788–98.

28. Fukagawa K, Knight DS, Hamilton KA, Tso P. Immunoreactivity for apolipoprotein A-IV in tanycytes and astrocytes of rat brain. *Neurosci Lett* 1995; **199**:17–20.

29. Harr SD, Uint L, Hollister R, Hyman BT, Mendez AJ. Brain expression of apolipoproteins E, J, and A-I in Alzheimer's disease. *J Neurochem* 1996; **66**:2429–35.

30. Eckel RH, Robbins RJ. Lipoprotein lipase is produced, regulated, and functional in rat brain. *Proc Natl Acad Sci USA* 1984; **81**:7604–7.

31. McConathy WJ, Alaupovic P. Isolation and partial characterization of apolipoprotein D: a new protein moiety of the human plasma lipoprotein system. *FEBS Lett* 1973; **37**:178–82.

32. Navarro A, Tolivia J, Astudillo A, del Valle E. Pattern of apolipoprotein D immunoreactivity in human brain. *Neurosci Lett* 1998; **254**:17–20.

33. Patel SC, Asotra K, Patel YC, McConathy WJ, Patel RC, Suresh S. Astrocytes synthesize and secrete the lipophilic ligand carrier apolipoprotein D. *Neuroreport* 1995; **6**:653–57.

34. Ong WY, He Y, Suresh S, Patel SC. Differential expression of apolipoprotein D and apolipoprotein E in the kainic acid-lesioned rat hippocampus. *Neuroscience* 1997; **79**:359–67.

35. Suresh S, Yan Z, Patel RC, Patel YC, Patel SC. Cellular cholesterol storage in the Niemann-Pick disease type C mouse is associated with increased expression and defective processing of apolipoprotein D. *J Neurochem* 1998; **70**:242–51.

36. Terrisse L, Poirier J, Bertrand P, *et al.* Increased levels of apolipoprotein D in cerebrospinal fluid and hippocampus of Alzheimer's patients. *J Neurochem* 1998; **71**:1643–50.

37. St Clair RW, Beisiegel U. What do all the apolipoprotein E receptors do? [Editorial; comment]. *Curr Opin Lipidol* 1997; **8**:243–45.

38. Linton MF, Gish R, Hubl ST, *et al.* Phenotypes of apolipoprotein B and apolipoprotein E after liver transplantation. *J Clin Invest* 1991; **88**:270–81.

39. Elshourbagy NA, Liao WS, Mahley RW, Taylor JM. Apolipoprotein E mRNA is abundant in the brain and adrenals, as well as in the liver, and is present in other peripheral tissues of rats and marmosets. *Proc Natl Acad Sci USA* 1985; **82**:203–7.

40. Ignatius MJ, Shooter EM, Pitas RE, Mahley RW. Lipoprotein uptake by neuronal growth cones in vitro. *Science* 1987; **236**:959–62.

41. Poirier J, Minnich A, Davignon J. Apolipoprotein E, synaptic plasticity and Alzheimer's disease. *Ann Med* 1995; **27**:663–70.

42. de Chaves EI, Rusinol AE, Vance DE, Campenot RB, Vance JE. Role of lipoproteins in the delivery of lipids to axons during axonal regeneration. *J Biol Chem* 1997; **272**:30766–73.

43. Goodrum JF, Bouldin TW, Zhang SH, Maeda N, Popko B. Nerve regeneration and cholesterol reutilization occur in the absence of apolipoproteins E and A-I in mice. *J Neurochem* 1995; **64**:408–16.

44. Mahley RW, Huang Y. Apolipoprotein E: from atherosclerosis to Alzheimer's disease and beyond. *Curr Opin Lipidol* 1999; **10**:207–17.

45. LaDu MJ, Lukens JR, Reardon CA, Getz GS. Association of human, rat, and rabbit apolipoprotein E with beta- amyloid. *J Neurosci Res* 1997; **49**:9–18.

46. Strittmatter WJ, Saunders AM, Goedert M, *et al*. Isoform-specific interactions of apolipoprotein E with microtubule-associated protein tau: implications for Alzheimer disease. *Proc Natl Acad Sci USA* 1994; **91**:11183–86.

47. DeMattos RB, Thorngate FE, Williams DL. A test of the cytosolic apolipoprotein E hypothesis fails to detect the escape of apolipoprotein E from the endocytic pathway into the cytosol and shows that direct expression of apolipoprotein E in the cytosol is cytotoxic. *J Neurosci* 1999; **19**:2464–73.

48. Montine TJ, Montine KS, Swift LL. Central nervous system lipoproteins in Alzheimer's disease. *Am J Pathol* 1997; **151**:1571–75.

49. Mulder M, Ravid R, Swaab DF, *et al*. Reduced levels of cholesterol, phospholipids, and fatty acids in cerebrospinal fluid of Alzheimer disease patients are not related to apolipoprotein E4. *Alzheimer Dis Assoc Disord* 1998; **12**:198–203.

50. Cassader M, Ruiu G, Gambino R, *et al*. Influence of apolipoprotein H polymorphism on levels of triglycerides. *Atherosclerosis* 1994; **110**:45–51.

51. Caronti B, Calderaro C, Alessandri C, *et al*. Beta2–glycoprotein I (beta2–GPI) mRNA is expressed by several cell types involved in antiphospholipid syndrome-related tissue damage. *Clin Exp Immunol* 1999; **115**:214–19.

52. Moestrup SK, Schousboe I, Jacobsen C, Leheste JR, Christensen EI, Willnow TE. Beta2–glycoprotein-I (apolipoprotein H) and beta2–glycoprotein-I- phospholipid complex harbor a recognition site for the endocytic receptor megalin. *J Clin Invest* 1998; **102**:902–9.

53. de Silva HV, Harmony JA, Stuart WD, Gil CM, Robbins J. Apolipoprotein J: structure and tissue distribution. *Biochemistry* 1990; **29**:5380–89.

54. Illingworth DR, Glover J. Lecithin: cholesterol acyl transferase activity in human cerebrospinal fluid. *Biochim Biophys Acta* 1970; **220**:610–13.

55. Jenne DE, Tschopp J. Clusterin: the intriguing guises of a widely expressed glycoprotein. *Trends Biochem Sci* 1992; **17**:154–59.

56. Danik M, Chabot JG, Hassan-Gonzalez D, Suh M, Quirion R. Localization of sulfated glycoprotein-2/clusterin mRNA in the rat brain by in situ hybridization. *J Comp Neurol* 1993; **334**:209–27.

57. Matsubara E, Frangione B, Ghiso J. Characterization of apolipoprotein J-Alzheimer's A beta interaction. *J Biol Chem* 1995; **270**:7563–67.

58. Zlokovic BV, Martel CL, Matsubara E, *et al*. Glycoprotein 330/megalin: probable role in receptor-mediated transport of apolipoprotein J alone and in a complex with Alzheimer disease amyloid beta at the blood–brain and blood–cerebrospinal fluid barriers. *Proc Natl Acad Sci USA* 1996; **93**:4229–34.

59. Koudinov AR, Koudinova NV. Alzheimer's soluble amyloid beta protein is secreted by HepG2 cells as an apolipoprotein. *Cell Biol Int* 1997; **21**:265–71.

60. Ben Zeev O, Doolittle MH, Singh N, Chang CH, Schotz MC. Synthesis and regulation of lipoprotein lipase in the hippocampus. *J Lipid Res* 1990; **31**:1307–13.

61. Huey PU, Marcell T, Owens GC, Etienne J, Eckel RH. Lipoprotein lipase is expressed in cultured Schwann cells and functions in lipid synthesis and utilization. *J Lipid Res* 1998; **39**:2135–42.

62. Smith KM, Lawn RM, Wilcox JN. Cellular localization of apolipoprotein D and lecithin:cholesterol acyltransferase mRNA in rhesus monkey tissues by in situ hybridization. *J Lipid Res* 1990; **31**:995–1004.

63. Shojania AM, Jain SK, Shohet SB. Hereditary lecithin-cholesterol acyltransferase deficiency. Report of 2 new cases and review of the literature. *Clin Invest Med* 1983; **6**:49–55.

64. Albers JJ, Tollefson JH, Wolfbauer G, Albright RE, Jr. Cholesteryl ester transfer protein in human brain. *Int J Clin Lab Res* 1992; **21**:264–66.

65. Jiang X, Francone OL, Bruce C, *et al*. Increased prebeta-high density lipoprotein, apolipoprotein AI, and phospholipid in mice expressing the human phospholipid transfer protein and human apolipoprotein AI transgenes. *J Clin Invest* 1996; **98**:2373–80.

66. Brown MS, Goldstein JL. A receptor-mediated pathway for cholesterol homeostasis. *Science* 1986; **232**:34–47.

67. Willnow TE. The low-density lipoprotein receptor gene family: multiple roles in lipid metabolism. *J Mol Med* 1999; **77**:306–15.

early, and in some cases even to intrauterine, death.

Clinical aspects and diagnosis

The clinical diagnosis of FH is based on typical physical signs, laboratory findings and the patient's medical history. The hallmark of the disease is an increased total- and LDL-cholesterol level, above the 95th percentile for sex and age (Table 6.1), with high density lipoprotein (HDL), very low density lipoprotein (VLDL) and triglycerides in the normal range. Total plasma cholesterol levels in FH het-

Age men (years)	Percentiles						
	5	10	25	50	75	90	95
5–9	3.25	3.41	3.67	3.98	4.37	4.76	4.91
10–14	3.22	3.41	3.74	4.16	4.50	4.89	5.25
15–19	3.07	3.20	3.54	3.95	4.37	4.76	4.97
20–24	3.07	3.28	3.69	4.13	4.65	5.12	5.51
25–29	3.38	3.56	4.00	4.58	5.17	5.80	6.08
30–34	3.69	3.95	4.45	4.95	5.54	6.16	6.71
35–39	3.82	4.08	4.58	5.07	5.77	6.45	6.94
40–44	3.90	4.16	4.65	5.30	5.95	6.53	6.76
45–49	4.24	4.45	4.89	5.46	6.11	6.71	7.15
50–54	4.08	4.37	4.91	5.49	6.16	6.84	7.12
55–59	4.19	4.47	4.89	5.56	6.14	6.76	7.28
60–64	4.24	4.42	4.97	5.59	6.16	6.81	7.46
65–69	4.32	4.52	4.99	5.54	6.50	7.15	7.49
70+	3.74	4.16	4.81	5.56	6.14	6.58	6.89
Age women (years)	Percentiles						
	5	10	25	50	75	90	95
5–9	3.41	3.54	3.93	4.26	4.58	4.94	5.12
10–14	3.25	3.41	3.69	4.13	4.45	4.97	5.33
15–19	3.07	3.28	3.64	4.08	4.58	5.15	5.38
20–24	3.15	3.43	3.82	4.29	4.85	5.72	6.16
25–29	3.38	3.69	4.11	4.63	5.15	5.64	6.01
30–34	3.46	3.67	4.11	4.63	5.17	5.59	5.93
35–39	3.61	3.87	4.29	4.84	5.43	6.06	6.47
40–44	3.80	4.06	4.47	5.02	5.72	6.27	6.73
45–49	3.85	4.21	4.73	5.30	6.01	6.66	6.97
50–54	4.24	4.45	4.89	5.56	6.24	6.94	7.31
55–59	4.34	4.73	5.23	5.95	6.53	7.23	7.64
60–64	4.47	4.84	5.38	5.88	6.53	7.33	7.80
65–69	4.34	4.65	5.51	6.06	6.73	7.33	7.57
70+	4.50	4.71	5.10	5.88	6.47	6.97	7.28

Table 6.1

Total plasma cholesterol levels (mmol/l) in men and women in the normal North American population.[16]

erozygotes vary between 7.5 and 13 mmol/l (290–500 mg/dl) and FH homozygotes have levels between 16 and 26 mmol/l (618–1005 mg/dl).

Increased LDL-cholesterol levels often result in cholesterol deposits, which can be recognised easily as xanthomas on the Achilles tendons (Figure 6.1) and extensor tendons of hands (Figure 6.2) and feet, tuberous xanthomas on the processus olecrani (Figure 6.3) and tibial tuberosity (Figure 6.4). Xanthomas in the initial stage are difficult to detect because they are usually not clearly visible. During careful examination of the extensor and Achilles tendons, xanthomas can be felt as hard irregularities on the tendon which do not move with the skin. In many cases, the Achilles tendon is thickened over the whole length. Very obvious clinical signs are xanthelasmas on the eyelids (Figure 6.5) and an arcus lipoides (or arcus cornealis) — a white deposit of lipids in the outer rim of the iris. Where the xanthomas are pathognomic for FH, with the exception of some extremely rare disorders of lipid metabolism,[17] the xanthelasmas and arcus cornealis are not. Xanthelasmas may be present in normolipidaemic persons, and are not uncommon in older persons. Often, an arcus can be seen in individuals over 60 years of age and it is then called an arcus senilis. Arcus lipoides is pathognomic for FH when it is found in persons below the age of 45 years. In FH patients the arcus lipoides starts to develop as a thin sickle-shaped white line on the upper or lower rim of the iris (Figure 6.6A) in one or both eyes and extends with age until the iris is completely surrounded (Figure 6.6B). These typical physical signs of FH are not present in all patients, especially not in younger patients, but the incidence of the signs increases with age. After surgical removal of xanthomas and xanthelasmas, these signs return quickly and are more pronounced.

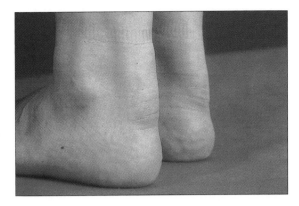

Fig. 6.1
Xanthoma on the Achilles tendon.

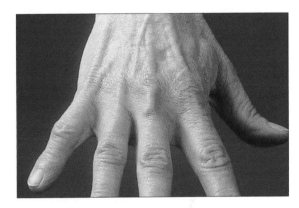

Fig. 6.2
Xanthoma on an extensor tendon of the hand.

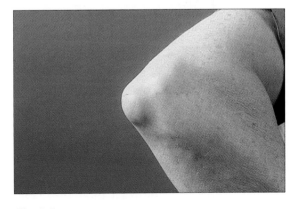

Fig. 6.3
Xanthomas on the processus olecrani.

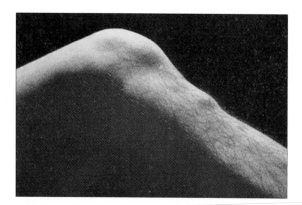

Fig. 6.4
Xanthomas on the tibial tuberosity.

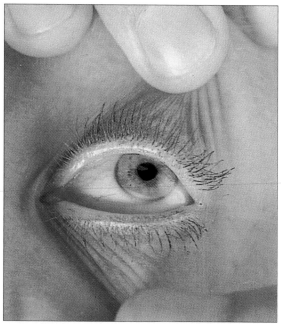

(A)

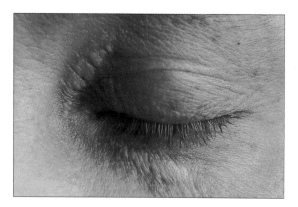

Fig. 6.5
Xanthelasmas on the eyelids.

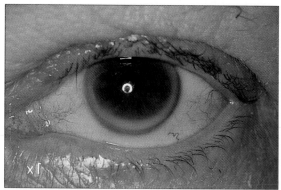

(B)

Fig. 6.6
Arcus cornealis: (A) initial stage; (B) fully developed.

There is a strong tendency to develop premature atherosclerosis in families affected by FH. Mainly coronary, but also cerebral and peripheral, arteries are affected. The possibility of a myocardial infarction before the age of 60 years is approximately five times higher in men with FH, compared with men without FH.[18] Female FH patients are four times more likely to suffer a myocardial infarction compared with women without FH, although the chance increases rapidly after menopause.[19]

Because FH exhibits an autosomal dominant mode of inheritance, a patient with FH consequently has one affected parent and often presents with a positive family history of premature cardiovascular disease. First degree relatives (children, parents, brothers and sisters of the patient) have a 50% chance of having FH.

Treatment
Diet

The first therapeutic measure in FH is the prescription of a cholesterol lowering diet that is low in cholesterol and saturated fats. The plasma cholesterol level depends on mainly the intracellular synthesis of cholesterol and the activity of LDL receptors, but also on the intake of cholesterol and saturated triglycerides. The bowel has a limited capacity for the uptake of cholesterol, approximately 1500 mg per day, including the re-absorbed bile acids, but the uptake of triglycerides is unlimited. In the production of very low density lipoproteins (VLDL), the liver adds a fixed amount of cholesterol for each unit of saturated triglycerides, hence dietary triglycerides have a direct cholesterol elevating effect. In spite of the fact that there is no scientific evidence that dietary measures have a favourable influence on morbidity and mortality rates of patients with FH, there is a general consensus of opinion that risk reduction in hypercholesterolaemic persons is possible by changes in diet.[20–22] Recently, evidence became available that the 'Mediterranean α-linolenic acid-rich diet' has a very favourable effect on the reduction of coronary heart disease mortality and non-fatal complications in myocardial infarction patients.[23] Therefore it is likely that patients with FH, who are exposed to the highest cardiovascular risk, will also benefit from such a diet. A diet low in saturated fats and cholesterol will result in a 10–15% reduction in the total plasma cholesterol level.

Medication

To lower the plasma LDL-cholesterol level in FH patients from an average of more than 6.5 mmol/l (250 mg/dl) to the recommended value of less than 3.5 mmol/l (135 mg/dl) in primary prevention, or less than 2.5 mmol/l (96 mg/dl) in secondary prevention, it is necessary to use medication in addition to a diet. As FH is characterised by an elevated LDL-cholesterol level only, and HDL-cholesterol and triglyceride levels are usually normal, the preferred drugs are those with a strong LDL reducing action. The bile acid sequestering resins and β-hydroxy-β-methylglutaryl-Coenzyme A (HMG-CoA) reductase inhibitors meet this requirement.

Bile acid sequestering resins

Bile acid sequestering resins, colestyramine and colestipol, are unresorbable basic polyanions which, when administered orally, reduce the enterohepatic recirculation of bile acids. Usually 95% of the bile acids are re-absorbed. When bile acid sequestering resins are applied, the quantity of bile acids in the gut is reduced. As a result, the production of bile acids by the liver increases. Cholesterol serves as a precursor molecule for bile acids and the liver will remove more LDL-cholesterol from the plasma by stimulation of LDL receptor activity. The effect of bile acid sequestering resins is made partially redundant by the increase of intracellular cholesterol synthesis and an increase in production of VLDL, the precursor of LDL. These latter effects are responsible for the upper limit of the maximal effective dose of bile acid sequestering resins.

HMG-CoA reductase inhibitors

The HMG-CoA reductase inhibitors represent a relatively new group of drugs. The prototype, mevastatin, was isolated in 1976 from a fungal culture of *Penicillium citrinum*.[24] Research on other fungal cultures resulted in lovastatin, a product obtained from *Aspergillus terreus* as well as *Monascus ruber*. Simvastatin and pravastatin were developed as fermentation derivatives of lovastatin.[25,26] In the following decade the synthetic products fluvastatin, atorvastatin and cerivastatin were developed. The HMG-CoA reductase inhibitors, or statins, act as reversible competitive inhibitors of HMG-CoA reductase, the rate limiting enzyme in the synthesis of cholesterol. Between 50 and 90% of any statin is bound to plasma protein and the half-life of most statins is approximately 2 hours, except that of atorvastatin, which is significantly longer. Excretion is mainly via the liver, and only a small amount passes through the kidneys. Administration of a statin at dosages between 10 and 80 mg results in more or less complete inhibition of intracellular cholesterol synthesis and a reduction of the cholesterol pool in the liver cell. This leads to enhancement of the production of LDL receptors, resulting in a decrease in the LDL-cholesterol level in the plasma. The individual properties of the statins differ substantially but at maximum dose, some can produce reductions in LDL-cholesterol levels of 55%.[27] Elevation of HDL-cholesterol levels by up to 15% and reduction of triglyceride levels by up to 30% are simultaneous effects of the statins.

In recent primary and secondary prevention trials with statins, involving a total of over 30 000 participants, significant reductions of up to 40% were seen in fatal and non-fatal coronary ischaemic events,[28–32] demonstrating that the statins must have other beneficial effects besides reduction of LDL-cholesterol levels.

Combination therapy

Patients with heterozygous FH have significantly elevated plasma LDL-cholesterol levels, and monotherapy with bile acid sequestering resins or HMG-CoA reductase inhibitors will not always result in the desired reduction of LDL-cholesterol levels to below 2.5 or 3.5 mmol/l (96 or 135 mg/dl). In the majority of FH patients the optimal value for LDL-cholesterol levels can be reached only by medication with a combination of HMG-CoA reductase inhibitors and bile acid sequestering resins. The intensity and frequency of side-effects of this combination does not differ from those caused by monotherapy.[33] Because bile acid sequestering resins can bind and inactivate a variety of drugs and other substances, there should be a time span of at least 4 hours between the intake of a resin and a statin.

Treatment of homozygous FH

Therapy for homozygous FH is more complicated. Since LDL receptor activity is completely absent, except in those rare cases where there is some residual activity, bile acid sequestering resins and HMG-CoA reductase inhibitors, which act by stimulation of LDL receptor activity, will not be effective.

There are some therapeutic regimens to treat homozygous FH patients. Plasmapheresis is used in homozygous patients, and occasionally also in heterozygous patients who do not respond to conventional therapies. In this procedure, which is usually performed once a week, the plasma is separated from the cells and subsequently replaced by a plasma substitute.[34] In general, the procedure is well tolerated, with an average decrease of 6–7 mmol/l (230–270 mg/dl) in total cholesterol level. Compared with untreated homozygous brothers and sisters, the expected life-span of treated patients can increase by more than 10 years. A disadvantage of replacing blood plasma is the removal of high density lipoproteins (HDL). As HDL plays an important role in reverse cholesterol transport and in protection against atherosclerosis, new techniques have been developed for selective removal of LDL from plasma.

LDL apheresis offers the advantage that LDL-cholesterol is removed selectively from the plasma and the original plasma is re-infused. Weekly LDL apheresis reduces the plasma LDL-cholesterol level by 40–70% and doubles the concentration of HDL-cholesterol.[35] LDL apheresis can be combined with HMG-CoA reductase inhibitors, which will increase the effect.

The most recent development is heparin extracorporeal LDL precipitation (HELP). In this technique, filtered plasma is mixed with a heparin buffer to decrease acidity. LDL precipitates at low pH and can be removed subsequently. On average, the LDL-cholesterol level is lowered by 30% and triglycerides by 20%, whereas HDL levels increase by 15%.[36] An additional advantage of all methods of extracorporeal removal of LDL is that lipoprotein(a) [Lp(a)] is removed from the plasma as well. Lp(a) is an independent risk factor for coronary heart disease for which there is no effective medication at this time.

The most definitive therapy that is possible at the moment is liver transplantation. This procedure been performed in only a few homozygous FH patients. The first successful transplantation was performed in 1984 on a 7-year-old girl with homozygous FH, serious coronary atherosclerosis and decompensatio cordis. The heart and liver were transplanted at the same time, following which the cholesterol level decreased from 25 mmol/l to 7 mmol/l (966 mg/dl to 270 mg/dl). Administration of lovastatin resulted in a return to normal LDL-cholesterol level.[37]

Molecular diagnosis

Medical management of lipoprotein disorders is directed at reduction of the cardiovascular risk and therefore accurate diagnosis is important for optimal treatment. FH is sometimes difficult to differentiate from hypercholesterolaemias of other origins, such as familial combined hyperlipidaemia or polygenic hypercholesterolaemia. The clinical characteristics may facilitate the diagnosis. By weighing the occurrence of these clinical signs, alone or in combination with others, a diagnostic scoring table can be constructed for FH (Table 6.2); but even here the diagnosis is not always unequivocal. In young FH patients not necessarily all of the clinical signs will have developed and cholesterol levels in the lower range for FH patients can coincide with the higher cholesterol levels observed in the general population.[38] Moreover another inherited disorder, familial defective apolipoprotein B (FDB), produces a clinical picture similar to FH.[39]

A highly accurate diagnosis of FH can be established by molecular diagnosis: the characterisation of the molecular defect in the LDL receptor gene that causes the disorder. Since clinical expression of FH and the cardiovascular risk is in part related to the nature of the mutation in the LDL receptor gene,[40] medical management can be optimised. Unfortunately, molecular diagnosis is not always possible.

In most populations, LDL receptor gene mutations and mutations causing FDB account for 15% at most of all FH cases. A complicating factor for routine molecular diagnosis is the enormous variety of mutations causing FH. At the moment more than 500 different mutations have been described worldwide[41] and the molecular basis of FH is very heterogeneous, as demonstrated by the 117 different mutations described in Dutch patients with FH.[42] At the present time, tools for simultaneous analysis of the large array of FH-causing mutations are not available, and a 'per-patient-per-mutation' protocol has to be followed.

have greatly expanded the therapeutic potential of gene therapy, but its application will probably remain limited to a few cases. Application in patients with less severe hypercholesterolaemia, such as heterozygous FH, will require a more efficient and safer approach for LDL receptor gene transfer to the liver. We await the resolution of not only a number of major technical problems, but also the medical ethical issues.

References

1. Fagge CH. Xanthomatous diseases of the skin. *Trans Pathol Soc London* 1873; 24:242–50.
2. Müller C. Xanthomata, hypercholesterolemia, angina pectoris. *Acta Med Scand* 1938; 89:75–83.
3. Wilkinson CF, Hand EA, Fliegelman MT. Essential familial hypercholesterolemia. *Ann Intern Med* 1948; 29:671–6.
4. Khachadurian AK. The inheritance of essential familial hypercholesterolemia. *Am J Med* 1964; 37:402–7.
5. Goldstein JL, Brown MS. Familial hypercholesterolemia: identification of a defect in the regulation of 3-hydroxy-3-methylglutaryl Coenzyme A reductase activity with overproduction of cholesterol. *Proc Natl Acad Sci USA* 1973; 70:2804–9.
6. Brown MS, Goldstein JL. Expression of the familial hypercholesterolemia gene in heterozygotes: mechanism for a dominant disorder in man. *Science* 1974; 185:61–3.
7. Anderson RGW, Goldstein JL, Brown MS. Localization of low density lipoprotein receptors on plasma membrane of normal human fibroblasts and their absence in cells from a familial hypercholesterolemia homozygote. *Proc Natl Acad Sci USA* 1976; 73:2434–8.
8. Brown MS, Goldstein JL. Receptor-mediated control of cholesterol metabolism. *Science* 1986; 191:150–4.
9. Kannel WB, Castelli WP, Gordon T, McNamara PM. Serum cholesterol, lipoproteins, and the risk of coronary heart disease. The Framingham Heart Study. *Ann Intern Med* 1971; 74:112.
10. Lipids Research Clinics Program. The Lipid Research Clinics coronary primary prevention trial results. *JAMA* 1984; 251:351–74.
11. Stamler J, Wentworth D, Neaton JD. Is relationship between serum cholesterol and risk of premature death from coronary heart disease continuous and graded? Findings in 356 222 primary screenees of the Multiple Risk Factor Intervention Trial (MRFIT). *JAMA* 1986; 256:2823–8.
12. Anderson KM, Castelli WP, Levy D. Cholesterol and mortality: 30 years of follow-up from the Framingham Study. *JAMA* 1987; 257:2176–80.
13. Frick MH, Elo O, Haapa K, *et al*. Helsinki Heart Study: primary prevention trial with gemfibrozil in middle-aged men with dyslipidemia. *N Engl J Med* 1987; 76:557–61.
14. Steinberg D, Witztum JL. Lipoproteins and atherogenesis, current concepts. *JAMA* 1990; 264:3047–52.
15. Okie S. Mortality: heart disease is the world's worst scourge. *Washington Post* 1990; April 30: A2.
16. American Heart Association Special Report. Recommendations for the treatment of hyperlipidemia in adults. *Circulation* 1984; 69:1067A–90A.
17. Cruz PD, East C, Bergstresser PR. Dermal, subcutaneous and tendon xanthomas: diagnostic markers for specific lipoprotein disorders. *J Am Acad Dermatol* 1988; 19:95–111.
18. Slack J, Nevin NC. Hyperlipidaemic xanthomatosis I: increased risk of death from ischaemic heart disease in first degree relatives of 53 patients with essential hyperlipidaemia and xanthomatosis. *J Med Genet* 1968; 5:4–8.
19. Beaglehole R. Oestrogens and cardiovascular disease. *Br Med J* 1989; 297:571–2.
20. American Heart Association. Diet and coronary heart disease. *Circulation* 1978; 58:762.
21. American Medical Association, Council on Scientific Affairs. Concepts of nutrition and health. *JAMA* 1979; 242:2335.
22. Expert Panel on Detection, Evaluation and Treatment of High Blood Cholesterol in Adults. Summary of the second report of the National Cholesterol Educational Program (NCEP). *JAMA* 1993; 269:3015–23.
23. De Lorgeril M, Salen P, Martin J-L, *et al*.

Mediterranean diet, traditional risk factors and the rate of cardiovascular complications after myocardial infarction: final report of the Lyon diet Heart Study. *Circulation* 1999; **99**:779–85.

24. Endo A, Kuroda M, Tsujita Y. ML-236A, ML-236B, and ML-236c, new inhibitors of choles-terogenesis produced by *Penicillium citrinum*. *J Antibiot* 1976; **29**:1346–8.

25. Endo A. Monacolin: a new hypocholes-terolemic agent produced by a *Monascus* species. *J Antibiot* 1979; **32**:852–4.

26. Alberts AW, Chen J, Kuron G, *et al.* Mevino-lin: a highly potent competitive inhibitor of hydroxy-methyl-glutaryl coenzyme A reductase and a cholesterol-lowering agent. *Proc Natl Acad Sci USA* 1980; **77**:3957–61.

27. Jones P, Kafonek S, Laurora I, Hunninghake D. Comparative dose efficacy study of atorvas-tatin versus simvastatin, pravastatin, lovastatin and fluvastatin in patients with hypercholes-terolemia (the CURVES study). *Am J Cardiol* 1998; **81**:582–6.

28. Scandinavian Simvastatin Survival Study Group. Randomised trial of cholesterol lower-ing in 4444 patients with coronary heart dis-ease: the Scandinavian Simvastatin Survival Study (4S). *Lancet* 1994; **344**:1383–9.

29. Shepherd J, Cobbe S, Ford I, *et al.* Prevention of coronary heart disease with pravastatin in men with hypercholesterolemia (WOSCOPS). *N Engl J Med* 1995; **333**:1301–7.

30. Sacks FM, Pfeffer MA, Moye LA, *et al.* The effect of pravastatin on coronary events in patients with average cholesterol levels (CARE). *N Engl J Med* 1996; **335**:1001–9.

31. Downs JR, Clearfield M, Weis S, *et al.* Primary prevention of acute coronary events with lovastatin in men and women with average cholesterol levels (AFCAPS/TexCAPS). *JAMA* 1998; **279**:1615–22.

32. The Long-Term Intervention with Pravastatin in Ischemic Disease (LIPID) Study Group. Pre-vention of cardiovascular events and death with pravastatin in patients with coronary heart disease and a broad range of initial cho-lesterol levels. *N Engl J Med* 1998; **339**:1349–57.

33. Emmerich J, Aubert I, Bauduceau B, *et al.* Effi-cacy and safety of simvastatin (alone or in association with cholestyramine). A 1-year study in 66 patients with type II hyperlipopro-teinaemia. *Eur Heart J* 1990; **11**:149–55.

34. Thompson GR, Barbir M, Okabayashi K, *et al.* Plasmapheresis in familial hypercholes-terolemia. *Arteriosclerosis* 1989; **9**:152–7.

35. Stoffel W, Borberg H, Greve V. Application of specific extracorporeal removal of low density lipoprotein in familial hypercholesterolemia. *Lancet* 1981; **2**:1005–7.

36. Eisenhauer T, Armstrong VW, Wieland H, *et al.* Selective removal of low density lipopro-teins (LDL) by precipitation at low pH: first clinical application of the HELP system. *Klin Wochenschr* 1987; **65**:161–8.

37. East C, Grundy SM, Bilheimer DW. Normal cholesterol levels with lovastatin (mevinolin) therapy in a child with homozygous familial hypercholesterolemia following liver transplan-tation. *JAMA* 1986; **256**:2843–8.

38. Nora JJ, Lortscher RM, Spangler RD, Bil-heimer DW. Familial hypercholesterolemia with 'normal' cholesterol in obligate heterozy-gotes. *Am J Med Genet* 1985; **22**:585–91.

39. Defesche JC, Pricker KL, Hayden MR, *et al.* Familial Defective Apolipoprotein B$_{100}$ is clini-cally indistinguishable from Familial Hyper-cholesterolemia. *Arch Intern Med* 1993; **153**:2349–56.

40. Sun X-M, Patel DD, Knight BL, Soutar AK. Influence of genotype at the low density lipoprotein (LDL) receptor gene locus on the clinical phenotype and response to lipid-lower-ing drug therapy in heterozygous familial hypercholesterolemia. *Atherosclerosis* 1998; **136**:175–85.

41. Varret M, Rabes JP, Thiart R, *et al.* LDLR Database (second edition): new additions to the database and the software, and results of the first molecular analysis. *Nucl Ac Res* 1998; **26**:248–52.

42. Redeker EJW, Defesche JC, Kastelein JJP, Mannens MMAM. Novel LDL-receptor muta-tions in Dutch Familial Hypercholesterolemia (abstract). Proceedings of the 70th meeting of the European Atherosclerosis Society; 1998: 159.

43. World Health Organisation, Human Genetics Program, Division of Non-communicable Dis-eases. Familial Hypercholesterolemia, report of

a WHO consultation. WHO/HGN/FH/CONS/ 98.7. Paris; October 1997.

44. World Health Organisation, Human Genetics Program, Division of Non-communicable Diseases. Familial Hypercholesterolemia, second report of a WHO consultation. WHO/HGN/FH/CONS/ [in preparation].

45. Bilheimer DW, Goldstein JL, Grundy SM, *et al*. Liver transplantation to provide low-density lipoprotein receptors and lower plasma cholesterol in a child with homozygous familial hypercholesterolemia. *N Engl J Med* 1984; **311**:1658–64.

46. Grossman M, Wilson JM. Frontiers in gene therapy: LDL-receptor replacement for hypercholesterolemia. *J Clin Lab Med* 1992; **119**:457–60.

47. Grosmann M, Rader DJ, Muller DWM, *et al*. A pilot study of ex vivo gene therapy for homozygous familial hypercholesterolemia. *Nature Med* 1995; **1**:1148–54.

48. Wilson JM, Jefferson DM, Chowdhury JR, *et al*. Retrovirus-mediated transduction of adult hepatocytes. *Proc Natl Acad Sci USA* 1988; **85**:3014–18.

49. Wu GY, Wu CH. Receptor-mediated in vitro gene transformation by a soluble DNA carrier system. *J Biol Chem* 1987; **262**:4429–32.

50. Nicolau C, Legrand A, Grosse E. Liposomes as carries for in vivo gene transfer and expression. *Methods Enzymol* 1988; **149**:157–76.

51. Kren BT, Bandyopadhyay P, Steer C. In vivo site-directed mutagenesis of the factor IX gene by chimeric RNA/DNA oligonucleotides. *Nature Med* 1998; **4**:285–90.

7

Fibrinogen: an independent coronary heart disease risk factor

Gordon DO Lowe

Introduction

There is increasing clinical and laboratory interest in measurement of plasma fibrinogen in prediction of coronary heart disease (CHD) and other arterial thrombotic events. There are several possible reasons for such interest. First, there is substantial evidence from prospective studies that plasma fibrinogen level is a strong, consistent predictor of such cardiovascular events in persons with or without clinically detectable arterial disease. In 'healthy' persons fibrinogen adds to the predictive value of major conventional risk predictors, such as smoking, blood pressure and serum cholesterol (Figure 7.1).[1-12] Second, there are several interactive, plausible, potential biological mechanisms through which increasing plasma fibrinogen levels (which are due to multiple gene–environment interactions) may promote ischaemic events. These include increased blood viscosity, atherogenesis and platelet–fibrin thrombogenesis (Figure 7.2). Third, the stability and practicability of measurement of fibrinogen in clinical and epidemiological studies is favourable. Fibrinogen assays are already available in many district hospitals for diagnosis of disseminated intravascular coagulation (DIC). However, as with assays of other major cardiovascular risk factors (smoking, blood pressure and serum cholesterol), those for fibrinogen need to be standardised.[13-19]

Clinical interest in plasma assays of fibrinogen may also increase, in the event that ongoing clinical trials of plasma fibrinogen reduction (for example with certain fibrates or ancrod) show that such treatments are beneficial.[20] This chapter will examine each of these aspects of fibrinogen in turn.

Fibrinogen as a predictor of arterial thrombotic events

Since the pioneering report of Meade *et al.* in 1980 from the Northwick Park Heart Study, which indicated that plasma fibrinogen was predictive of cardiovascular death,[21] over 30 prospective studies have reported on its association with incident clinical ischaemic events. Ernst and Resch[1,22] performed a meta-analysis of seven prospective studies, in which most subjects were free of clinically detectable vascular disease at baseline. They observed that the relative risk of cardiovascular events in persons in the upper third of plasma fibrinogen level was 2.45 (95% CI, 2.05–2.93) compared to the lower third.[22] In a more recent meta-analysis of 18 studies (including studies of persons with pre-existing cardiovascular disease), which considered only CHD endpoints, Danesh *et al.*[6] observed that the relative risk of CHD in persons in the upper third of plasma fibrinogen level was 1.8 (95% CI, 1.6–2.0). This relative risk was calculated after

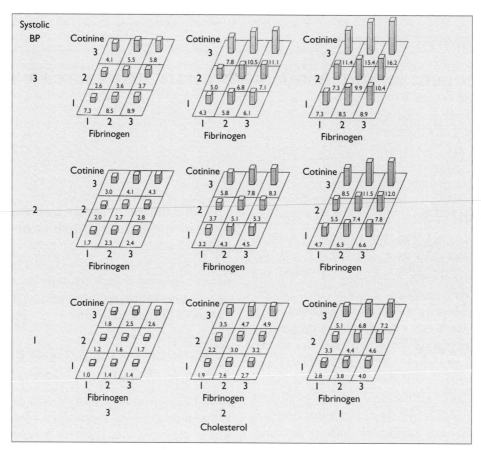

Fig. 7.1
Hazard ratios for coronary events (coronary death, MI or coronary artery surgery) in 4235 men aged 40–59 years at 8-year follow-up in the Scottish Heart Health Study. The hazard ratios are shown by thirds (1,2,3) for serum cholesterol, systolic blood pressure, smoking (serum cotinine) and plasma fibrinogen (Clauss assay) and are all relative to the lowest third of all four variables (hazard = 1). Each of these four variables is adjusted for the other three and for age. At any level of coronary risk predicted by the three classical risk predictors (cholesterol, blood pressure, smoking), fibrinogen increases risk prediction. Reproduced with permission.[7]

adjustments for potential confounders where these had been performed in individual studies. The relative risk was similar in persons with and without baseline evidence of cardiovascular disease.

In other prospective studies, plasma fibrinogen has been associated with significant increased risk of stroke,[4,23–25] peripheral arterial disease,[4,26] atrial fibrillation,[4] heart failure,[4]

restenosis following angioplasty,[27,28] or bypass grafting,[9,29] as well as progression of arterial narrowing.[30,31]

It is therefore clear that plasma fibrinogen is a strong and consistent predictor of clinical CHD and non-coronary ischaemic events (most of which are caused by arterial thrombosis). The increased risk for CHD is approximately two-fold in persons in the upper third

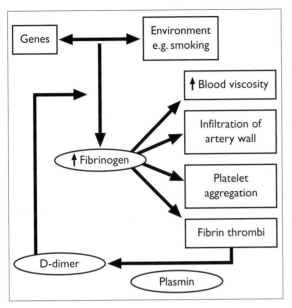

Fig. 7.2
Possible biological mechanisms through which increasing plasma fibrinogen levels (which are caused by gene–environment interactions) may promote ischaemic events. The formation of plasma D-dimer from fibrinogen is also indicated, as is its ability to increase plasma fibrinogen level through stimulation of hepatic synthesis.

of plasma fibrinogen values compared to persons in the lower third. This increased risk is similar in men and women, and in those with and without clinical evidence of baseline vascular disease,[7] and it is additive to that of the major conventional risk predictors, such as smoking, blood pressure and serum cholesterol.[7]

The latter point is illustrated by results from the Scottish Heart Health Study (see Figure 7.1).[7,32–35] This study is unique, in that it is a random sample of men and women aged 40–59 years from general practitioner lists in 50% of the local government districts in a single country (Scotland). As such, this cohort is as representative a sample of middle-aged persons in a nation as can be achieved. The study

methods were those of the internationally standardised WHO-MONICA Study. We assayed fibrinogen by the commonly used Clauss assay in a semi-automated coagulometer, with satisfactory internal and external quality control. Figure 7.1 shows that, given any combination of the three major conventional risk factors (smoking, blood pressure and cholesterol), fibrinogen added to the prediction of coronary risk in men (after age adjustment). These data are consistent with those of other studies.[1,6] Furthermore, fibrinogen was a much stronger predictor of both cardiovascular mortality and total mortality than blood pressure or cholesterol in the Scottish Heart Health Study.[7,35]

Because of the large size of the Scottish Heart Health Study, we were able to establish that there were no statistically significant interactions (that is, multiplicative effects) between fibrinogen and these other major predictors of CHD risk.[7] Smoking dose-dependently increases both CHD risk and plasma fibrinogen levels, hence it is not surprising that there are links between smoking, fibrinogen and CHD risk. However, the association between fibrinogen and prospective CHD risk is not 'explained' by smoking: conversely, the association between smoking and prospective CHD risk is only partially explained by fibrinogen.[7,15]

Thus, there is increasing evidence that fibrinogen could usefully be added to the standard cardiovascular risk profile for CHD prediction.[1–7] The European Atherosclerosis Society included fibrinogen in its 1992 guidelines for treating dyslipidaemia,[36] and this suggestion is supported in the current 'statin era' by our finding that fibrinogen was a predictor of CHD and mortality in the West of Scotland Coronary Prevention Study of pravastatin in primary prevention of CHD in moderately hypercholesterolaemic men.[37] On the basis of the Framingham Heart Study data, a multiplicative adjustment

Fibrinogen level (g/l)	Multiplication factor for multivariate CHD risk	
	Men	Women
<2.35	0.83	0.77
2.35–3.35	1.00	1.00
>3.35	1.20	1.30

Table 7.1
Adjustment to the American Heart Association multivariate risk profile formulation for coronary heart disease (CHD) to include the independent effect of fibrinogen[5,38]

factor to the American Heart Association coronary risk formulation has been calculated,[38] to allow fibrinogen to be taken into account when estimating the multivariate risk of a coronary event (Table 7.1).[5] Future collaborative analyses should refine the place of fibrinogen in multivariate risk prediction of cardiovascular events, especially if they can access individual data rather than grouped data.

Biological links between fibrinogen and ischaemic events

Figure 7.2 illustrates some potential biological mechanisms through which increasing plasma fibrinogen levels may promote ischaemic events.[1,3,15] Fibrinogen is an important determinant of plasma viscosity and of red cell aggregation, and hence of whole blood viscosity. All three of these rheological variables (which influence blood flow, especially at sites of atherogenesis and thrombogenesis) are predictors of cardiovascular events and stroke,[15,24,37] as recently confirmed in a meta-analysis of prospective studies.[39] Data from the Caerphilly and Speedwell studies suggest that about 50% of the predictive value of plasma viscosity for CHD events may be

'explained' by plasma fibrinogen.[40] Fibrinogen is also atherogenic, infiltrating the arterial wall and contributing to atherogenesis through several potential mechanisms including deposition of fibrinogen or fibrin and stimulation of cell proliferation. Fibrinogen may also contribute to atherogenesis through its effect on blood viscosity, and hence shear effects on the arterial wall.[31]

Fibrinogen also plays a role in thrombogenesis, first through promoting platelet aggregation by linking GP IIb/IIIa receptors on adjacent platelets,[3] and second as the precursor of fibrin. There is evidence that thrombi formed from plasma with high levels of fibrinogen are larger, and more likely to persist (by being less deformable and more resistant to lysis by plasmin) than thrombi formed from plasma with low levels of fibrinogen.[3]

Practicability of fibrinogen assays in predicting arterial thrombotic events

Plasma fibrinogen assays are now widely available for hospital diagnosis of DIC. However several practical issues have to be addressed before they can be applied to prediction of arterial thrombotic events. It is important to define the best assay in terms of predictive value, laboratory precision, standardisation and clinical utility. Several types of assay are used in clinical practice, including clotting, immunological and precipitation methods.[41,42] The most commonly used assays in haematology laboratories are the Clauss (clotting rate) and prothrombin-time (PT)-derived methods, which are usually performed in automated coagulometers. These assays require citrated plasma samples (either fresh, or rapidly centrifuged and frozen) and measure only the clottable fraction of fibrinogen. Standardisation of clottable fibrinogen assays has been aided by the introduction of an International Fibrinogen Standard,[14] but there are still variations between assays due to differences in commercial standards, reagents and coagulometers[17-19] and these have implications for categorisation of persons at risk of cardiovascular events, for example by thirds of the population distribution of fibrinogen.[19] Effects of high fibrin degradation product (FDP) levels, anticoagulant therapy or thrombolytic therapy on such assay discrepancies have been described[42] but these are unlikely to be relevant in risk prediction samples from healthy subjects. Further work is required in standardisation of clottable fibrinogen assays.

In contrast to haematology laboratories, biochemistry laboratories usually assay fibrinogen by immunological methods, such as immunonephelometry or precipitation methods (e.g. heat precipitation nephelometry). Not surprisingly, such assays do not correlate well with clottable fibrinogen assays in samples taken from the general population, which again has implications for risk categorisation in the general population.[19] Sweetnam et al.[16] noted a tendency among reported studies for improved prediction of CHD by such assays of 'total' fibrinogen in comparison with clottable fibrinogen assays, and in the only direct, prospective comparison reported to date, showed that the heat-precipitation nephelometric assay was a significantly better predictor of CHD events in the Caerphilly–Speedwell studies than the Clauss assay.[16] This may reflect partly higher precision, and partly the likelihood that total (rather than clottable) fibrinogen is more relevant to most potential pathogenic roles of fibrinogen in CHD (viscosity, atherogenesis, platelet aggregation), whereas clottable fibrinogen may be related only to its roles in fibrin formation (see Figure 7.2). Again, further work is required to compare different types of fibrinogen assay in cardiovascular risk prediction. However, biochemical assays of total fibrinogen have the practical advantage that they can be measured in the same K_2 edetate-anticoagulated samples that are routinely sent to biochemistry laboratories for lipoprotein assays in cardiovascular risk prediction.[15]

One should also consider biological variation in plasma fibrinogen, for example the effects of age, sex, hormones and other risk factors,[43,44] as well as longitudinal variation[45] including seasonal variation. It has been proposed that accurate classification of an individual's fibrinogen level may require several measurements over several weeks,[45] as is commonly performed for other major cardiovascular risk factors such as blood pressure or serum cholesterol.[15]

Does fibrinogen play a causal role in CHD?

While plasma fibrinogen is a risk predictor for arterial thrombosis, and potentially may promote arterial disease as discussed previously, its causal role in CHD can be established only by clinical trials of fibrinogen reduction.[15] Acute fibrinogen reduction, which lowers plasma and blood viscosity, is achieved by thrombolytic therapy (which may add to the benefits of coronary thrombolysis in treatment of acute myocardial infarction) and by defibrinogenation with ancrod, which has shown promising results in treatment of acute ischaemic stroke.[15] Chronic reduction in fibrinogen can be achieved by stopping smoking, which lowers fibrinogen level by 10% and lowers CHD risk in parallel with the decrease in fibrinogen level.[32] Alcohol (any) lowers fibrinogen level by about 10%.[32,44] The antiplatelet drug, ticlopidine, also lowers plasma fibrinogen level by about 10%;[46] whether or not its derivative, clopidogrel has a similar effect is not established. Oral hormone replacement therapy also lowers fibrinogen level by about 10%.[33] Certain fibrates (e.g. bezafibrate, clofibrate, fenofibrate) lower fibrinogen levels by about 13%, while others (e.g. gemfibrozil) increase fibrinogen levels by a similar amount.[48] While clofibrate reduced risk of myocardial infarction in the WHO primary prevention study, it increased mortality.[49] Bezafibrate is currently under study in secondary prevention of CHD in survivors of myocardial infarction[48] and in patients with intermittent claudication.[48] Fibrates are also being studied in CHD prevention in diabetic subjects. In general, statins do not appear to alter fibrinogen levels,[37,50] although there are recent reports of elevation by atorvastatin,[51] which requires confirmation in large trials.

Acknowledgements

Our studies in these areas are supported by the British Heart Foundation and by the Chief Scientist Office, The Scottish Office.

References

1. Ernst E, Resch KL. Fibrinogen as a cardiovascular risk factor: a meta-analysis and review of the literature. *Ann Intern Med* 1993; **118**:956–63.
2. Heinrich H, Balleisen L, Schulte H, *et al*. Fibrinogen and factor VII in the prediction of coronary risk. Results from the PROCAM Study in healthy men. *Arterioscler Thromb* 1994; **14**:54–59.
3. Lowe GDO. *Fibrinogen. A cardiovascular risk factor*, 2nd edn. Mannheim: Boehringer Mannheim; 1997.
4. Kannel WB, D'Agostino RB, Belanger AJ. Update of fibrinogen as a cardiovascular risk factor. *Ann Epidemiol* 1992; **2**:457–66.
5. Kannel WB. Influence of fibrinogen on cardiovascular disease. *Drugs* 1997; **54**: S32–S40.
6. Danesh J, Collins R, Appleby P, Peto R. Fibrinogen, C-reactive protein, albumin or white cell count: meta-analyses of prospective studies of coronary heart disease. *JAMA* 1998; **279**:1477–82.
7. Woodward M, Lowe GDO, Rumley A, Tunstall-Pedoe H. Fibrinogen as a risk factor for coronary heart disease and mortality in middle aged men and women: The Scottish Heart Health Study. *Eur Heart J* 1998; **19**:55–62.
8. Lowe GDO, Rumley A. Use of fibrinogen and fibrin D-dimer in prediction of arterial thrombotic events. *Thromb Haemost* 1999; **82**:667–72.
9. Woodburn KR, Rumley A, Lowe GDO, *et al*. Clinical, biochemical and rheologic factors affecting the outcome of infrainguinal bypass grafting. *J Vasc Surg* 1996; **24**:639–46.
10. Smith FB, Lee AJ, Fowkes FGR, *et al*. Hemostatic factors as predictors of ischemic heart disease and stroke in the Edinburgh Artery Study. *Arterioscler Thromb Vasc Biol* 1997; **17**:3321–25.
11. Smith FB, Rumley A, Lee AJ, *et al*. Haemostatic factors and prediction of ischaemic heart disease and stroke in claudicants. *Br J Haematol* 1998; **100**:758–63.
12. Maresca G, Di Blasio A, Marchioli R, Di Minno G. Measuring plasma fibrinogen to predict stroke and myocardial infarction: an update. *Arterioscler Thromb Vasc Biol* 1999; **19**:1368–77.
13. Furlan M, Felix R, Escher N, Lämmle B. How high is the true fibrinogen content of fibrinogen standards? *Thromb Res* 1989; **56**:583–92.

14. Gaffney PJ, Wong MY. Collaborative study of proposed international standard for plasma fibrinogen measurement. *Thromb Haemost* 1992; **68**:428–32.

15. Lowe GDO. Haemostatic risk factors for arterial and venous thrombosis. In: Poller L, Ludlam CA, eds. *Recent Advances in Blood Coagulation, 7*. Edinburgh: Churchill Livingstone, 1997: 69–96.

16. Sweetnam PM, Yarnell JWG, Lowe GDO, *et al*. The relative power of heat-precipitation nephelometric and clottable (Clauss) fibrinogen in the prediction of ischaemic heart disease: the Caerphilly and Speedwell studies. *Br J Haematol* 1998; **100**:582–88.

17. Lawrie AS, Mackie IJ, Kitchen S, *et al*. An evaluation of popular Clauss and prothrombin time derived fibrinogen assay reagents. *Blood Coag Fibrinol* 1999; **10**:S101–S102.

18. Mackie IJ, Lawrie AS, Howarth D, *et al*. The impact of commercial reference preparations on fibrinogen assays. *Blood Coag Fibrinol* 1999; **10**:S102.

19. Rumley A, Woodward M, Hoffmeister A, *et al*. Comparison of three plasma fibrinogen assays in a random population sample. *Blood Coag Fibrinol* 1999; **10**:S102.

20. Lowe GDO. Agents lowering blood viscosity, including defibrinogenating agents. In: Verstraete M, Fuster V, Topol EJ, eds. *Cardiovascular Thrombosis*, 2nd edn. Philadelphia: Lippincott-Raven, 1998: 321–33.

21. Meade TW, North WRS, Chakrabarti R, *et al*. Haemostatic function and cardiovascular death: early results of a prospective study. *Lancet* 1980; **i**:1050–54.

22. Resch KL, Ernst E. The complex impact of fibrinogen on atherosclerosis-related disease. In: Koenig W, Hombäck V, Bond MG, Dramsch DM, eds. *Progression and Regression of Atherosclerosis*. Vienna: Blackwell MZV, 1995: 36–40.

23. Wilhelmsen L, Svardsudd K, Korsan-Bengsten K, *et al*. Fibrinogen as a risk factor for stroke and myocardial infarction. *N Engl J Med* 1984; **311**:501–5.

24. Lowe GDO, Lee AJ, Rumley A, *et al*. Blood viscosity and risk of cardiovascular events: the Edinburgh Artery Study. *Br J Haematol* 1997; **96**:168–73.

25. Tanne D, Benderly M, Boyko V, *et al*. Fibrinogen is an independent predictor of stroke-TIA in patients with coronary heart disease [abstract]. *Blood Coag Fibrinolysis* 1994; **5**:0–52.

26. Bainton D, Sweetnam P, Baker I, *et al*. Peripheral vascular disease. Consequence for survival and association with risk factors in the Speedwell Prospective Heart Disease Study. *Br Heart J* 1994; **72**:128–32.

27. Montalescot G, Ankri A, Vicant E, *et al*. Fibrinogen after coronary angioplasty as a risk factor for restenosis. *Circulation* 1995; **92**:31–38.

28. Stein D, Schoebel FC, Heins M, *et al*. Lipoprotein(a) and fibrinogen in restenosis after percutaneous transluminal coronary angioplasty. *Clin Hemorheol* 1995; **15**:737–47.

29. Wiseman S, Kenchington G, Dain R, *et al*. Influence of smoking and plasma factors on patency of femoropopliteal vein grafts. *Br Med J* 1989; **299**:643–46.

30. Grotta JC, Yatsu TM, Pettigrew LC, *et al*. Prediction of carotid stenosis progression by lipid and hematologic measurements. *Neurology* 1989; **39**:1325–31.

31. Lee AJ, Mowbray PI, Lowe GDO, *et al*. Blood viscosity and elevated carotid intima-media thickness in men and women: the Edinburgh Artery Study. *Circulation* 1998; **97**:1467–73.

32. Lee AJ, Smith WCS, Lowe GDO, Tunstall-Pedoe H. Plasma fibrinogen and coronary risk factors: the Scottish Heart Health Study. *J Clin Epidemiol* 1990; **43**:913–19.

33. Lee AJ, Lowe GDO, Smith WCS, Tunstall-Pedoe H. Plasma fibrinogen in women; relationships with oral contraception, the menopause and hormone replacement therapy. *Br J Haematol* 1993; **83**:616–21.

34. Lee AJ, Lowe GDO, Woodward M, Tunstall-Pedoe H. Fibrinogen in relation to personal history of prevalent hypertension, diabetes, stroke, intermittent claudication, coronary heart disease and family history: the Scottish Heart Health Study. *Br Heart J* 1993; **69**:338–42.

35. Tunstall-Pedoe H, Woodward M, Tavendale R, *et al*. Comparison of the prediction by 27 different risk factors of coronary heart disease and death in men and women of the Scottish

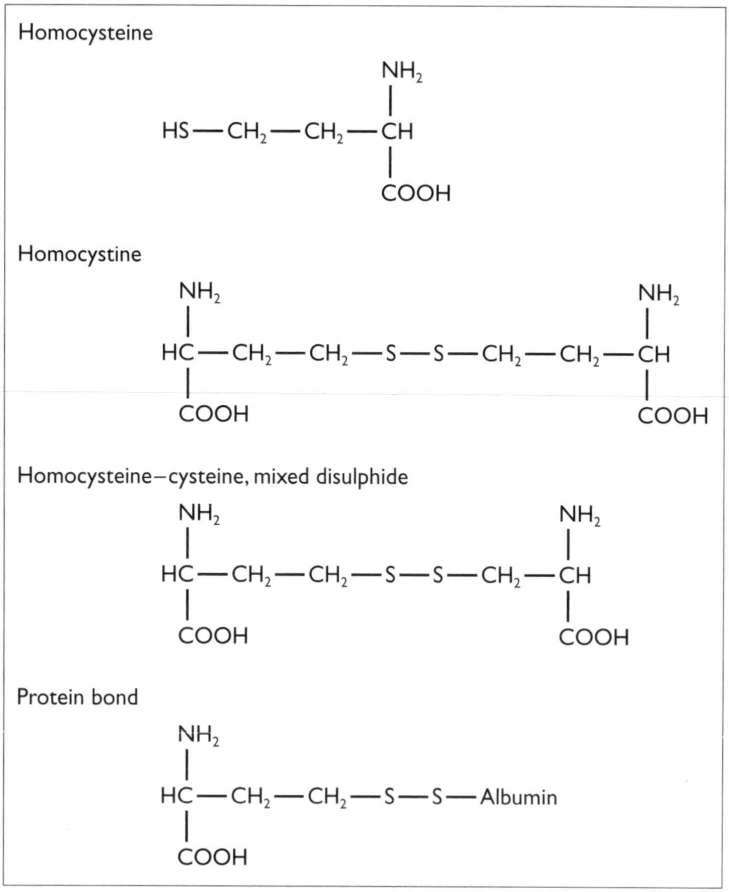

Fig. 8.1
Homocysteine species found in plasma.

means is presented, possible clinical and public health benefits considered and current randomised control trials outlined. The third question may be addressed satisfactorily when data from large randomised control trials are available.

Throughout the chapter, the abbreviation Hcy refers generically to the various species of homocysteine; tHcy, now accepted as standard, refers to plasma *total* homocysteine which is inclusive of all homocysteine species, whether free, protein-bound, mixed disulphide (homocysteine-cysteine) and pure disulphide (homocystine) (Figure 8.1).

Homocystinuria as a model for the study of vascular disease

Homocystinuria refers to the excretion in urine of the sulphur amino acid dimer homocystine as a result of severely elevated plasma Hcy levels. First described in 1962 by Carson in Northern Ireland,[2] this autosomal recessive inborn error of metabolism was detected while screening for metabolic defects among mentally retarded children. By 1964, deficiency of the enzyme cystathionine β-synthase (CBS) in the liver biopsy of a typical patient was reported.[3] The correct location of this defec-

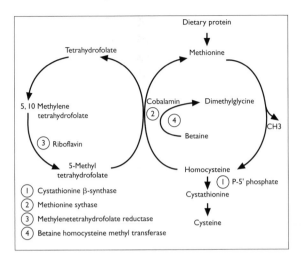

Fig. 8.2
*Methionine metabolism and the
transsulphuration and remethylation of
homocysteine.*
*Note that vitamin B6 is a cofactor for
cystathionine β-synthase, vitamin B12 is a
cofactor for methionine synthase and folate is a
cosubstrate for methylenetetrahydrofolate
reductase. Modified with permission.[4]*

tive enzyme in the metabolic pathway had been predicted on the basis of the biochemical findings of hypermethioninaemia, elevated plasma Hcy and low plasma cysteine levels (Figure 8.2). Since then, it has become clear that the inheritance on chromosome 21 of two defective alleles of CBS or, more rarely, severe deficiency of methylenetetrahydrofolate reductase (MTHFR), or defects of cobalamin metabolism can each result in homocystinuria.[3]

Clinically, subjects with homocystinuria are characterised by skeletal, connective tissue, neuropsychological and vascular defects. The high frequency of vascular events in such subjects is striking. Thrombotic events occur in 30% of untreated subjects by the age of 20 years and constitute the most common cause

of death.[5] Prognosis is worse in subjects with defective CBS, which is unresponsive to vitamin B6, compared with those who are B6 responsive.[3] While studying the autopsy findings of two subjects with homocystinuria attributed to different enzyme defects, McCully noted the shared features of premature vascular disease and a raised plasma Hcy level. This suggested that a raised plasma Hcy, rather than any other metabolite, was the cause of the vascular disease, and led to the proposal that milder elevations of plasma Hcy might also be associated with increased risk of vascular disease.[6] An examination of this putative relationship had to await the development of assays capable of measuring plasma Hcy levels significantly lower than those found in homocystinuria. Since that time, the relationship between such moderately elevated plasma levels of Hcy and risk of vascular disease has been established, and many genetic, nutritional and other determinants have been defined.

Homocysteine metabolism

Hcy is a sulphur amino acid with a reactive free sulphydryl group derived from the metabolism of the essential amino acid, methionine (see Figures 8.1 and 8.2). The daily intake of methionine is 15–35 mg/kg and the daily requirement is 10–40 mg/kg.[7] Methionine, through conversion to S-adenosylmethionine, acts as a methyl donor to many acceptors, including hormones, nucleic acids, neurotransmitters and creatinine.

Once formed, Hcy has two possible fates. It may condense with serine to be irreversibly transsulphurated by CBS to form cystathionine, which is further metabolised by cystathionine γ-synthase to form cysteine. Alternatively, it may be remethylated to methionine in a reaction requiring 5-methyltetrahydrofolate as a methyl donor, cobalamin as a methyl carrier, and the enzyme methionine synthase (5-methyltetrahydrofolate-homocysteine methyltransferase). An alternative pathway utilises betaine as methyl donor to reconstitute methionine in an irreversible reaction involving betaine-homocysteine methyltransferase. This latter pathway is thought to have a relatively minor role in humans.[3]

The activity of each metabolic pathway is dependent on cofactor nutrients; in particular, CBS utilises vitamin B6 (as pyridoxal 5-phosphate) and methionine synthase utilises vitamin B12 (as methylcobalamin) as cofactors. To provide bioavailable intracellular folate, vitamin B6 acts with serine hydroxymethyltransferase to convert tetrahydrofolate to 5,10 methylenetetrahydrofolate. In a subsequent reaction that requires folate as cosubstrate, this is further reduced to 5-methyltetrahydrofolate (5-MTHF) by 5,10-methylenetetrahydrofolate reductase (MTHFR); 5-MTHF is then demethylated, the methyl group being carried by the cobalamin-methionine synthase complex and subsequently transferred to homocysteine, thus reconstituting methionine. Therefore in vitamin B12 deficiency, folate bioavailability is impaired and 5-methyltetrahydrofolate accumulates intracellularly. This process is often referred to as the folate 'trap' hypothesis.[7]

Based on the above, an elevated plasma tHcy level may arise from deficient intake of folate, vitamin B12, or B6, or from defects in the enzymes CBS, MTHFR or methionine synthase, or from defects in cobalamin metabolism.

Species of homocysteine, measurement and variability

Of the homocysteine in plasma, 70–80% is protein bound. Of the non-protein-bound species, 1% is free Hcy and the remainder exists as homocystine (10%) or homocysteine-cysteine mixed disulphide (10%)[3] (see Figure 8.1). In freshly taken blood, levels of free (non-protein-bound) species of Hcy decline progressively as binding to plasma proteins occurs.[3] Therefore as a measurement, plasma tHcy level is more reproducible than free Hcy level and is preferable in clinical studies. When a blood sample has been taken for Hcy assay, placement on ice is recommended to reduce protein binding until the plasma sample has been prepared by centrifugation.

The advantages and disadvantages of a variety of methods of derivatisation, separation and detection of tHcy have been described in detail by Ueland et al.[7] Most are based on chromatographic methods. A more recent immunoassay is likely to make tHcy measurements more widely available.

Homocysteine levels appear to be relatively stable over time. Garg and colleagues noted little variability in Hcy levels over 1 month.[8] In a healthy elderly population, both seasonal and intra-individual variation were small (~1 µmol/l) over a 1-year period.[9] However, it was estimated that this small degree of variability could account for a 10–15% underestimation of any association between Hcy and risk of vascular disease.[9]

Fasting and post-methionine load homocysteine

Impaired transsulphuration due to defective CBS activity may not result in raised fasting plasma tHcy, but it may be unmasked by means of a methionine loading test.[7] This involves oral administration of a standardised methionine load (100 mg/kg) after which plasma tHcy is measured, usually 2–6 hours after the dose ('post-load tHcy'). It is thought that elevated post-load tHcy reflects defective transsulphuration, while elevated fasting tHcy reflects defective remethylation.[7] In rats, folate deficiency was associated with an elevated fasting plasma tHcy level but not with post-load elevation, whereas vitamin B6 deficiency was associated with marked methionine intolerance but had no effect on the fasting tHcy level.[10] Further support comes from a study involving patients taking the vitamin B6 antagonist, theophylline; these individuals were found to have higher post-load Hcy levels than healthy controls in response to methionine loading.[11]

Determinants of plasma homocysteine levels

While age, sex, lifestyle factors and drugs may all affect tHcy levels, the major determinants in most people, as with plasma cholesterol, are nutritional and genetic (Table 8.2).

Age, sex and the menopause

Plasma tHcy levels increase with age.[12] This may reflect age-related impairment of renal function, decline in CBS activity, or both.[13] Although independent of serum vitamin level, the effects may be increased by inadequate intake of B vitamins in the elderly.[14]

Plasma tHcy levels tend to be higher in men than in women.[13,15] Since Hcy formation is associated with the formation of creatine-creatinine, the higher plasma tHcy in males may reflect their larger skeletal muscle mass.[3] In the elderly, the male–female difference may also be explained by differences in vitamin level.[14]

Some (but not all) studies report higher Hcy levels in post-menopausal women compared with those who are premenopausal. In a European case–control study that involved more women than earlier studies, post-menopausal women had higher post-methionine load plasma tHcy levels than men of similar age.[15]

Genetic factors

Hyperhomocysteinaemia that is severe enough to cause homocystinuria occurs in homozygous deficiency of CBS and MTHFR, and in cobalamin mutations. Even the commonest of these, CBS deficiency, occurs in only 1 in 300 000 subjects, with wide geographic variation.[3] Heterozygous CBS deficiency occurs in up to 1% of the general population. It is associated primarily with increased tHcy levels after methionine loading. The most frequent known mutation affecting Hcy metabolism is the C677T mutation in the MTHFR gene, with an allele frequency of about 40% and a homozygous frequency of about 10% in the Caucasian population.[13] It is associated with thermolability and reduced enzyme activity. However, it is probably only associated with hyperhomocysteinaemia in subjects with poor folate status.[16,17]

Conventional cardiovascular risk factors

Data from the Norwegian Hordaland community study have allowed an exploration of relationships between conventional cardiovascular risk factors and plasma tHcy level.[12] Plasma tHcy levels were higher in smokers and showed a linear dose–response effect.[12] Although tHcy levels did not differ significantly between non-smokers and former smokers, the tHcy level increased with the duration of smoking in former smokers. The mechanism by which smoking raises plasma tHcy is unclear but may relate to lower serum, plasma, red cell and buccal mucosa folate levels, as well as lower vitamin B12 and B6 blood levels observed in smokers compared with non-smokers.[18]

1. PERSONAL CHARACTERISTICS
Increasing age ↑
Male gender ↑
Menopause ↑

2. GENETIC
Enzyme defects
Homozygous/heterozygous defects in cystathionine β-synthase ↑↑↑
Homozygous/heterozygous defects in methylenetetrahydrofolate reductase ↑↑↑
Thermolabile methylenetetrahydrofolate reductase ↑↑
Methionine synthase ↑
Cobalamin transport and metabolism ↑↑↑

3. ACQUIRED
Nutritional deficiency of:
Folate ↑↑
Vitamin B12 ↑↑
Vitamin B6 ↑
Disease states
Renal impairment ↑↑
Hypothyroidism ↑
Liver disease ↑
Diabetic retinopathy ↑
Psoriasis ↑
Acute lymphoblastic leukaemia ↑
Convalescent period following myocardial infarction ↑
Convalescent period following stroke ↑
Drugs
Nitrous oxide ↑↑
Anticonvulsants — phenytoin, carbamazepine ↑
Theophylline ↑
Methotrexate ↑
Tamoxifen ↓
Azarabine ↑
Nicotinic acid ↑
Oral contraceptive ↓
Fish oil ↓
Penicillamine ↓
Lifestyle characteristics
Tobacco smoking ↑
Sedentary lifestyle ↑
Caffeinated coffee ↑
Alcohol ↑↓

↓, reduced plasma tHcy level; ↑, mildly increased plasma Hcy level (<15 µmol/l); ↑↑, moderate hyperhomocysteinaemia (15–30 µmol/l); ↑↑↑, severe hyperhomocysteinaemia (>30 µmol/l).

Table 8.2
Determinants of plasma homocysteine level

Plasma tHcy levels have been positively related to both systolic and diastolic blood pressure and to serum total cholesterol and triglyceride levels.[12] These relationships were weaker after adjustment for other factors and rendered non-significant in the case of plasma triglyceride level.[12]

Plasma tHcy concentration was also found to relate inversely to the level of physical activity, although again, this relationship was weakened by multivariate analysis.[12] The biological significance of any relationships between tHcy, blood pressure or physical activity remains unclear.

Nutritional determinants

Figure 8.2 illustrates the dependence of the plasma level of tHcy upon vitamin B12, vitamin B6 and folate concentrations. An inverse relationship between tHcy and the plasma level of such nutrients has been documented in many studies including one of an elderly American population[14] and one of a younger European population.[19] This inverse relationship also held for vitamin B6 and folate *intake* in the Framingham study.[14]

From a therapeutic perspective, it is noteworthy that tHcy levels begin to rise at plasma levels of folate, vitamin B12 and vitamin B6 that are regarded as being within the low–normal range and that surrogate markers of vitamin B12 deficiency such as raised methylmalonic acid and methyl citric acid levels are evident at such levels.[20] These findings suggest suboptimal intracellular tHcy metabolism even at low–normal plasma folate and B12 levels, and that current recommended daily allowances for these vitamins may require revision.

Diseases and drugs affecting plasma homocysteine

As well as age, gender and vitamin level, numerous disease states are associated with altered levels of plasma tHcy. Hcy is metabolised by the kidney, relates to serum creatinine, and is markedly raised in renal failure, perhaps contributing to the aggressive vascular disease associated with this condition.[21] Plasma tHcy levels are increased in hypothyroidism, liver disease, diabetic retinopathy, psoriasis and other proliferative disorders such as acute lymphoblastic leukaemia.[7,13]

Anti-folate agents such as anticonvulsant drugs and methotrexate, nitrous oxide (which inactivates methionine synthase), and lipid lowering agents have been associated with elevated plasma tHcy levels (see Table 8.2).[13] Oral contraceptives, tamoxifen, fish oils and aminothiols such as penicillamine and acetylcysteine have been associated with a reduction in plasma tHcy levels.[13]

Possible mechanisms of vascular injury by homocysteine

It seems that Hcy is a toxic substance with the potential to damage the endothelium, possibly to promote the oxidation of lipids, and to interact with both platelets and coagulation factors. However, no clear unifying hypothesis has emerged from the plethora of proposed mechanisms of vascular damage.[22] Some experiments used supraphysiological concentrations of Hcy or derivatives such as Hcy thiolactone which, *in vivo*, is not present in high concentration and consequently its use has been the subject of criticism.[13,22] These experiments, which have been reviewed extensively elsewhere,[7,13,22] require replication under more physiological conditions. However, more recent work has examined the possible role of homocysteine in endothelial dysfunction, lipid peroxidation, smooth muscle cell and platelet dysfunction. If significant, these mechanisms may be susceptible to therapeutic manipulation.

Endothelial dysfunction

In a comparison of homocystinuric subjects with their heterozygous relatives and controls using flow-mediated dilatation as a marker of endothelial function, evidence of endothelial dysfunction was found in homozygotes only.[23] Heterozygotes had a similar response to control subjects. A second study of elderly subjects with mild to moderate elevation of plasma tHcy levels (mean $\pm$SE = 19 µmol/l $\pm$0.8) has also indicated impaired endothelial function.[24] One further study using flow-mediated dilatation detectable on ultrasound has shown a rapidly impaired endothelial response in healthy subjects following methionine loading.[25] An inverse and linear relationship between dilatation and plasma tHcy level was detected.[25] The implication of such work is that nitric oxide (NO) release may be impaired by levels of tHcy found commonly in patients with vascular disease. Short-term exposure of healthy endothelial cells to thiols may result in NO release and the formation of S-nitrosothiols, which have vasodilatory and antiplatelet properties. With long-term exposure, the capacity of the endothelium to generate NO may decline, thereby setting up a cycle of endothelial injury resulting from unopposed Hcy effects.[13] While nitroso-Hcy formation attenuates the adverse effects of Hcy, the reaction results in the generation of a peroxynitrite ($OONO^-$) and a reduction in bioavailable NO. Apart from its antiplatelet and vasodilatory properties, NO combines with the sulphydryl group of Hcy and limits hydrogen peroxide generation, resulting in less oxidative damage. This finding of endothelial dysfunction in association with exposure to Hcy has been corroborated by two further studies.[22,24]

The intravenous administration of 5-MTHF, which is known to be essential in remethylating Hcy (see Figure 8.2), restored endothelial function in subjects with familial hypercholesterolaemia.[26] However, the authors of this study suggest that the mechanism of action of 5-MTHF may be through supporting the synthesis of NO by endothelial NO synthase (eNOS).[26]

Lipid peroxidation

The oxidation of LDL is considered to be aetiologically important in atherogenesis and LDL oxidation by Hcy has been proposed as a mechanism by which Hcy might induce atherothrombosis.[22] However, despite evidence of free radical generation by Hcy *in vitro*, evidence of lipid peroxidation *in vivo* is lacking[27] and low levels of peroxidation products have been found. *In vivo*, Hcy already exists largely (95%) in oxidised form, while *in vitro* studies used predominantly reduced Hcy which readily underwent auto-oxidation.[13,22]

Platelet effects

In animal models and humans, evidence of enhanced platelet activation with increased thromboxane biosynthesis and lipid peroxidation products has been demonstrated.[13] Such in vivo platelet activation may explain in part the high risk of atherothrombotic events in subjects with homocystinuria but its relevance to patients with more moderately elevated plasma Hcy levels remains unclear.

Homocysteine and thrombosis

Recently, it has been suggested that the increased risk of thrombosis associated with homocystinuria is mediated through an interaction between inherited protein C (factor V Leiden) resistance and greatly elevated plasma tHcy levels.[13,22] This biological interaction effect has also been noted in non-homocystinuric subjects with venous thrombotic disease and moderately elevated plasma tHcy levels.[13,22]

A large number of studies have demonstrated effects of Hcy on the coagulation cascade. These include enhanced tissue factor activity, reduced von Willebrand factor secretion and inhibition of tissue plasminogen activator binding to endothelial cells.[13] Fibrinogen and Hcy concentrations correlate and the affinity of lipoprotein (a) [Lp(a)] for fibrin may be enhanced by Hcy concentrations as low as 8 μmol/l.[13] Lp(a) may compete with plasminogen for binding to fibrin and Hcy may enhance this binding.[13] The precise nature of the interaction between Hcy and these coagulation factors remains unclear.

Smooth muscle cell growth

Hcy has been found to enhance vascular smooth muscle cell growth and collagen production.[13] This represents a further mechanism whereby homocysteine may be atherogenic.

Epidemiological evidence for a relationship between homocysteine and cardiovascular risk

The majority, but by no means all of the published epidemiological data indicate an association between elevated plasma Hcy and cardiovascular disease.[28,29] The relationship seems stronger in cross-sectional, case–control[29] and some cohort studies of subjects with established disease[30] than in certain prospective studies of initially healthy subjects.[29]

Interpretation and comparison of these studies is limited by substantial discrepancies in design and methodology:[31]

- variable criteria for selection of cases and controls;

- variable definitions of an elevated plasma Hcy level, 'hyperhomocysteinaemia';
- the measurement of different species of Hcy;
- variations in the inclusion and exclusion criteria;
- variations in the recording of risk factors;
- differences in data analysis.

Figure 8.3, based on the metaanalysis by Danesh and Lewington,[29] indicates the relative strength of the relationship between homocysteine and cardiovascular disease as found in retrospective and prospective studies. Metaanalysis of individual subject data could be of further help in determining the strength of the relationship[29] but since there are such fundamental differences in the results of the prospective studies, Law has suggested that metaanalysis is inappropriate.[32]

The strength of the relationship

Case–control studies cannot prove causality but can contribute to its assessment by allowing an estimate of the strength and independence of an association between a risk factor and a disease. Thus, the European Concerted Action Project 'Homocysteine and Vascular Disease'[33] which addressed some of the methodological problems of earlier studies, confirmed that the relationship between a raised plasma tHcy level and risk of coronary, cerebral and peripheral vascular disease in both men and women was independent of classical cardiovascular risk factors. However, case–control studies may overestimate a relationship between a risk factor and disease if the putative risk factor is modified by the disease. Such may be the case for Hcy, the plasma level of which rises after a stroke or myocardial infarction, although it is not known if this rise represents a return to pre-stroke or pre-infarction levels.[34] This could

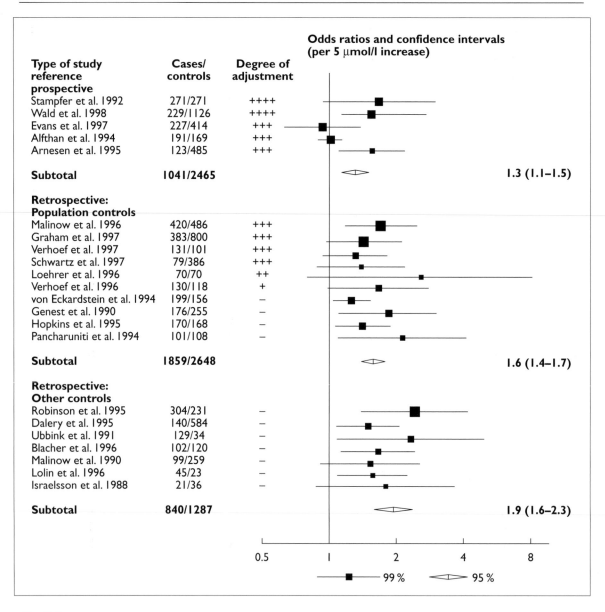

Fig. 8.3
Metaanalysis of case–control and prospective epidemiological studies up to 1998. Odds ratios in epidemiological studies of plasma total homocysteine and coronary heart disease. Odds ratios compare a 5 µmol/l increase in baseline concentration of plasma total homocysteine in the different studies. Black squares indicate the odds ratio in each study plotted on a doubling scale, with the square size proportional to the number of cases and the horizontal lines representing the 99% confidence intervals (CI). The combined odds ratio in each subtotal and its 95% CI are indicated by unshaded diamonds. Degree of adjustment for confounders denoted as:– for no adjustment at all, + for age and sex only, ++ for age and sex plus smoking, +++ for these plus some other standard vascular risk factors, ++++ for these plus markers of social class. Adapted with permission.[29]

explain in part the stronger relationship found in many case–control studies compared with cohort studies.[29] However, this reverse causality hypothesis has no biological foundation.[34]

Conversely, if a putative risk factor is lethal, a case–control study (which can only examine survivors) would underestimate its impact on risk. In addition, while many prospective studies have confirmed the relationship with regard to coronary heart disease and stroke, others have failed to do so thus calling into question the role of Hcy in the aetiology of vascular disease.[29] However most of the studies reported did not allow for the effect of regression dilution bias, which means that the reported relationships are underestimates rather than overestimates of risk.[32]

Recalling the model of homocystinuria suggests that, at least in the severe genetic forms of hyperhomocysteinaemia, the presence of an elevated plasma Hcy level must precede the onset of vascular disease. In addition, there is limited evidence for atherosclerotic plaque regression in a small number of patients treated with Hcy-lowering B vitamins.[34] Finally, supporting a temporal relationship between risk factor and disease outcome, both dietary induced and post-methionine load hyperhomocysteinaemia have led to vascular dysfunction in animals[34] and humans.[22,24,25]

In the European Concerted Action Project, a tHcy level at or above the top quintile of the control distribution (fasting = 12 μmol/l, post-methionine load = 38 μmol/l) compared with the remaining four-fifths conferred a significant two-fold increase in risk.[33] This risk estimate approximated to that associated with a systolic blood pressure of 160 mmHg or greater, a diastolic pressure of 95 mmHg or greater, or a serum total cholesterol level of 250 mg/dl (6.5 mmol/l) or greater.[33]

Prospective studies are not prone to the biases of a case–control study. For example

the US physician's health study which, at five years' follow up reported an adjusted relative risk of MI of 3.4 (95% CI = 1.3–8.8) comparing the top fifth percentile with the bottom 90th percentile of plasma tHcy.[35] A ten-year follow up of the same population indicated no significant risk attributable to elevated plasma tHcy level.[36] For subjects with stable angina in the same study population, the relative risk derived by comparing the top fifth with the bottom fifth of plasma tHcy concentration was non-significant at 1.7 (95% CI = 0.7–3.5) after adjustment for other risk factors.[37] This discrepancy in findings from the same study population may relate to the fact that angina pectoris is representative of an atherosclerotic process whereas Hcy may be related more to atherothrombotic events.[12]

The differences in mean ages (patients in retrospective studies were younger than those in cohort studies), choice of different cut-off points, and definitions of raised plasma tHcy in these studies makes direct comparison of risk difficult. In addition, the range of cut-off points in published work suggests that these were not chosen until the data had been explored and that some degree of post-hoc analysis was carried out.[28,29] Furthermore, the population impact of a study demonstrating increased risk based on the top fifth percentile is limited.[35]

One further study type, the clinical cohort study of subjects with established vascular disease, has provided relevant data on disease *recurrence*. These studies suggest a two- to three-fold increase in risk of disease recurrence associated with an elevated plasma tHcy level[30,38] and consistent findings have been reported in prospective studies of patients with end-stage renal disease who are at high risk of vascular events.[34] Therefore, while the strength is variable and methodologies differ, for many reasons the relationship remains robust.

Dose–response effect

While one study found only a weak relationship between elevated plasma tHcy level and extracranial carotid artery disease in CBS obligate heterozygotes, an association between tHcy concentration and significant (greater than 25%) extracranial carotid stenosis in the Framingham cohort and in an elderly Dutch population has been documented.[13] In a further study of asymptomatic subjects, the plasma level of tHcy correlated with the carotid intimal–medial wall thickness which was used as a marker of pre-atherosclerotic vascular disease.[13] The relationship demonstrated in this prospective study is of particular interest as plasma tHcy levels could not have been influenced by therapy or lifestyle changes.[12] Such changes made after a vascular event may act as a source of bias in case–control studies.[13] Although weaker, some of the clinical cohort studies also indicate a dose–response effect.[30,34]

More significant support for a dose–response relationship between plasma Hcy and vascular disease risk is found in large prospective community-based studies. In the Tromsø study, the unadjusted relative risk for a 4 µmol/l increase in serum tHcy level was 1.41 (95% CI = 1.16–1.71).[13] Adjustment for possible confounders reduced this risk to 1.32 (95% CI = 1.05–1.65), an odds ratio similar to that of 1.6 (95% CI = 1.4–1.7) per 5 µmol/l increment in plasma tHcy level.[28] No threshold effect could be defined.

Similarly, the British Regional Heart Study demonstrated a graded increase in the relative risk of stroke from the second to fourth quartiles of the plasma tHcy distribution (relative risk = 1.6; 95% CI = 1.7–2.5).[13,28] Adjustment for cigarette smoking and systolic blood pressure did not significantly alter this association.

In a metaanalysis published in 1995, summary odds ratios (95% confidence interval) per 5 µmol/l increment in tHcy level (an increment that matches the risk associated with an increase in serum total cholesterol of 1.93 mg/dl or 0.5 mmol/l) were derived.[28] These were 1.7 (1.5–1.9) for coronary artery disease, 2.5 (2.0–3.0) for cerebrovascular disease, and 6.8 (2.9–15.8) for peripheral vascular disease. In terms of risk of coronary disease for men alone, the odds ratio (95% confidence interval) was 1.6 (1.4–1.7) and that for women was 1.8 (1.3–1.9).[28] Additional data reported in a further metaanalysis have indicated, for the same increment in plasma tHcy level, an odds ratio of 1.3 (1.1–1.5) for prospective studies, 1.6 (1.4–1.7) for retrospective studies with population controls and 1.9 (1.6–2.3) for retrospective studies with opportunistically recruited controls (see Figure 8.3).[29] More recent data, not included in these metaanalyses, have also indicated significant increases in cardiovascular risk associated with increasing plasma Hcy levels.[38–40]

In the US physician's health study alluded to above, a possible threshold effect was seen with risk of MI increasing above the 95th percentile of the tHcy distribution.[35] Intrinsic differences in the populations studied may explain these findings. The mean plasma tHcy level in US physician controls was 10.5 µmol/l ±2.8 (cases = 11.1 µmol/l ±4.0)[35] while that of Tromsø controls was 11.3 µmol/l ±3.7 (cases = 12.7 µmol/l ±4.7).[13] In addition, the age ranges differed in the two studies: 34–61 years in Norway (mean = 51.2 years ±7.3)[13] and 40–84 years in the US (mean = 58.9 ±8.5).[35] The issue of age has also been raised when examining the stronger relationship observed in retrospective case–control studies, in which subjects were young, compared to that in prospective studies, in which subjects tended to be older.[32] Apart from these measured differences, lifestyle differences between a highly selected population of health-conscious US physicians and an unselected rural Norwegian community are likely and may prove to be important.

Is the relationship independent of confounding factors?

The Hordaland study has indicated the important factors that influence plasma Hcy concentration and might act as confounders in epidemiological studies.[12] Many studies indicate an independent relationship between Hcy and vascular disease risk but the degree to which adjustment for the many confounding factors was made in these studies varies. Thus, the European Concerted Action Project indicated a relationship that was independent of the traditional cardiovascular risk factors smoking, hypertension and hypercholesterolaemia.[33] Other studies adjusted for many more factors and a significant relationship was still evident.[39] In spite of this additional adjustment, observational studies cannot exclude confounding by other dietary and non-dietary factors and reliance for proof of causality must be placed upon randomised controlled trials.[41]

Interaction effects between homocysteine and conventional cardiovascular risk factors

Interaction effects between elevated plasma tHcy and other cardiovascular risk factors have been described.[33] In particular, the risk of vascular disease in subjects who shared elevated plasma tHcy and elevated plasma cholesterol levels, tobacco smoking or elevated blood pressure was substantially higher (and often multiplicative) than that in subjects who had one risk factor alone (Figure 8.4). No conclusions regarding biological interaction are possible on the basis of these findings but the clinical implication is that substantial modification of risk may be achieved in subjects who

have combined risk factors by lowering plasma tHcy concentrations.[33]

Fasting and post-methionine load total homocysteine measurements: are they equally predictive of risk?

While methionine loading is inconvenient in clinical practice, the exclusive use of a fasting tHcy measurement may lead to diagnostic loss.[13] The use of fasting or post-methionine load tHcy measurements identifies different individuals, some with both elevated fasting and post-load levels and others with elevation of one level only. In the European Concerted Action Project, 12% of the controls defined as having elevated tHcy levels would not have been so classified if fasting tHcy alone was measured.[33] An elevated tHcy level in this study was defined as being at or above the top quintile of the control distribution for either fasting or post-load tHcy level. The rise [Δ] in tHcy following methionine loading was also used to classify individuals with an abnormal response to methionine loading and the top quintile of this distribution in controls was used to define normality.[33] Only a further 2% of controls were identified as having a significantly elevated rise after methionine loading and would not have been so classified if only fasting and post-load levels had been used. The use of fasting and Δ measurements was inclusive of a greater number of subjects with elevated tHcy levels. However, in terms of the risk attributed to each measurement, fasting and post-load tHcy, unlike a high Δ, are equal and independent predictors of risk. On this basis, the use of absolute fasting and post-load tHcy is still necessary and the use of Δ contributes little to risk prediction.[33]

One earlier study used a 4-hour post-load tHcy measurement and the 90th percentiles of the fasting, post-load and Δ tHcy distributions

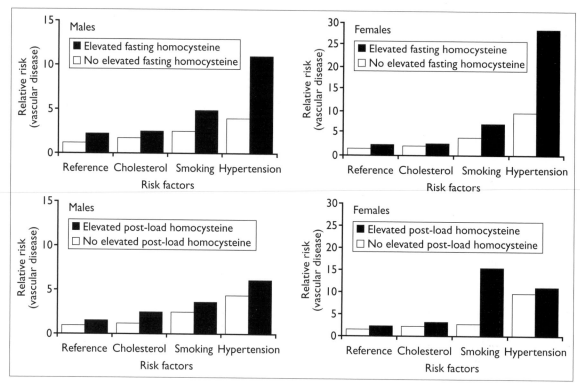

Fig. 8.4

Relative risk of vascular disease in groups defined by the presence or absence of classical risk factors and elevated plasma total homocysteine. Adjusted for age, sex and centre. Adapted with permission.[33]

as the cut-off points to operationally define normality.[13] Of all subjects with an elevated tHcy level, 57% had an abnormal fasting tHcy, 36% had an abnormal post-load response (but normal fasting tHcy), and 7% had an abnormal Δ tHcy.[13] Thus, over 40% of subjects would have been misclassified if methionine loading had not been carried out. Both studies[13,33] argue in favour of retaining the post-load tHcy measurement.

Gene–environment interaction

Sibling studies suggest a significant genetic contribution to a moderately elevated plasma Hcy level.[13] In monozygotic twins, the correlation coefficient between shared Hcy levels was approximately 0.50, indicating that genetic factors contribute by about one-quarter to the Hcy level. In older subjects the correlation coefficient was smaller, indicating the importance of the other modulating factors.[12]

In considering gene–environment interactions in individuals with elevated Hcy levels, parallels can be drawn with hypercholesterolaemia. In each disorder, severe genetic defects resulting in homocystinuria or familial hypercholesterolaemia lead to virtually universal severe and premature atherothrombotic and sclerotic vascular disease. Although at very high risk, these subjects are greatly outnumbered by those with milder elevations of Hcy or cholesterol. In such subjects, nutritional and milder genetic disorders may be relevant to varying degrees.

Initially, attention focused on homocystinuria[3] and on the importance of defects in CBS, MTHFR and cobalamin metabolism.[7,13] However, population gene frequency calculations indicate that defects of CBS are too rare (1–2%) to account for the observed prevalence of elevated plasma Hcy levels or for much of the associated increase in risk.[41] In the Irish population, the most frequent CBS mutation among the first degree relatives of subjects with homocystinuria is G307S with an observed allele frequency of 71%.[13] This 'Celtic' mutation, originally found in a subject of French-Scottish ancestry, was not present in 111 Irish vascular disease cases but was found at the expected allele frequency of 1% among the 105 control subjects.[4] Therefore, the contribution of defective CBS alleles to elevated plasma tHcy levels and to vascular disease risk is likely to be negligible.[4]

More recently, attention has shifted to the remethylation enzyme MTHFR and to a thermolabile variant arising from a single amino acid substitution.[13] The relationship between elevated plasma tHcy level, cardiovascular disease risk and the mutation has been examined.[42] Homozygosity for this defect is significantly associated with elevated plasma tHcy levels[13] and with cardiovascular risk in many[13] but not all[42] studies. Heterozygotes may also have significantly elevated plasma Hcy levels.[4,13] The prevalence of the defective allele varies among populations, ranging from 29% to 44%, as does the frequency of the homozygous state among cases (7–20%), and controls (4–18%).[13]

Genetic studies indicate that the region of thermolabile MTHFR coded for by the mutation is involved in folate binding and is stabilised in the presence of adequate folate levels.[13] Among subjects with plasma folate levels less than the median (15.4 nmol/l) of one study population, those homozygous for the thermolabile defect had tHcy levels 24% greater than levels of normal subjects.[16] No difference between the genotypes was found among individuals with folate levels above the median.[16] In healthy men, serum folate levels,[17] and in subjects with late-onset vascular disease, plasma folate levels[4] were lowest in thermolabile homozygotes. Thus, thermolabile MTHFR homozygotes may have a higher folate requirement than other subjects[13,16,17] and current dietary folate recommendations may require revision.[4] In addition, while thermolabile MTHFR homozygotes demonstrate resistance to low-dose folate therapy[13] they are sensitive to higher doses.[4,13]

In studies where no clear relationship between genotype, folate and risk has been demonstrated,[4,13,42] it is possible that subjects may have been folate replete and the range of intake may have been too narrow to allow for a definitive exclusion of significant interaction effects. Such gene–environment interactions may account, at least in part for the relationship between elevated plasma Hcy levels and vascular disease risk.

Using risk to identify a normal range of plasma total homocysteine

Plasma Hcy concentrations in the range 5–15 μmol/l[13,34] have been cited as normal for fasting plasma tHcy in healthy populations. However, differences in laboratory methods in the measurement of tHcy and difficulty in correcting for inter-individual variation in those determinants of tHcy (see Table 8.2) suggest that a reference range so derived may be of limited value. Statistical or operational definitions of normality based on means, standard deviations or percentiles are also limited. Such definitions are arbitrary [a fixed proportion of the population is always abnormal and disease prevalence is constant] and meaningless if Hcy has a continuous relationship with risk. If treatment above a certain level of plasma tHcy were proven to be of benefit, a normal range that is not based on a statistical definition of normality but that is 'desirable for health' could be derived. However so far, no randomised control trial of tHcy lowering therapy with clinical endpoints has been completed.

In terms of what is 'ideal for health', a reference range can be inferred from observational data. Subjects with a plasma tHcy level exceeding the 95th percentile (15.8 µmol/l) in a prospective study had a relative risk of MI three times that of subjects at or below the 90th percentile.[35] Case–control data indicate that at fasting plasma tHcy levels ⩾12 µmol/l, the risk of vascular disease is doubled.[33] Therefore, choosing a level of plasma tHcy that is identified with a particular risk rather than one that is based on the assumption of statistical normality is less arbitrary and clinically more useful. This implies that different reference ranges will probably be required for primary and secondary prevention strategies, assuming such intervention is beneficial.

Potential for the reduction of vascular risk

Homocystinuric subjects with severe MTHFR deficiency are resistant to many forms of treatment except betaine,[3] while subjects with CBS deficiency require a low methionine-cysteine diet with supplements of vitamin B6 and folic acid.[3] Subjects responsive to vitamin B6 therapy have a better prognosis with a reduced incidence of vascular events compared with subjects who are non-responsive.[3] The mecha-

nism for this is unclear but vitamin B6 (*in vitro*) may be antithrombotic.[11] Evidence from *in vivo* experiments is lacking.

In subjects with moderately elevated plasma tHcy levels, the presence of a likely continuous graded relationship with risk suggests possible benefit from plasma tHcy reduction. Pancharuniti, in a case–control study, related the risk of CHD to plasma folate level.[43] Upon adjustment for plasma tHcy level, the relationship disappeared suggesting that the total risk was mediated through the elevated plasma tHcy level.[43] A further study demonstrated a relationship between serum folate and fatal CHD events over a 20-year period.[44] Similarly, European[33] and American[45] users of vitamin supplements (containing folate, B6 or B12) were apparently protected from vascular disease, an effect partly mediated by lower tHcy levels. The possible influence of unaccounted variables suggests that the data should not be over-interpreted. Some case–control studies[19] have demonstrated increased risk of CHD in vitamin B6-deficient subjects, an effect found to be independent of Hcy.[19]

As tHcy and B vitamin levels are related continuously and inversely to each other, defining a vitamin deficiency level is problematic. Once defined, such a level determines the prevalence of each vitamin deficiency. In a study of the Framingham cohort, a strong inverse relationship between tHcy level and plasma folate level was demonstrated with weaker inverse relationships for vitamins B6 and B12.[14] In addition, plasma tHcy level was inversely related to intake of vitamin B6 and folate but not to B12 intake.[14] The optimal folate intake level (400 µg daily), in other words that associated with the lowest plasma tHcy level, was present in only 40% of subjects.[14]

A higher prevalence of vitamin deficiency may exist than can be estimated on the basis of measured plasma vitamin levels alone and plasma/serum levels may not reflect tissue levels. Vitamin B12 (1 mg), folate (1.1 mg) and vitamin B6 (5 mg) supplements given to elderly subjects with normal serum vitamin concentrations produced improvements in the profile of markers of tissue vitamin deficiency.[20] Markers such as methylmalonic acid may be useful in identifying subjects who might benefit from vitamin supplementation.[13]

Based on the assumption that lowering Hcy levels will reduce progression of atherosclerosis and CHD mortality,[34] the benefit of increasing dietary intake of folate, both from supplements and from fortified flour and cereal was estimated.[28] A programme resulting in a 40% increase in intake of folate-rich fruit and vegetables was predicted to prevent about 2% of CHD deaths.[28] Folic acid supplements, if 50% effective, would prevent about 4% of CHD deaths and fortification of flour and cereals would prevent about twice this percentage.[28] These different effects probably relate to the reduced bioavailability of natural compared to synthetic folate.[46] The US Food and Drug Administration initiated flour fortification with 140 µg folate in 100 g flour in 1997 and significant effects in terms of Hcy reduction have been reported.[46] Observed increases in risk caused by interaction effects between Hcy and conventional risk factors suggest a public health benefit from a reduction in plasma tHcy levels, especially in smokers and in hypertensive subjects.[33]

Vitamin trials of homocysteine-lowering therapy: surrogate and clinical endpoints

Many trials of Hcy lowering therapies have been performed.[13,47] Most of these have involved vitamin therapies and, in about half, no estimate of fasting tHcy level was made. The doses of folic acid ranged from 0.65 mg to 5 mg. Doses of vitamin B6 ranged from 7.2 mg to 250 mg. In general, folic acid reduced fasting and post-load Hcy levels while vitamin B6 reduced post-load levels. Folate also reduced Hcy levels deemed to be within a normal range[13] and the response to folate supplementation depended on MTHFR genotype.[4,13]

A metaanalysis of trials of Hcy lowering therapy involving 1114 subjects has indicated that daily folate supplementation of 0.5–5 mg will reduce tHcy levels by 25% and an additional 0.5 mg vitamin B12 daily will achieve a further 7% reduction.[47]

While it is clear that Hcy reduction is possible, the impact on cardiovascular disease occurrence and recurrence is unknown. Many B vitamin trials with clinical endpoints are currently underway (Table 8.3).[41] These involve combinations of vitamins B6, B12 and folate and two involve blood pressure lowering and lipid lowering agents. Although folate fortification, already underway in the United States,[46] may reduce the likelihood of clear findings from randomised control trials, these trials remain the best method for addressing the uncertainty surrounding Hcy as a causal cardiovascular risk factor.

Conclusion

Of the criteria required to conclude that raised plasma Hcy causes cardiovascular disease, many have been fulfilled. The relationship is strong, consistent, independent of other risk factors, likely graded, and probably biologically plausible. Data are largely consistent within and between scientific disciplines but causality cannot be inferred beyond reasonable doubt until the question of whether lowering plasma Hcy levels reduces vascular disease risk has been systematically addressed.

Trial title	Patient population	Sample size	Vitamin therapy
VISP Vitamin Intervention in Stroke Prevention	Stroke	3600	Folic acid 2.5 mg + B6 25 mg + B12 400 µG versus Folic acid 200 µg + B6 200 µg + B12 60 µg
WACS Women's Antioxidant and Cardiovascular Disease Study	Vascular disease or high risk	6–8000	Folic acid 2.5 mg + B6 50 mg + B12 1 mg versus placebo
SEARCH Study of the Effectiveness of Additional Reductions in Cholesterol and Homocysteine	Myocardial infarction	12 000	Folic acid 2 mg + B12 1 mg versus placebo in a 2 × 2 factorial design with simvastatin 80 mg versus 20 mg
NORVIT Norwegian Study of Homocysteine Lowering with B-vitamins in Myocardial Infarction	Myocardial infarction	3000	Folic acid 5 mg × 2 weeks + 800 µg + B12 400 µg versus placebo in a 2 × 2 factorial design with B6 40 mg versus placebo.
BERGEN VITAMIN STUDY	Coronary Heart Disease	2000	Folic acid 5 mg × 2 weeks + 800 µg + B12 400 µg versus placebo in a 2 × 2 factorial design with B6 40 mg versus placebo.
PACIFIC Prevention with a combined ACE inhibitor and Folate in Coronary Heart Disease	High risk or previous vascular disease	10 000	Folic acid 200 µg or 2 mg versus placebo in 2 × 2 factorial design with omapatrilat
CHAOS-2 Cambridge Heart Antioxidant Study	Myocardial infarction or unstable angina	4000	Folic acid 5 mg versus placebo

Modified with permission.[41]

Table 8.3
Vitamin trials to evaluate the relationship between elevated plasma homocysteine and cardiovascular disease risk

So far, no randomised-controlled trials of the effect of reducing plasma tHcy levels on vascular disease events have been reported. Trials of Hcy lowering vitamin therapy are underway. Whether nutritional changes or food supplementation, as recently introduced in the United States for neural tube defect prevention, should also be recommended to reduce population tHcy levels and possibly vascular disease risk is of fundamental public health importance. Whether to target at-risk groups or to prescribe for the entire community remains a contentious issue. In the context of advice on neural tube defect prevention, recommendations regarding increased intake of folic acid from dietary sources may be impractical as insufficient bioavailable folic acid is obtained and supplements in the form of tablets are required to achieve target levels of folate intake.[13] However, a flour fortification programme resulting in an extra 100 μg folate per day, if taken continuously, may still have significant public health benefits.[28,34,46]

References

1. Hill AB. The environment and disease: association or causation? *Proc R Soc Med* 1965; **58**:295–300.

2. Carson NAJ, Neill DW. Metabolic abnormalities detected in a survey of mentally backward individuals in Northern Ireland. *Arch Dis Child* 1962; **37**:505–13.

3. Mudd SH, Levy HL, Skovby F. Disorders of transsulphuration. In: Scriver CR, Beaudet AL, Sly WS, Valle D, eds. *The metabolic and molecular basis of inherited disease.* New York: Mc Graw Hill, 1995: 1279–327.

4. Meleady RA, Graham IM. Homocysteine and vascular disease: Nature or nurture? *J Cardiovasc Risk* 1998; **5**(4):233–8.

5. Mudd SH, Skovby F, Levy HL, *et al.* The natural history of homocystinuria due to cystathionine B-synthase deficiency. *Am J Hum Genet* 1985; **37**:1–31.

6. McCully KS, Wilson RB. Homocysteine theory of arteriosclerosis. *Atherosclerosis* 1975; **22**:215–27.

7. Ueland PM, Refsum H, Brattstrom L. Plasma homocysteine and cardiovascular disease. In: Francis RB, ed. *Atherosclerotic Cardiovascular Disease, Hemostasis and Endothelial Function.* New York: Marcell Dekker, 1992: 183–235.

8. Garg UC, Zheng Z-J, Folsom AR, *et al.* Short-term and long term variability of plasma homocysteine measurement. *Clin Chem* 1997; **43**:141–5.

9. Clarke R, Woodhouse P, Ulvik A, *et al.* Variability and determinants of total homocysteine concentrations in plasma in an elderly population. *Clin Chem* 1998; **44**:102–107.

10. Miller JW, Nadeau MR, Smith D, Selhub J. Vitamin B_6 deficiency vs folate deficiency: comparison of responses to methionine loading in rats. *Am J Clin Nutr* 1994; **59**:1033–9.

11. Ubbink JB, van der Merwe A, Delport R, *et al.* The effect of a subnormal vitamin B_6 status on homocysteine metabolism. *J Clin Invest* 1996; **98**:177–84.

12. Nygård O, Vollset SE, Refsum H, *et al.* Total plasma homocysteine and cardiovascular risk profile. The Hordaland homocysteine study. *JAMA* 1995; **274**:1526–33.

13. Refsum H, Ueland PM, Nygård O, Vollset SE. Homocysteine and cardiovascular disease. *Ann Rev Med* 1998; **49**:31–62.

14. Selhub J, Jacques PF, Wilson PWF, *et al.* Vitamin status and intake as primary determinants of homocysteinemia in an elderly population. *JAMA* 1993; **270**:2693–8.

15. Verhoef P, Meleady R, Daly LE, *et al.* and the European Concerted Action Project. Homocysteine, vitamin status and risk of vascular disease; effects of gender and menopausal status. *Eur Heart J* 1999; **20**:1234–45.

16. Jacques PF, Bostom AG, Williams RR, *et al.* Relation between folate status, a common mutation in methylenetetrahydrofolate reductase, and plasma homocysteine concentrations. *Circulation* 1996; **93**:7–9.

17. Harmon DL, Woodside JV, Yarnell JWG, *et al.* The common "thermolabile" variant of methylenetetrahydrofolate reductase is a major determinant of mild hyperhomocysteinaemia. *Q J Med* 1996; **89**:571–7.

18. Piyalthilake CJ, Macaluso M, Hine RJ, *et al.*

Local and systemic effects of cigarette smoking on folate and vitamin B_{12}. *Am J Clin Nutr* 1994; **60**:559–66.

19. Robinson K, Arheart K, Refsum H, *et al.* and the European Concerted Action Group. Low circulating folate and vitamin B_6 concentrations: risk factors for stroke, peripheral vascular disease and coronary artery disease. *Circulation* 1998; **97**:437–43.

20. Naurath HJ, Joosten E, Reizler R, *et al.* Effects of vitamin B_{12} folate, and vitamin B_6 supplements in elderly people with normal serum vitamin concentrations. *Lancet* 1995; **346**:85–9.

21. Bostom AG, Lathrop L. Hyperhomocysteinemia in end stage renal disease (ESRD): prevalence, etiology and potential relationship to arteriosclerotic outcomes. *Kidney Int* 1997; **52**:10–20.

22. Welch GN, Loscalzo J. Homocysteine and atherothrombosis. *N Engl J Med* 1998; **338**:1042–50.

23. Celermayer DS, Sorensen K, Ryalls M, *et al.* Impaired endothelial function occurs in the systemic arteries of children with homozygous homocystinuria but not in their heterozygous parents. *J Am Coll Cardiol* 1993; **22**:854–58.

24. Tawakol A, Omland T, Gerhard M, *et al.* Hyperhomocyst(e)inemia is associated with impaired endothelium-dependent vasodilation in humans. *Circulation* 1997; **95**:1119–21.

25. Chambers JC, McGregor A, Jean-Marie J, Kooner JS. Acute hyperhomocysteinaemia and endothelial dysfunction. *Lancet* 1998; **351**: 36–7.

26. Verhaar MC, Wever RMF, Kastelein JJP, *et al.* 5-Methyltetrahydrofolate, the active form of folic acid, restores endothelial function in familail hypercholesterolemia. *Circulation* 1998; **97**:237–41.

27. Blom HJ, Kleinveld HA, Boers GHJ, *et al.* Lipid peroxidation and susceptibility of low-density lipoprotein to *in vitro* oxidation in hyperhomocysteinemia. *Eur J Clin Invest* 1995; **25**:149–54.

28. Boushey C, Beresford SAA, Omenn G, Motulsky A. A quantitative assessment of plasma homocysteine as a risk factor for vascular disease. Probable benefits of increasing folic acid intakes. *JAMA* 1995; **274**:1049–57.

29. Danesh J, Lewington S. Plasma homocysteine and coronary heart disease: systematic review of published epidemiological studies. *J Cardiovasc Risk* 1998; **5**:229–32.

30. Nygard O, Nordrehaug JE, Refsum H, *et al.* Plasma homocysteine levels and mortality with coronary artery disease. *N Engl J Med* 1997; **337**:230–6.

31. Graham IM. Homocysteine as a risk factor for cardiovascular disease. *Trends Cardiovasc Med* 1991; **1**:244–9.

32. Wald NJ, Watt HC, Law MR, *et al.* Homocysteine and Ischaemic Heart Disease. Results of a prospective study with implications regarding prevention. *Arch Intern Med* 1998; **158**:862–7.

33. Graham IM, Daly LE, Refsum HM, *et al.* Plasma homocysteine as a risk factor for vascular disease. The European Concerted Action Project. *JAMA* 1997; **277**:1775–81.

34. Malinow MR, Bostom AG, Krauss RM. Homocyst(e)ine, diet and cardiovascular diseases. A statement for healthcare professionals from the nutrition committee, American Heart Association. *Circulation* 1999; **99**: 178–82.

35. Stampfer MJ, Malinow R, Willet WC, *et al.* A prospective study of plasma homocyst(e)ine and risk of myocardial infarction in US physicians. *JAMA* 1992; **268**:877–881.

36. Chasan-Taber L, Selhub J, Rosenberg IH, *et al.* A prospective study of folate and vitamin B_6 and risk of myocardial infarction in US physicians. *J Am Coll Nutr* 1996; **15**:136–43.

37. Verhoef P, Hennekens CH, Allen RH, *et al.* Plasma total homocysteine and risk of angina pectoris with subsequent coronary artery bypass surgery. *Am J Cardiol* 1997; **79**:799–801.

38. Hoogeveen EK, Kostense PJ, Beks PJ, *et al.* Hyperhomocysteinaemia is associated with an increased risk of cardiovascular disease, especially in non-insulin dependent diabetes mellitus. A population based study. *Arteriosclerosis Thromb Vasc Biol* 1998; **18**:133–8.

39. Ridker PM, Manson JE, Buring JE, **et al.** Homocysteine and risk of cardiovascular disease among postmenopausal women. *JAMA* 1999; **281**:1817–21.

40. Bostom AG, Silbershatz H, Rosenberg IH, *et al.* Non-fasting plasma total homocysteine levels and all-cause and cardiovascular mortality

in elderly Framingham men and women. *Arch Intern Med* 1999; **159**:1077–80.

41. Clarke R, Collins R. Can dietary supplements with folic acid or vitamin B$_6$ reduce cardiovascular disease risk. Design of clinical trials to test the homocysteine hypothesis of vascular disease. *J Cardiovasc Risk* 1998; **5**:249–55.

42. Brattstrom L, Wilcken DE, Ohrvik J, Brudin L. Common methylenetetrahydrofolate reductase gene mutation leads to hyperhomocysteinemia but not to vascular disease: the result of a meta-analysis. *Circulation* 1998; **98**: 2520–6.

43. Pancharuniti N, Lewis CA, Sauberlich HE, *et al.* Plasma homocyst(e)ine, folate, and vitamin B$_{12}$ concentrations and risk for early-onset coronary artery disease. *Am J Clin Nutr* 1994; **59**:940–8.

44. Morrison HI, Schaubel D, Desmeules M, Wigle DT. Serum folate and risk of fatal coronary heart disease. *JAMA* 1996; **275**:1893–6.

45. Rimm EB, Willett WC, Hu FB, *et al.* Folate and vitamin B$_6$ from diet and supplements in relation to risk of coronary heart disease among women. *JAMA* 1998; **279**:359–64.

46. Jacques PF, Selhub J, Bostom AG, *et al.* The effects of folic acid fortification on plasma folate and total homocysteine concentrations. *N Engl J Med* 1999; **340**:1449–54.

47. Homocysteine Triallists' Collaboration. Lowering blood homocysteine with folic acid based supplements: meta-analysis of randomised trials. *Br Med J* 1998; **316**:894–8.

9

Chronic infection and coronary heart disease: potential for new therapies?

Sandeep Gupta and Juan Carlos Kaski

Atherogenic risk factors and CHD: *an incomplete explanation*

Atherosclerotic-related disorders, in particular coronary heart disease (CHD), remain a major cause of morbidity and mortality worldwide, with approximately 12 million deaths annually.[1] Although there has been a 20–40% decline in CHD mortality in many industrialised countries over the last two decades, countries in Eastern Europe and in south Asia are witnessing a striking rise in CHD morbidity and mortality rates.

Established risk factors for CHD include cigarette smoking, hypercholesterolaemia, diabetes mellitus and hypertension. However, variations in the presence or severity of these factors probably account for no more than half of the known differences in prevalence and severity of CHD.[2,3] In addition, up to 30% of patients presenting with myocardial infarction (MI) have none of these risk factors.[4]

Several 'novel' risk factors are thought to contribute to the atherosclerotic process and are the focus of intense current research (and will be discussed at various points in this book). Such factors include hyperhomocysteinaemia,[5] elevated Lp(a) levels and genetic predispositions and polymorphisms.[6] Defining whether, and to what extent, such mechanisms play a role in atherothrombosis requires further investigation. Chronic infection, in particular with the organism *Chlamydia pneumoniae*, is a major factor that is implicated increasingly in the pathogenesis of atherosclerosis and is the focus of this review.[7]

Infection, inflammation and atherosclerosis

The revised 'response-to-injury' hypothesis emphasises the importance of endothelial dysfunction and denudation as the first steps to atherogenesis and plaque development.[8] Possible causes of endothelial dysfunction and vessel injury include elevated and modified LDL-cholesterol, free radicals caused by cigarette smoking, hypertension and diabetes mellitus, genetic predisposition, elevated plasma homocysteine, microorganisms, or combinations of these and other factors. In particular, the involvement of infective agents could explain the presence or progression of local inflammatory processes in the atheromatous lesions and/or the elevation in systemic markers of inflammation. The idea that infection could be a causal factor in the pathogenesis of atherosclerosis is not new. Indeed, Osler and others first proposed such a mechanism as long ago as 1908.[9] Until recently, however, the suggestion had been largely dismissed. Fresh

Disease	Infective agent
Peptic ulcers	*Helicobacter pylori*[11]
Rheumatoid arthritis	*Herpesviruses*[12]
Crohn's disease	*Mycobacterium paratuberculosis*[13]
Multiple sclerosis	*Herpesviruses*[14]
Sarcoidosis	*Mycobacterium*[15]

Table 9.1
The potential association between chronic inflammatory diseases and infection.

debate now focuses on whether or not common chronic infections contribute to the development and progression of atherosclerotic disease. In addition, *in vitro* experiments, animal studies, pathological examinations and clinical observations provide supporting evidence for associations between infectious diseases and atherosclerosis.[10]

It is interesting to observe how an increasing number of chronic inflammatory conditions have been associated with infective aetiologies, although the weight of supporting evidence varies markedly from disease to disease (Table 9.1). Although several infective agents have been implicated in atherosclerosis (including herpesviruses such as cytomegalovirus [CMV], *Helicobacter pylori* and bacteria from chronic dental sepsis) on current evidence, *C. pneumoniae* is the microorganism most clearly linked with atherosclerosis and CHD.

Herpesvirus infections
Animal models

An elegant animal model of infection-induced atherosclerosis was demonstrated by Fabricant *et al.*[16,17] Inoculation of chickens with Marek's disease virus led to aggressive lipid deposition within the walls of the animals' coronary arteries. When the animals were concomitantly fed a cholesterol-enriched diet the vascular lesions changed, becoming fibroproliferative in appearance and very similar to human atherosclerotic plaques. Moreover, vaccination of chickens (with a turkey vaccine) before inoculation with the Marek's disease virus led to the formation of fewer than expected atherosclerotic lesions.

Cytomegalovirus in humans

Cytomegalovirus infection is very common. In the USA, for example, the prevalence of antibodies to CMV is about 10–15% in the adolescent population, rising to 40–50% by age 35 years, and to over 60–70% in adults over 65 years of age. This age-related pattern resembles that of atherosclerosis.[18] As with other herpesviruses, infection with CMV can become chronic and 'latent', although the site of such dormancy remains unclear. Periodic reactivation of the infection may occur, particularly in immunosuppressed patients. The finding of herpesvirus-induced atherosclerosis in chickens stimulated research into a possible analogous role of such viruses in humans.

In 1983, Melnick *et al.* reported the presence of CMV in smooth muscle cells cultured from arterial specimens taken from patients who had undergone carotid endarterectomy.[19] Several groups subsequently pursued this line of investigation. Overall, in 16 published studies on CMV in vascular pathology samples, there were only small differences in the proportion of atheromatous and non-atheromatous blood vessels positive for CMV (47% versus 39%) with a weighted odds ratio of 1.4.[20] It is possible that in some cases CMV may have initiated the atherosclerotic process but subsequently became difficult to detect.

A significantly higher prevalence of anti-CMV antibodies and higher antibody titres have been observed among patients with vascular disease compared with controls matched for hyperlipidaemia, age, ethnicity and socioeconomic background. A role for CMV in restenosis following coronary angioplasty has also been investigated. In one study, patients with serological evidence of previous CMV infection had a high rate of restenosis after coronary angioplasty — 43% of those with anti-CMV IgG antibodies compared with 8% of seronegative patients ($P < 0.002$).[21] It is proposed that in certain patients, angioplasty-induced injury to the vessel wall may reactivate a latent CMV infection and enhance the smooth muscle cell proliferation typically seen in restenotic lesions. Stronger evidence of a role for CMV in atherogenesis and atherosclerosis comes from studies of the infection's association with the development of the accelerated allograft vasculopathy often seen in recipients of cardiac transplants.[22] This atherosclerotic process usually comprises diffuse smooth muscle proliferation, perivascular inflammation and collagen accumulation, with classical atheromatous plaques being uncommon.[23]

A recent meta-analysis of the epidemiological associations between CMV and CHD identified several studies reporting odds ratios of 2 or higher.[20] However, many of the studies considered involved small sample sizes, inadequate adjustments for known confounders and exploratory statistical analyses. In addition, fewer than 400 of the 1600 cases in these studies were defined as 'native' coronary atherosclerosis, with the majority involving cases of coronary artery restenosis, development of accelerated transplant atherosclerosis after transplantation, or disease in arteries other than coronary arteries.

Helicobacter pylori

In a case–control study conducted in London, UK, seropositivity to *H. pylori* correlated significantly with angiographically-diagnosed CHD.[24] The same investigators went on to show that seropositivity to *H. pylori* was associated with serum cardiovascular risk markers and postulated that this association with markers of cell activation and inflammation suggested mechanisms by which common infections could play a part in atherogenesis.[25]

Subsequent, larger studies (incorporating prospective data and better defined control subjects) have been unable to demonstrate any independent association between this infection and CHD.[26,27] These studies also suggested that lower socioeconomic status is a major confounding variable in any relationship between *H. pylori* infection and atherosclerotic disease. No current evidence exists to suggest that *H. pylori* is directly involved in the pathogenesis of atherosclerotic plaques. Indeed in a recent study, aortic plaque tissue was taken from 51 patients undergoing abdominal aortic aneurysm surgery.[28] Although 92% of the patients had serum antibodies to *H. pylori*, polymerase chain reaction techniques revealed no evidence of the organism in the aortic specimens.

A meta-analysis of 18 epidemiological studies, involving a total of over 10 000 patients, found no correlations between evidence of *H. pylori* infection and blood pressure, leucocyte count, or serum concentrations of total cholesterol, fibrinogen, triglycerides or C-reactive protein.[29] It has been suggested that the earlier claims of correlation between *H. pylori* seropositivity and certain vascular risk factors were largely, or wholly, due to chance or preferential publication of positive results.

In summary, the early case–control study[24] that observed an association between *H. pylori*

Consistent link between anti-*C. pneumoniae* antibodies and CHD
Identified and cultured from atheroma
Infects vascular cells *in vitro*
Induces atherosclerosis in animal models
Analogy with the pathogenesis of trachoma
Anti-chlamydial antibiotics show potential benefit in CHD

Table 9.2
Lines of evidence linking C. pneumoniae *with atherosclerosis.*

and CHD has been superseded by larger prospective investigations.[26,27] The latter studies indicate that the organism is unlikely to have a major independent role in atherogenesis or development of CHD. Whether or not a subgroup of seropositive subjects (say, those infected with particularly virulent strains of *H. pylori*[30]) mount abnormal immune or inflammatory responses (which could, in theory, trigger cardiac events) is not known.

Dental infections

A clear relationship between dental health and CHD has emerged in observational studies.[31] However, confirmatory prospective data are lacking, and the association between dental hygiene and CHD may simply reflect general health habits rather than a causal relationship between dental sepsis and atherosclerosis. Whether dental disease simply mirrors other lifestyle factors more clearly associated with CHD, such as diet, exercise and smoking, needs further clarification.

Chlamydia pneumoniae

Chlamydia pneumoniae is thought to be the strongest candidate infectious agent implicated in CHD.[32] It is an intracellular pathogen and a common cause of benign respiratory symptoms. It is estimated that by the age of 50 years, 50% of the population will have been exposed to the organism.[33] *Chlamydia pneumoniae* is very difficult to grow in culture and diagnosis of infection has relied hitherto on indirect serological tests.[34] Accordingly, *C. pneumoniae* had been regarded, until recently, as a rather obscure infective agent which was clinically significant only as a potential cause of atypical pneumonia.[35] The evidence supporting its association with atherosclerosis and CHD is based on several different lines of investigation (Table 9.2) which are now briefly discussed.

Epidemiological studies

In 1988, Saikku *et al.* were the first investigators to describe an apparent association between *C. pneumoniae* and CHD.[36] They had conducted a case–control study in which 26 of 38 (68%) consecutive males presenting with acute MI had a significantly high antibody titre against an epitope of chlamydial lipopolysaccharide. A similar titre was present in only 3% of a control group and absent in patients with chronic CHD. Furthermore, IgG and IgA antibody titres against *C. pneumoniae* (measured using an microimmunofluorescence assay) were significantly elevated in the patients with acute MI or chronic CHD compared with titres in the controls. On this evidence, the investigators suggested that acute MI might be associated with an exacerbation of an underlying chronic *C. pneumoniae* infection.

Work based at a UK institution demonstrated an association between seropositivity to *C. pneumoniae* and prevalent CHD in a community cross-sectional survey.[37] In particular, the study found evidence of a strong correlation between the presence of an elevated anti-*C. pneumoniae* IgG titre (1/64 and greater) and CHD that was independent of conventional cardiovascular risk factors, age and social class.

To date, over 20 studies performed by different groups in different countries and investigating patients with various degrees of CHD have found a consistently increased risk of prevalent CHD in patients who are seropositive to *C. pneumoniae*.[38] However, such serological studies can be criticised in certain respects: how their control groups have been chosen, the borderline statistical significances of many of the results, and the anti-*C. pneumoniae* antibody titre cut-off points arbitrarily used to indicate seropositivity.[39] Also, it is by no means clear whether an elevated antibody titre is a reliable indicator of underlying *C. pneumoniae* infection, of past exposure to infection, or simply of antigenic cross-reactivity.[40] Establishing the existence of a causal association between such titres and CHD is also hampered by the wide variation in antibody responses to the organism, which might result from variations in the original infective dose, the mode of infection or any previous exposure. As a further complication, a few negative serology-based studies have been published.[41,42] For example, Danesh *et al.* have shown a lack of association between serological markers of infection with *C. pneumoniae*,

H. pylori or CMV and evidence of CHD in a case–control study involving 288 patients with prevalent CHF and 704 age- and sex-matched controls.[42]

More recently, the debate of a causative link between anti-*C. pneumoniae* antibodies and CHD has been rekindled. A prospective longitudinal study by Strachan *et al.* demonstrated (for the first time) that seropositivity to *C. pneumoniae* (presence of IgA antibodies) was predictive of subsequent mortality and incidence of CHD over a 13-year follow-up period in 1773 males (age 45–59 years).[43]

Plaque studies

Stronger evidence for an association between *C. pneumoniae* and atherosclerosis has come from examination of arterial plaque tissue. The first report of identification of the organism within such lesions was published by Shor *et al.* in 1992.[44] In the following year investigators in Seattle, USA, examined coronary plaque lesions obtained at autopsy for the presence of *C. pneumoniae*, using molecular and immunohistochemical techniques.[45] Of 36 subjects who had died from non-cardiac causes, the organism was detected in 20 (56%) using one or both methods. *Chlamydia pneumoniae* was found only within sites of tissue damage, including necrotic areas and the lipid-rich core of atheromatous plaques and smooth muscle cells within the plaque. The organisms were not detectable in normal tissue adjacent to the sclerotic lesions or in normal coronary arteries from 11 control cases. More recently, Muhlestein *et al.* tested for the presence of *Chlamydia* species using direct immunofluorescence in plaque specimens obtained from 90 patients undergoing coronary atherectomy for symptomatic angina;[46] they also examined 24 autopsy control specimens from patients without atherosclerosis. A markedly higher proportion of the atheromatous tissue

(A)

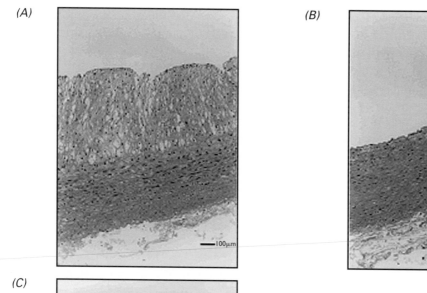

(B)

(C)

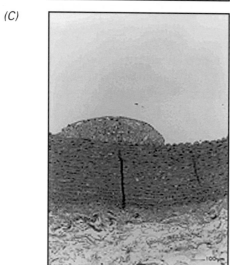

Fig. 9.1
Photomicrographs of representative aortic sections from (A) animals in the infected/untreated group, (B) the control (uninfected/untreated) group, and (C) the infected/treated group. Haematoxylin and eosin-stained section; original magnification × 100. Reproduced with permission.[53]

specimens from the patients with CHD were positive for *Chlamydia* spp. when compared with those from controls (79% versus 4%, P < 0.001).

Several published studies have now demonstrated that *C. pneumoniae* can localise in atherosclerotic coronary, aortic, carotid or peripheral arteries.[47] By contrast, the organism has been identified only rarely in 'healthy' control arteries. In a recent meta-analysis of stud-

ies that looked for *C. pneumoniae* in human pathology samples, evidence of the organism within endovascular tissue (defined by the presence of chlamydial DNA, antigens, or elementary bodies) was found in 52% of atheromatous lesions but in only 5% of control non-atheromatous samples of arterial tissue (overall odds ratio = 10; 95% CI = 5–22).[29]

A further important development has been the recent successful isolation and culture of viable *C. pneumoniae* organisms from atheromatous vessels, as reported by several independent investigators.[48–50]

Animal models

A rabbit model of *C. pneumoniae*-induced atherosclerosis has been developed. When deliberately infected with the organism, these animals develop fatty streaks and grade III atherosclerotic and inflammatory lesions in the aorta, as well as pneumonia.[51–53] In the largest animal model study to date,[53] rabbits were given repeated intranasal inoculations of either *C. pneumoniae* or saline at 3-week intervals, and fed a diet supplemented with cholesterol. After the final inoculation, infected and control rabbits were randomised to a 7-week course of azithromycin antibiotic or no therapy. The results of subsequent pathology studies showed that intimal thickening of the aorta was much more obvious in the infected animals than in control animals; however, such changes did not occur in infected animals given azithromycin (Figure 9.1). While these results are intriguing, it would, of course, be premature to assume that they necessarily have direct implications for atherogenesis in humans.

Proposed mechanisms of damage

Despite the evidence presented above, how *C. pneumoniae* enters atheromatous plaques and whether it has a direct causal role in atherogenesis remains unclear.[54] *Chlamydia pneumoniae* as a primary respiratory pathogen has to be conveyed from the lung to the coronary arteries before vascular infection can occur. One possibility is that the microorganism gains entry to, and is transported within the bloodstream via the macrophage–monocyte system.[39] Indeed, there is evidence to suggest that *C. pneumoniae* can reproduce within phagocytic cells (including macrophages).[55] In theory, there are several possible consequences of uptake of *C. pneumoniae* by macrophages. The organism may simply rest within such cells without causing any harmful effects (in other words, act as an innocent bystander), and any association between the organism and CHD may be purely coincidental. Alternatively, chronic macrophage infection may contribute directly to local inflammation, development of atheromatous plaques and plaque instability, leading to acute coronary events. This scenario may be analogous to the pathogenesis of trachoma, in which the closely related *C. trachomatis* causes blindness as a result of the fibrosis and scarring that follows conjunctival infiltration by macrophages and lymphocytes.[56] Another suggestion is that *C. pneumoniae* infection may induce chronic immune activation which contributes to direct chronic endothelial cell damage or stimulates the synthesis of acute phase proteins, such as fibrinogen[57] and C-reactive protein.[58] The process of lipid peroxidation may be enhanced by infection and lead to vascular damage and plaque disruption — a mechanism that merits further investigation.[59] Finally, chronic *C. pneumoniae* infection may produce a hypercoaguable state, with an accompanying increased risk of coronary thrombosis, perhaps through activation of the monocyte-derived procoagulant, tissue factor.[60]

Other mechanisms of damage may also be relevant. *Chlamydia pneumoniae* may have a direct role in atherogenesis, as suggested by recent *in vitro* studies in which infection induced foam cell formation.[61] The demonstration that chlamydial heat shock protein 60 (HSP60) co-localises with its homologue, human HSP (which is associated with atherosclerosis), within atherosclerotic plaque macrophages[62] supports an indirect autoimmune mechanism of action. Both *Chlamydia* HSP60 and human HSP60 have also been shown to stimulate enhanced mouse macrophage production of TNF-alpha (a pro-inflammatory cytokine) and matrix metallo-proteinase-9 (an enzyme that can degrade connective tissue).

That *C. pneumoniae* infection interacts with certain atherogenic risk factors may be an important prerequisite for the microorganism to contribute to pathogenesis of atherosclerosis. Elevated antibodies to *C. pneumoniae* are positively associated with hypertension,[63] an atherogenic lipid profile[64] and cigarette smoking.[65] Furthermore, seropositivity to *C. pneumoniae* is associated with elevated levels of fibrinogen[66] and C-reactive protein[67] in patients with CHD.

Koch's postulates

By convention, for an infective agent to be implicated as a direct cause of CHD, it would need to fulfil Koch's postulates.[68] The microorganism would be present in all, or nearly all, cases of the disease; inoculations of its pure cultures would produce disease (for example, when injected into susceptible animals); it would be obtainable from these diseased states, and it could then be propagated in pure culture. So far the first — and, possibly, the second — of these postulates appear to be fulfilled with respect to *C. pneumoniae* in CHD. However, some workers have argued that Koch's postulates may lack sufficient sensitivity to be used for dismissing the possibility of a causal link between an infectious agent and a given chronic disease.[69] Interestingly, *H. pylori* does not completely satisfy the requirements of Koch's postulates for a causative organism for peptic ulceration.[70]

Antibiotic therapy in CHD

The results of preliminary anti-chlamydial antibiotic intervention studies in CHD[71,72] has triggered widespread interest in the potential role of antimicrobial therapy in CHD and deserves discussion.

St George's study: azithromycin in male survivors of MI

In a randomised, placebo-controlled study, the new-generation macrolide antibiotic, azithromycin was given (500 mg once daily for 3 or 6 days) to a series of male survivors of MI with stable elevated anti-*C. pneumoniae* antibody titres (that is, two raised IgG titres of 1/64 and above, taken 3 months apart).[73] The primary hypothesis under test was that *C. pneumoniae* infection may have a pathogenetic role in atherogenesis via enhanced activation of serum and monocyte markers.[74] A reduction in the levels of such activation markers following treatment with an anti-chlamydial antibiotic could provide indirect evidence that *C. pneumoniae* does indeed act through such a mechanism. The study also assessed whether an elevated anti-*C. pneumoniae* antibody titre predicted further adverse cardiovascular events (at a mean follow up of 18 months) in a consecutive series of 220 men who had had an MI (from whom the antibiotic intervention trial participants were drawn). The incidence of future cardiovascular events was also observed in the subgroup of patients with elevated titres who were randomised (in a double-blind fashion) to azithromycin or placebo.

By 6 months the anti-*C. pneumoniae* antibody titre had fallen to less than 1/16 in 43% (17/40) of patients who received azithromycin compared with only 10% (2/20) of patients taking placebo ($P = 0.02$).[71] Subjects receiving azithromycin had a significant fall in levels of certain serum and monocyte activation markers (monocyte integrins CD11b/CD11c, fibrinogen and leucocyte count; $P < 0.05$).[73]

Group	Total CV events (%)	Unadjusted OR (95%CI)	Adjusted OR (95%CI)
Cp −ve (n = 59)	4 (7)		
Cp-I (n = 74)	11 (15)	2.4 (0.7–8.0)	2.0 (0.6–6.8)
Cp +ve-NR/P (n = 40)	11 (28)	5.2 (1.5–17.8)*	4.2 (1.2–15.5)†
Cp +ve-A (n = 40)	3 (8)	1.1 (0.2–5.3)‡	0.9 (0.2–4.6)§

*P = 0.008, †P = 0.03
‡P = 0.03 versus Cp +ve-R/P group
§P = 0.03 versus Cp +ve-R/P group

Comparison of cardiovascular events (CV) for all groups relative to Cp −ve group [expressed as OR (95%CI)]. Adjusted OR was calculated after controlling for variables: age, diabetes mellitus, smoking status, hypertension, dyslipidaemia and previous coronary revascularisation. Cp −ve indicates seronegative group of patients; Cp-I, group with intermediate antibody titres (IgG = 1/8–1/31); Cp +ve-NR/P, group with elevated antibody titres (IgG > 1/64) either randomised to placebo or not randomised; Cp +ve-A, group with elevated antibody titres (IgG ≥ 1/64) randomised to azithromycin. Reproduced with permission.[71]

Table 9.3
Odds ratios for cardiovascular events in seropositive patients relative to seronegative patients.

These findings help support the hypothesis that *C. pneumoniae* contributes to the progression of atherosclerosis via up-regulation of inflammatory markers.

The study also showed that the higher the baseline anti-*C. pneumoniae* antibody titre, the greater the risk of experiencing an adverse cardiovascular event, an association which persisted following correction for potential confounding variables. There was a fourfold higher risk of experiencing adverse cardiovascular events among the group with elevated *C. pneumoniae* titres compared with the group with negative serology (odds ratio 4.2 [95% CI = 1.2–15.5; P = 0.03]). For the high-titre group receiving antibiotic therapy, the adjusted odds ratio was 0.9 (0.2–4.6; P = NS) (Table 9.3).

The ROXIS study

In the Roxithromycin in Ischaemic Syndromes (ROXIS) study, another pilot randomised intervention trial, the aim was to assess whether the anti-chlamydial antibiotic, roxithromycin (150 mg twice daily, for 30 days) was more effective than placebo in decreasing the incidence of recurrent ischaemic events in 205 patients presenting with acute coronary syndromes.[72] At day 31, the cumulative number of ischaemic events was significantly lower in the patients randomised to roxithromycin compared with the placebo group (2 versus 9 events, P = 0.03 unadjusted, P = 0.06 adjusted). One postulated mechanism by which roxithromycin may have acted in this clinical setting is by an anti-inflammatory, 'plaque-stabilising' effect. Alternatively, roxithromycin therapy may have suppressed reactivation of a chronic C. *pneumoniae* infection within the atherosclerotic plaque.

Large randomised antibiotic trials

The first two pilot studies of macrolide therapy in the prevention of cardiovascular events have prompted the large-scale, prospective antibiotic trials currently underway.[7] Further justification for carrying out these trials has been provided by the results of a large, recently published case–control study. Meier *et al.* showed that 3315 patients presenting with a first MI were significantly less likely to have taken antibiotics with anti-chlamydial activity (tetracyclines or quinolones) in the preceding 3 years, compared with age, sex and time-matched controls (n = 13 139).[75]

It is of additional interest that some investigators have noted that there is a positive epidemiological correlation between the introduction of anti-chlamydial antibiotics and the decline in cardiovascular disease (CVD) mortality seen in certain countries over the last 3–4 decades. For example, Ånestad *et al.* compared mortality rates from CVD in Norway with some lifestyle risk factors (dietary fat intake and cigarette smoking) and the consumption of tetracycline.[76] They showed that CVD mortality rates peaked in 1961–65, but both fat intake and smoking rates in the community remained high for at least another decade. On the other hand, increasing usage of tetracycline after the drug was licensed in Norway in 1954 mirrored a temporal fall in CVD mortality. Saikku *et al.* have made similar observations, relating the declining mortality from CHD in Finland to the introduction of erythromycin and other macrolides (P. Saikku, personal communication).

The Weekly Intervention with Zithromax in Atherosclerotic-Related Disorders (WIZARD) study has recruited around 3500 patients (who have had an MI more than 6 weeks previously and who have positive anti-C. *pneumoniae* serology) to receive either an acute 3-day course of azithromycin followed by a chronic 3-month course of the antibiotic or of placebo. The primary aim of the study is to assess whether the antibiotic reduced total cardiovascular events over a 2.5-year follow-up period. Results of this trial are expected towards the end of the year 2000 (M. Dunne, personal communication).

A further prospective antibiotic trial is the UK-based Might Azithromycin Reduce Bypass List Events? (MARBLE) study. This aims to randomise around 1200 patients on a waiting list for coronary artery bypass surgery (CABG) to a 3-month course of weekly azithromycin (irrespective of baseline anti-C. *pneumoniae* antibody titre), and to assess whether total cardiovascular events can thereby be reduced during the period waiting for CABG. At time of operation, a proportion (20–25%) of these patients will undergo coronary endarterectomy procedures. Samples of coronary arteries taken at this time will be examined for presence of C. *pneumoniae*, and correlations sought with serology, inflammatory markers and any effects of antibiotic treatment. The results of the MARBLE study, if positive, may provide data on the relationship between antibiotic treatment and effects of infection within coronary arteries, but moreover could have socioeconomic and political ramifications. Other interventional studies include South Thames Antibiotics in Myocardial Infarction and Angina (STAMINA), Azithromycin in Coronary Artery Disease: Elimination of Myocardial Infection with *Chlamydia* (ACADEMIC), Croatian Azithromycin In Atherosclerosis Study (CROAATS) and Azithromycin and Coronary Events Study (ACES).

Whilst there exists an understandable drive to complete the large antibiotic intervention trials promptly, certain important issues need addressing. Such points include difficulties in confirming chronic *C. pneumoniae* infection, precise characterisation of any subgroups of patients likely to benefit from (or to be harmed by) antibiotic therapy, potential effects of reinfection with *C. pneumoniae* and the possible confounding by other infections.[77] The potential implications of widespread use of broad-spectrum antibiotics in the community and the risk of increased antibiotic resistance, a very topical issue,[78] also needs careful consideration and risk–benefit evaluation. Despite their limitations, the ongoing antibiotic trials are likely to increase our understanding of the role of infection and antimicrobials in CHD. Macrolides may exhibit beneficial (anti-inflammatory[79]) properties independent of their antimicrobial action. Should the trials confirm the results of the pilot studies, antibiotic treatment of chronic *C. pneumoniae* infection could have major therapeutic implications and potentially help reduce the burden of the epidemic of CHD which persists, despite other advances in risk-factor modification and coronary interventions.

Conclusions

Inflammation plays a central role in atherosclerosis. Accumulating epidemiological, laboratory and preliminary clinical trial evidence suggests that *C. pneumoniae* (a potential contributor to the inflammatory process) may have a pathogenetic role in CHD. On this basis, large interventional trials are now attempting to establish whether treatment with antibiotic therapy can improve the clinical outlook in patients with CHD. Together with parallel, laboratory-based investigations, such studies may also help to indicate exactly how *C. pneumoniae* might produce deleterious effects in the setting of atherosclerosis. While this research is obviously exciting, it should not be allowed to sanction premature use of anti-chlamydial therapy outside the context of controlled studies. Although an infectious basis to atherosclerosis is plausible (at least in part), proof of a definitive causal link is still awaited. An answer is expected early in the next millennium and, if positive, will have profound implications for public health worldwide. In the meantime our attention remains focused on targeting and treating the established risk factors for CHD.

References

1. Yusuf S, Ounpuu S, Anand S. The global burden of cardiovascular disease: a review of the evidence. *Cardiologist* 1999; **2**:1–11.
2. Nieminen MS, Mattila K, Valtonen V. Infection and inflammation as risk factors for myocardial infarction. *Eur Heart J* 1993; **14(suppl. K)**:12–16.
3. Buja LM. Does atherosclerosis have an infectious eitology? *Circulation* 1996; **94**:872–3.
4. Sumpter MT, Dunn MI. Is coronary artery disease an infectious disease? *Chest* 1997; **112**: 302–3.
5. Malinow MR. Homocysteine and arterial occlusive diseases. *J Intern Med* 1994; **236**: 603–17.
6. Harrap SB, Watt GCM. Genetics and risk of coronary heart disease. *Med J Aust* 1992; **156**: 594–6.
7. S Gupta. Chronic infection in the aetiology of atherosclerosis — focus on *Chlamydia pneumoniae* ('The John French Memorial Lecture'). *Atherosclerosis* 1999; **143**:1–6.
8. Ross R. Atherosclerosis – an inflammatory disease. *N Engl J Med* 1999; **340**:115–26.
9. Osler W. Diseases of the arteries. In: Osler W, ed. *Modern Medicine: Its Practice and Theory.* Philadelphia: Lea & Febiger, 1908: 429–47.

10. Gupta S, Camm AJ. Is there an infective aetiology to atherosclerosis? *Drugs Aging* 1998; **13**: 1–7.

11. Marshall BJ. *Helicobacter pylori* in peptic ulcer: Have Koch's postulates been fulfilled? *Ann Med* 1995; **27**:565–8.

12. Silman AJ. Is rheumatoid arthritis an infectious disease? *Br Med J* 1991; **303**:200–1.

13. Sanderson JD, Moss MT, Tizard ML, Hermon-Taylor J. *Mycobacterium paratuberculosis* DNA in Crohn's disease tissues. *Gut* 1992; **33**:890–6.

14. Soldan SS, Bertri R, Salem N, *et al.* Association of human herpes virus 6 (HHV-6) with multiple sclerosis: increased IgG response to HHV-6 early antigen and detection of serum HHV-6 DNA. *Nature Med* 1998; **3**:1394–7.

15. Saboor SA, Johnson N, McFadden J. Detection of mycobacterial DNA in sarcoidosis and tuberculosis with polymerase chain reaction. *Lancet* 1992; **339**:1012–15.

16. Fabricant CG, Fabricant J, Litrenta MM, Minick CR. Virus-induced atherosclerosis. *J Exp Med* 1978; **148**:335–40.

17. Fabricant CG, Fabricant J, Minick CR, Litrenta MM. Herpesvirus-induced atherosclerosis in chickens. *Fed Proc* 1983; **42**:2467–9.

18. Melnick JL, Adam E, Debakery ME. Cytomegalovirus and atherosclerosis. *Eur Heart J* 1993; **14(suppl. K)**:30–8.

19. Melnick JL, Petrie BL, Dreesman GR, *et al.* Cytomegalovirus antigen within human arterial smooth muscle cells. *Lancet* 1983; **2**:644–7.

20. Danesh J, Collins R, Peto R. Chronic infections and coronary heart disease: is there a link? *Lancet* 1997; **350**:430–6.

21. Zhou YF, Leon MB, Waclawiw MA. Association between prior cytomegalovirus infection and the risk of restenosis after coronary atherectomy. *N Engl J Med* 1996; **335**:624–30.

22. Grattan MT. Accelerated graft atherosclerosis following cardiac transplantation: Clinical perspectives. *Clin Cardiol* 1991; **14(suppl. II)**: 16–20.

23. Johnson DE, Gao SZ, Schroeder JS, *et al.* The spectrum of coronary artery pathological findings in human cardiac allografts. *J Heart Transplant* 1989; **8**:349–59.

24. Mendall MA, Goggin PM, Molineaux N, *et al.* Relation of *Helicobacter pylori* infection and coronary heart disease. *Br Heart J* 1994; **71**:437–9.

25. Patel P, Mendall MA, Carrington D, *et al.* Association of *Helicobacter pylori* and *Chlamydia pneumoniae* infections with coronary heart disease and cardiovascular risk factors. *Br Med J* 1995; **311**:711–14.

26. Murray LJ, Bamford KB, O'Reilly DP, *et al. Helicobacter pylori* infection: relation with cardiovascular risk factors, ischaemic heart disease, and social class. *Br Heart J* 1995; **74**:497–501.

27. Wald NJ, Law MR, Morris JK, Bagnall AM. *Helicobacter pylori* infection and mortality from ischaemic heart disease: negative results from a large, prospective study. *Br Med J* 1997; **315**:1199–201.

28. Blasi F, Denti F, Erba M, *et al.* Detection of *Chlamydia pneumoniae* but not *Helicobacter pylori* in atherosclerotic plaques of aortic aneurysms. *J Clin Microbiol* 1996; **34**:2766–9.

29. Danesh J, Peto R. Risk factors for coronary heart disease and infection with *Helicobacter pylori*: meta-analysis of 18 studies. *Br Med J* 1998; **316**:1130–2.

30. Pasceri V, Cammarota G, Patti G, *et al.* Association of virulent *Helicobacter pylori* strains with ischemic heart disease. *Circulation* 1998; **97**:1675–9.

31. Mattila KJ, Nieminen MS, Valtonen VV, *et al.* Association between dental health and acute myocardial infarction. *Br Med J* 1989; **298**:779–82.

32. Gupta S, Camm AJ. Chronic infection in the aetiology of atherosclerosis – the case of *Chlamydia pneumoniae*. *Clin Cardiol* 1997; **20**:829–36.

33. Saikku P. The epidemiology and significance of *Chlamydia pneumoniae*. *J Infect* 1992; **25**: 27–34.

34. Grayston JT, Wang SP, Campbell LA, *et al.* Current knowledge on *Chlamydia pneumoniae* strain TWAR, an important cause of pneumonia and other acute respiratory diseases. *Eur J Clin Microbiol Infect Dis* 1989; **8**: 191–202.

35. Kauppinen M, Saikku P. Pneumonia due to *Chlamydia pneumoniae*: prevalence, clinical features, diagnosis and treatment. myocardial infarction. *Clin Infect Dis* 1995; **21**: S244–S252.

36. Saikku P, Leinonen M, Mattila K, *et al.* Serological evidence of an association of a novel *Chlamydia*, TWAR, with chronic coronary heart disease and acute myocardial infarction. *Lancet* 1988; 2:983–86.

37. Mendall MA, Carrington D, Strachan D, *et al. Chlamydia pneumoniae*: risk factors for serpositivity and association with coronary heart disease. *J Infect* 1995; 30:121–8.

38. Wong Y-K, Gallagher PJ, Ward PE. *Chlamydia pneumoniae* and atherosclerosis. *Heart* 1999; 81:232–8.

39. Gupta S, Camm AJ. *Chlamydia pneumoniae* and coronary heart disease: coincidence, association or causation? *Br Med J* 1997; 314:1778–9.

40. Gupta S, Leatham EW. The relation between *Chlamydia pneumoniae* and atherosclerosis. *Heart* 1997; 77: 7–8.

41. Kark J, Leinonen M, Paltiel O, *et al. Chlamydia pneumoniae* and acute myocardial infarction in Jerusalem. *Int J Epidemiol* 1997; 26:730–8.

42. Danesh J, Wong Y-K, Ward M, *et al.* Chronic infection with *Helicobacter pylori*, *Chlamydia pneumoniae* or cytomegalovirus: population based study of coronary heart disease. *Heart* 1999; 81:245–7.

43. Strachan DP, Carrington D, Mendall MA, *et al.* Relation of *Chlamydia pneumoniae* serology to mortality and incidence of ischaemic heart disease over 13 years in the Caerphilly prospective heart disease study. *Br Med J* 1999; 318:1035–40.

44. Shor A, Kuo CC, Patton DL. Detection of *Chlamydia pneumoniae* in coronary arterial fatty streaks and atheromatous plaques? *S Afr Med J* 1992; 82:158–61.

45. Kuo CC, Shor A, Campbell LA, *et al.* Demonstration of *Chlamydia pneumoniae* in atherosclerotic lesions of coronary arteries. *J Infect Dis* 1993; 167:841–9.

46. Muhlestein JB, Hammond EH, Carlquist JF, *et al.* Increased incidence of *Chlamydia* species within the coronary arteries of patients with symptomatic atherosclerotic versus other forms of cardiovascular disease. *J Am Coll Cardiol* 1996; 27:1555–61.

47. Ong G, Thomas BJ, Mansfield AO, *et al.* Detection and widespread distribution of *Chlamydia pneumoniae* in the vascular system and its possible implications. *J Clin Pathol* 1996; 49:101–6.

48. Ramirez JA. Isolation of *Chlamydia pneumoniae* from the coronary artery of a patient with coronary atherosclerosis. The *Chlamydia pneumoniae* Atherosclerosis Study Group. *Ann Intern Med* 1996; 125:979–82.

49. Jackson LA, Campbell LA, Kuo C-C, *et al.* Isolation of *Chlamydia pneumoniae* (TWAR) from a carotid atherosclerotic plaque specimen. *J Infect Dis* 1997; 176:292–5.

50. Maass M, Bartels C, Engel PM, *et al.* Endovascular presence of viable *Chlamydia pneumoniae* is a common phenomenon in coronary artery disease. *J Am Coll Cardiol* 1998; 31:827–32.

51. Fong IW, Chiu B, Viira E, *et al.* Rabbit models for *Chlamydia pneumoniae* infection. *J Clin Microbiol* 1997; 35:48–52.

52. Laitinen K, Laurila A, Pyhälä L, *et al. Chlamydia pneumoniae* induces inflammatory changes in the aortas of rabbits. *Infect Immun* 1997; 65:4832–5.

53. Muhlestein JB, Anderson JL, Hammond EH, *et al.* Infection with *Chlamydia pneumoniae* accelerates the development of atherosclerosis and treatment with azithromycin prevents it in a rabbit model. *Circulation* 1998; 97:633–6.

54. Gupta S, Kaski JC. *Chlamydia* and coronary heart disease: an inflammatory idea? *Acute Coronary Syndromes* 1999; 2:34–40.

55. Kaukoranta-Tolvanen SS, Teppo AM, Laitinene K, *et al.* Growth of *Chlamydia pneumoniae* in cultured human peripheral blood mononuclear cells and induction of a cytokine response. *Microbiol Pathog* 1996; 21:215–21.

56. Holland MJ, Bailey RL, Ward ME, *et al.* Cell mediated responses to *Chlamydia trachomatis* in scarring trachoma. *Proc Europ Soc Chlamydial Res* 1992; 2:134 [abstract].

57. Patel P, Carrington D, Strachan DP, *et al.* Fibrinogen: a link between chronic infection and coronary heart disease. *Lancet* 1994; 343: 1634–5 [letter].

58. Mendall MA, Patel P, Balla L, *et al.* C reactive protein and its relation to cardiovascular risk factors: a population based cross sectional study. *Br Med J* 1996; 312:1061–5.

59. Kaski JC, Smith DA. *Chlamydia pneumoniae*

and atherosclerosis: mechanisms of vascular damage. coronary disease. In: Allegra L, Blasi F, eds. *Chlamydia pneumoniae: the lung and the heart*. Milan: Springer-Verlag, 1999: 152–62.

60. Leatham EW, Bath PM, Tooze JA, *et al*. Increased monocyte tissue factor expression in coronary disease. *Br Heart J* 1995; **73**:10–13.

61. Kalayoglu MV, Byrne GI. Induction of macrophage foam cell formation by *Chlamydia pneumoniae*. *J Infect Dis* 1998; **177**:725–9.

62. Kol A, Sukhova GK, Lichtman AH, Libby P. Chlamydial heat shock protein 60 localizes in human atheroma and regulates macrophage tumour necrosis factor-α and matrix metallo-proteinase expression. *Circulation* 1998; **98**: 300–7.

63. Cook PJ, Lip GY, Davies P, *et al*. *Chlamydia pneumoniae* antibodies in severe essential hypertension. *Hypertension* 1998; **31**:589–94.

64. Laurila A, Bloigu A, Näyhä S, *et al*. Chronic *Chlamydia pneumoniae* infection is associated with a serum lipid profile known to be a risk factor for atherosclerosis. *Arteriosclerosis Thromb Vasc Biol* 1997; **17**:2910–13.

65. Hahn DL, Golubjatnikov R. Smoking is a potential confounder of the *Chlamydia pneumoniae*-coronary artery disease association. *Arterioscler Thromb* 1992; **12**:255–60.

66. Toss H, Gnarpe J, Gnarpe A, *et al*. Increased fibrinogen levels are associated with persistent *Chlamydia pneumoniae* infection in unstable coronary artery disease. *Eur Heart J* 1998; **19**:570–7.

67. Biasucci LM, Luizzo G, Grillo RL, *et al*. Elevated levels of C-reactive protein at discharge in patients with unstable angina predicts recurrent instability. *Circulation* 1999; **99**:855–60.

68. Moxon ER. Microbes, molecules and man. The Mitchell Lecture 1992. *J R Coll Physicians Lond* 1993; **27**:169–74.

69. Fredericks DN, Relman DA. Sequence-based identification of microbial pathogens a reconsideration of Koch's postulates. *Clin Microbiol Rev* 1996; **9**:18–33.

70. Marshall BJ. *Helicobacter pylori* in peptic ulcer: have Koch's postulates been fulfilled? *Ann Med* 1995; **27**:565–8.

71. Gupta S, Leatham EW, Carrington D, *et al*. Elevated *Chlamydia pneumoniae* antibodies, cardiovascular events and azithromycin in male survivors of myocardial infarction. *Circulation* 1997; **96**:404–7.

72. Gurfinkel E, Bozovich G, Darcoca A, *et al*. Randomised trial of roxithromycin in non-Q-wave coronary syndromes: ROXIS pilot study. *Lancet* 1997; **350**:404–7.

73. Gupta S, Leatham EW, Carrington D, *et al*. The effect of azithromycin in post myocardial infarction patients with elevated *Chlamydia pneumoniae* antibody titers. *J Am Coll Cardiol* 1997; **755**:209 [abstract].

74. Gupta S. *Chlamydia pneumoniae*, monocyte activation and antimicrobial therapy in coronary heart disease. MD thesis, University of London; 1999.

75. Meier CR, Derby LE, Jick SS, *et al*. Antibiotics and risk of subsequent first-time acute myocardial infarction. *JAMA* 1999; **281**:427–31.

76. Ånestad G, Scheel G, Hugnes O. Chronic infections and coronary heart disease. *Lancet* 1997; **350**:1028 [letter].

77. Gupta S, Kaski JC, Camm AJ. Antibiotic therapy for coronary heart disease: hype versus hope. *Br J Cardiol* 1998; **5**:65–6.

78. Hart CA. Antibiotic resistance: an increasing problem? *Br Med J* 1998; **316**:1255–6.

79. Martin D, Bursill J, Qui MR, *et al*. Alternative hypothesis for efficacy of macrolides in acute coronary syndromes. *Lancet* 1998; **351**:1858–9.

10

Lipids and non-coronary vascular disease
Anthony F Winder

Introduction

There are clear data associating lipid profiles with accelerated development of coronary heart disease (CHD), and evidence of anatomical and clinical benefit by modifying those profiles. The benefits of lipid intervention are particularly evident in secondary prevention, but also apply in primary prevention, and these various studies are backed up by convincing cellular and animal studies which establish the importance of lipids in the pathogenesis of arterial disease. The key clinical data have come mainly from the statin trials which used agents that are particularly effective at controlling LDL, and from trials with some recruitment bias towards patients with above average levels of low density lipoprotein (LDL) in plasma, and at most limited hypertriglyceridaemia.

CHD mortality and morbidity are the most evident and most investigated clinical associations with adverse lipid profiles, but atheromatous arterial disease can express at a range of extracoronary sites, particularly at sites of flow turbulence such as branch points. The range of potential extracoronary sites includes cerebral vessels (manifesting as stroke and transient ischaemic attacks), but most available data are from the iliac-femoral tree for which involvement is commonly defined as peripheral vascular disease (PVD). Important

practical questions are whether similar pathological processes operate at all vulnerable arterial sites, whether significant differences arise through specific local circumstances, and what place lipid data might have in risk stratification and then management in the primary and secondary prevention of the various patterns of extracoronary vascular disease.

Lipid profiles and non-coronary vascular disease

Associations can be assessed by follow-up studies of disease-free patients with lipid

---

Some established facts:

- Patients present as arteriopaths, with a spectrum of clinical events and coronary, cerebrovascular and other extracoronary disease.
- Lipid profiles adverse for age/gender are reported for all manifestations of atherosclerotic vascular disease.
- Whatever the presenting vascular feature, there is an increased risk of coronary events including death.
- Outcome is also related to other risk associations.

Table 10.1
Lipid profiles and extracoronary disease.

profiles recorded at entry, or through recording lipid profiles or the results of lipid intervention in patients with established disease. Most data on associations before treatment were collected from small groups of patients with PVD presenting as intermittent claudication (IC) or other established femoral disease, and from a very wide spectrum of clinical manifestations from reduced ankle–brachial pressure index (ABPI) but no symptoms, to critical limb ischaemia and amputation for vascular insufficiency. Some patterns of association emerge, with reported lipid abnormalities in serum or plasma in comparison with comparable clinically disease-free patients.[1,2] The major associations are: low levels of high density lipoprotein (HDL), mainly of the larger HDL_2 fraction, and raised levels of triglyceride showing some association with levels of intermediate density lipoprotein (IDL), the atherogenic remnant lipoproteins. Levels of total cholesterol or of LDL may be increased or within the reference range but there may be some shift from the larger less dense fractions towards the smaller denser fractions within LDL. Levels of apoB may be increased even if levels of cholesterol are not, consistent with an increase in apoB lipoproteins as LDL and very low density lipoproteins (VLDL) and remnant IDL.[3] Low birthweight is also associated with above average risk of CHD and stroke in later life, and similarly to the prevalence and severity of carotid arteriosclerosis, with a further but non-significant association with PVD.[4] Extracoronary vascular disease is thus apparently influenced by fetal growth, as are levels of total- and LDL-cholesterol although that association is not known to be causal. Fatty streak development in fetal aorta has also been linked to maternal hypercholesterolaemia.[5]

The circulating LDL may show or be more vulnerable to oxidative change[6,7] and levels of circulating antibody to oxidised LDL may also be increased.[8] Mean or median levels of lipoprotein(a) [Lp(a)] may also be increased and the increase compared with control series may be greater than that predicted from the molecular size of the apo(a) isoform patterns present.[9–11] The overall scatter is wide with considerable overlap with data from clinically unaffected patients, and is not significantly different from that recorded from patients with CHD. Patients with end-stage renal disease (ESRD) have high levels of Lp(a), which are associated with the number of sites affected by plaques in the extracranial carotid arteries, as well as with a history of angina, previous myocardial infarction and cerebrovascular events.[12] Lp(a) levels are also associated with both the presence of clinical CHD and the presence and extent of carotid intimal thickening and degree of obstruction in patients with heterozygous familial hypercholesterolaemia. As for CHD, marked elevation of Lp(a) levels can act as a risk factor for cerebrovascular disease as defined by carotid wall thickening, particularly in association with raised LDL levels.[13]

Many studies have examined these issues: those discussed below are of particular interest.

- Low HDL mainly of the HDL_2 fraction.
- High triglycerides, maybe characteristically as IDL.
- LDL not in excess but may have bias to small dense LDL.
- Moderately raised levels of lipoprotein(a).
- Maybe adverse lipoprotein oxidation status.

Table 10.2
Associations between lipid profiles and extracoronary disease.

The Framingham Study

The Framingham Study has reported on associations between cardiovascular risk factors for atherosclerotic and cardiovascular outcomes in different arterial territories after up to 36 years of follow-up of the original cohort of 5209 men and women.[4] The major recognised cardiovascular risk factors were associated with clinical outcomes for all vascular territories up to the age 65 years. The associations for serum total cholesterol (TC) but not the HDL/TC ratio attenuated with age: the relationship between a history of cigarette smoking and PVD persisted with age.

The Lipid Research Clinics Protocol follow-up study

This study recorded mortality over 10 years for 565 male and female patients with a mean age of 66 years, and peripheral arterial disease (PAD) status defined by Rose questionnaire, ABPI and flow Doppler techniques.[15] In the group with PAD at entry there were 21 out of 34 deaths in men and 11 out of 33 deaths in women versus 31 out of 183 deaths in men and 28 out of 225 deaths in women without PAD. After various adjustments, the relative risk for death from all causes or any cardiovascular or coronary artery disease ranged from 3.1 to 6.6. There was a 15-fold increase in mortality from any cardiovascular cause including CHD in those patients with large-vessel PAD that was both severe and symptomatic at entry. The clear conclusion was that patients with large-vessel PAD have a high risk of death from cardiovascular causes.

The Edinburgh Artery Study

This study addressed the issue of whether certain risk factors in the general population were more strongly related to the development of PAD than CHD, using data on ABPI and reactive hyperaemia, and responses to the WHO-PVD questionnaire, collected for 1592 men and women aged 55–74 years.[16,17] A further PVD questionnaire with increased sensitivity was also developed.[18] PAD was strongly related to lifetime smoking habit (apparently in a stronger association than for CHD), and to the recognised established CVD risks, including levels of triglycerides, HDL, cholesterol, diabetes and systolic blood pressure. On multiple regression analysis, extent of smoking was the only consistent difference for PVD versus CHD. Unexpectedly, diabetes was not a stronger risk factor for PVD than it was for CHD. Smoking was also the most significant risk association for the development of abdominal aortic aneurysm.[19] Follow-up showed that claudicants defined by questionnaire had an increased risk of developing CHD as angina, and that asymptomatic PVD defined by ABPI had a similar incidence of cardiovascular events and death compared with the claudicant group. This study has also reported that PVD in non-diabetic patients can be associated with higher levels of insulin after a glucose load,[20] although smoking habit may be confounding.

Lipid-lowering trials

The relevance of lipid profiles to the development and progression of extracoronary vascular disease is emphasised by the growing evidence of clinical and anatomical benefits of lipid intervention.[21] Many data have come from interventional trials in the primary or secondary prevention of CHD, but some direct studies of extracoronary disease of the femoral and carotid arteries, and of stroke and TIA have also reported. From a range of studies, those discussed below are of particular interest.

The St Thomas' trial of femoral atherosclerosis progression

This first reported controlled trial of lipid lowering directed specifically at femoral arteries,[22] studied 24 mostly male patients with a mean age of 55–56 years and cholesterol levels at or greater than 251 mg/dl (6.5 mmol/l) and/or triglycerides at or greater than 157 mg/dl (1.8 mmol/l). On two occasions patients were randomised to usual care or usual care plus various combinations of lipid-lowering agents. Patients had a history of at least 6 months of stable IC from femoropopliteal disease but not hypertension or diabetes: smokers were included but given support, and there were no differences or changes in habit between groups. Mean lipid levels at entry were cholesterol levels of 297–309 mg/dl (7.7–8.0 mmol/l), and triglyceride levels of 269–287 mg/dl (3.1–3.3 mmol/l). The treated group achieved a reduction of 20% in cholesterol level, 37% in triglyceride levels. Aortography at entry and at 19 months showed fewer progressing segments, a reduction in the mean increase of plaque area and of edge irregularity, and overall 60% fewer progressing segments. For usual care and lipid-treated groups, progression correlated with levels of LDL, with a further weak non-significant inverse correlation with levels of HDL. From this first trial of lipid lowering in PVD the investigators concluded that therapy affected the process of atherosclerosis on a per-segment basis. However, this attractive result did involve four patients with variant apoE isoforms and familial (type III) dysbetalipoproteinaemia. This genetic disorder of very variable expression has a predilection to accelerate peripheral arterial disease, but lipid levels are markedly responsive to lipid therapy. Three type III patients were allocated to treatment, one to the usual care group, with possible bias to the result.

The Cholesterol Lowering Atherosclerosis Study (CLAS)

This study cohort was men aged 40–59 years, post-coronary artery bypass graft and either non-smokers or ex-smokers for at least 6 months. The investigators addressed primarily CAD progression in 82 patients randomised to diet/placebo compared with 80 patients given colestipol and niacin for 2 years.[23] Femoral atherosclerosis was also assessed through angiographic segmental measurement, and other imaging procedures including an annual progression rate of computer-estimated atherosclerosis. Progression of femoral atherosclerosis per segment, and on an overall National Heart Lung and Blood Institute (NHLBI) per-patient score was less marked in the drug-treated group but the difference from placebo was less than that seen in native and bypass coronary grafts.

Program on the Surgical Control of Hyperlipidemias (POSCH)

A cohort of 838 mostly male survivors of a first myocardial infarct, aged 30–64 years (mean age 51 years) was randomised to partial ileal bypass or usual care outside hospital.[24] After a mean follow-up of 9.7 years and a mean 38% reduction in LDL levels, various endpoints were reviewed. These included PVD as defined by arteriography and scored segmental analysis, Doppler ultrasonography and ABPI, and the need for vascular surgery. Expression of disease as PVD-related events or peripheral pulse analysis was significantly more frequent in the control group. The overall incidence of all cerebrovascular events was not significantly different between groups.

The Probucol Quantitative Swedish Regression Trial (PQRST)

In this study, 79 men and 57 women (mean age 55 years) who had been referred for management of hyperlipidaemia were randomly allocated to treatment with diet, cholestyramine and probucol, or diet and cholestyramine alone as a relative placebo group.[25] The study included asymptomatic and symptomatic patients in primary and secondary prevention: diabetes and familial (type III) dysbetalipoproteinaemia were specifically excluded. Levels of cholesterol were reduced from around 350 to around 270 mg/dl (9–7 mmol/l) over 3 years. Computer image analysis of femoral atheroma and progression over 3 years included quantitation of edge roughness and minimum and maximum diameters, plus digital pulse plethysmography. Clinical state was essentially unchanged for 2 years, but some benefits were inferred for the placebo group. Thus probucol was ineffective when added to cholestyramine and diet in reducing indices of femoral atherosclerosis, but there was significant evidence of improvement in the group prescribed diet plus cholestyramine alone, a difference possibly related to the fall in levels of HDL resulting from probucol.

The Scandinavian Simvastatin Survival Study (4S)

In this landmark study of the benefits of significant lipid lowering,[26] 4444 male and female patients with established CAD, raised cholesterol and LDL but not triglyceride levels (for which the exclusion limit was 217 mg/dl, or 2.5 mmol/l) were randomly allocated to usual care and placebo or simvastatin predominantly at 20 or 40 mg od for a mean follow-up period of 5.4 years. The primary objectives addressed aspects of CHD but clinical assessment included evaluation of femoral and carotid bruit. Most of the data recording PVD were derived from the adverse experience forms, recording new or worsening intermittent claudication. Thus femoral disease was recorded for 81 usual care and 52 simvastatin

cases (3.6 versus 2.2%) — a reduction of 38% (CI = 0.44–0.88; mean = 0.62; $P = 0.008$).

The Kuopio Atherosclerosis Prevention Study (KAPS)

A small study of patients with heterozygous familial hypercholesterolaemia who were receiving therapy had previously shown that plaque development in the carotid and femoral arteries was significantly greater than for a matched control group.[27] B-mode ultrasound data also showed that carotid intimal medial thickness (IMT) correlated well with the prevalence of plaque in the carotid and femoral arteries and suggested that it could be used as a general marker of the extent of atherosclerosis. In KAPS,[28] men with moderate excess baseline lipids were recruited from a population survey of risk factors for coronary and extracoronary atherosclerosis and their outcome. Final data were obtained for 424 men aged 44–65 years (mean age = 57 years), less than 10% of whom had a prior myocardial infarction, after random allocation to diet plus placebo or 40 mg pravastatin once daily. Various assessments, including high resolution B-mode ultrasonography, were made of the carotid tree and femoral arteries over a 3-year period. The rate of overall progression and the annual rate of change in IMT was reduced for carotid arteries but there was no significant difference in femoral arteries. However a significant improvement in composite carotid plus femoral score was found in those who received lipid treatment.

The Pravastatin, Lipids and Atherosclerosis in the Carotid arteries Study (PLAC-II)

A cohort of 151 patients with proven CHD and cholesterol and LDL-cholesterol levels significantly above population means were randomly allocated to treatment with placebo or pravastatin at a dose adjusted by response

(40 mg once daily in most cases), maintained for 3 years.[29] The main specified endpoint was carotid IMT at various sites and overall, determined by B-mode ultrasound. Maximal IMT was determined at 12 sites, averaged to the mean maximum IMT index which showed a non-significant reduction in progression over 3 years. However, there was a significant reduction in progression at specific sites, including the common carotid artery. Cardiovascular events were also significantly reduced. Thus the potential to retard progression of atheromatous disease in elements of the carotid tree was shown in the 4S[26] and PLAC-II[29] studies, which recruited patients with established CHD, and in the KAPS study[28] which demonstrated primary prevention. However the response at specified arterial segments remains rather variable, in a manner that is not yet understood.

These results are supported by the ongoing Asymptomatic Carotid Atherosclerosis Progression Study (ACAPS),[30] a prospective investigation of changes in carotid IMT defined by serial B-mode ultrasound at 12 sites. The study cohort is asymptomatic men and women with levels of LDL between the 60th and 90th percentiles, randomly allocated to treatment with placebo or lovastatin. Initial results show that progression was significantly retarded by statin treatment.

Lipid-lowering trials with the potential to report data on PVD

The Cholesterol and Recurrent Events (CARE) study of patients with CHD but average levels of cholesterol showed that peripheral arterial status at baseline was not obviously associated with cholesterol:[31] further analysis of outcome data is awaited. Carotid and femoral B-mode data were collected but have not yet been reported for the REGRESS trial,[32] as is the case with data on intermittent claudication

- Long-term follow-up, e.g. 36 years of Framingham and 10-year LRC studies show significant clustering of CVD events.
- Patients with extracoronary atherosclerosis then treated for lipids have fewer coronary events.
- Patients with coronary disease given lipid treatment have fewer carotid and femoral events, e.g. 4S study.
- Other evidence of benefit by lipid lowering, e.g. St Thomas's study, POSCH, CLAS, and PQRST.

Table 10.3
Lipid profiles and extracoronary outcomes: the present.

from the WOSCOPS, LIPID and LCAS studies.[33-35] No data of this type are expected from the WHO-clofibrate primary prevention trial,[36] or the Helsinki Heart Study.[37]

Trials investigating other specific extracoronary syndromes

Numerous small studies have addressed the differences in risk factors associated with specific extracoronary presentations. One study of 169 patients with supra-aortic and peripheral atherosclerosis, in which some effort was made to exclude patients with detectable CHD, again confirmed associations with smoking, diabetes and low HDL.[38] In smokers, the habit of frequent small meals (nibbling or grazing) is reported to be associated with a much reduced expression of PVD: however, lipid profiles are also less adverse.[39] The larger epidemiological studies from Framingham[14] and the Multiple Risk Factor Intervention Trial (MRFIT)[40] clearly show that high levels of cholesterol and LDL are associated with the risk of subsequent stroke, but in a weaker relationship than that for CHD. The confounding issue, which also relates to any benefits of lipid lowering,[41,42] is that haemorrhagic rather than thrombotic stroke shows a relative increase at naturally low levels of cholesterol, as shown in the MRFIT study. The issue is complicated because this pattern of stroke is mostly associated with rupture of the smaller intracranial arteries, and it is seen in hypertensive patients who, through alcoholism, may also have low levels of cholesterol. Data from the Honolulu Heart Study, indicate that hypertension may be the key issue, not low cholesterol.[43] The association between alcohol consumption and risk of stroke has recently been extended to intakes of over 14 units a week.[44] Transient ischaemic attacks and minor ischaemic strokes show a strong association with hypertension and smoking, and not with large artery atherosclerosis or defined metabolic risk associations including hypercholesterolaemia and diabetes.[45] Levels of Lp(a) have been shown in several but not all studies to be associated with stroke and transient ischaemic attacks but, as with cholesterol, high levels of Lp(a) are associated with an enhanced risk of CHD which is itself a risk factor for thrombotic stroke.[46] Levels of cholesterol, particularly in association with raised levels of Lp(a), are also associated with the presence and severity of carotid stenosis.[4]

Unique factors in the distribution of atheromatous vascular disease

An immediate difficulty in assessing extracoronary vascular disease is that similar relationships between lipid profiles and clinical or anatomical extracoronary atherosclerotic disease have also been reported for patients pre-senting with or subsequently developing CHD, which has a high attendant mortality and morbidity and is the most comprehensively investigated aspect of atheromatous vascular disease. Patients with an initial clinical presentation of extracoronary disease have a high probability of significant disease at other sites and particularly of coronary events including death. The combination of CHD and PVD manifestations carries a particularly severe prognosis.[15,47] Is the individual presentation unique or the tip of a wide atherosclerotic iceberg? In disentangling these various presentations and any predominant causal or promotional influences and consequent policies for management, a real difficulty is that assessment of extracoronary status is not routine practice in cardiac units. Silent coronary disease or vascular status other than at the presenting site, for example carotid stenosis in patients presenting for management of PVD, is also not routinely assessed in surgical vascular units, and even when considered it may not be significantly pursued: a wider screening strategy is recommended.[47–49] Thus, the issue of whether all these presentations reflect generalised arteriopathy is not resolved, and is further clouded by the wide range of diagnostic criteria applied to PVD, from acute limb ischaemia through intermittent claudication to determination of pulse pressures and various imaging techniques.

What could be involved in any localised atherosclerotic change? Most data for extracoronary disease are measures of PVD, and in most surveys the most obvious risk associations are smoking history, blood pressure and diabetes, followed by aspects of the lipid profile. The selective development of vascular disease could reflect the operation of systemic risk factors which have different effects at local sites through unique local conditions. Haemodynamic influences, patterns of laminar and turbulent flow, and associated shear stresses differ within the vascular tree and atherosclerotic changes are emphasised at sites of turbulence. Possible mechanisms of selective local effects are now coming out through recent, very attractive developments in vascular biology.[50,51] Endothelium can be activated by local humoral factors, in response to local flow conditions.[50,52] Endothelial changes can lead to altered vascular reactivity and spasm, permeability to lipoproteins, adhesion and penetration of monocytes and altered growth patterns within the arterial wall. The further demonstration of increased mRNA levels implies gene activation: a shear stress response element has been identified in the promoter of several vascular factors of interest, including platelet-derived growth factor β (PDGF-β).[52] Therefore any unique site-specific pathology of extracoronary vascular atherosclerotic disease could involve interaction between systemic risk factors including lipid profiles and local haemodynamic, endothelial humoral and gene-dependent effects.

- Need to clarify the overlaps, if any, between presentations of arterial disease at different sites, through agreed diagnostic criteria and validated multisite assessment.
- Lipid control does seem to have benefits but specific targets and best agents are not defined.
- Why should ECVD be different from CHD? Developing issues of haemodynamics, local responses and gene activation.

Table 10.4
Lipid profiles and extracoronary outcomes: the future.

Conclusion

Dyslipoproteinaemia is associated with a wide-ranging expression of atherosclerotic vascular disease and related events. Modification of associated lipid profiles has a significant impact on progression, morbidity and mortality in relation to a range of sites. A wider interest in the diagnosis and treatment of vascular disease and attendant risk factors at sites other than that of presentation seems important, both for patient care and to advance understanding of the extent to which individual influences and local processes are involved. Rapid developments in vascular biology and control of local gene expression are likely to extend understanding of the pathology and progression of extracoronary disease and provide opportunities for intervention but, based on present evidence, an interest in lipid profiles and their treatment as part of a whole-patient approach is appropriate.

References

1. Mowat BF, Skinner ER, Wilson HM, *et al.* Alteration in plasma lipids, lipoproteins and high density lipoprotein subfractions in peripheral arterial disease. *Atherosclerosis* 1997; **131**:161–6.
2. Pedro-Botet J, Rubies-Prat J, Senti M. A little more on lipoprotein profile in peripheral arterial disease. *Atherosclerosis* 1998; **136**:403–4.
3. Powell JT, Edwards RJ, Worrell PC, *et al.* Risk factors associated with the development of peripheral arterial disease in smokers: a case-control study. *Atherosclerosis* 1997; **129**:41–8.
4. Martyn CN, Gale CR, Jespersen S, Sherriff SB. Impaired fetal growth and atherosclerosis of carotid and peripheral arteries. *Lancet* 1998; **352**:173–8.
5. Napoli C, D'Armient FP, Mancini FP, *et al.* Fatty streak formation occurs in human fetal aortas and is greatly enhanced by maternal hypercholesterolemia. Intimal accumulation of low-density lipoprotein and its oxidation pre-

cede monocyte recruitment into early atherosclerotic lesions. *J Clin Invest* 1997; **100**:2680–90.

6. Sanderson KJ, van Rij AM, Wade CR, Sutherland WHF. Lipid peroxidation of circulating low density lipoproteins with age, smoking and in peripheral vascular disease. *Atherosclerosis* 1995; **118**:45–51.

7. Andrews B, Burnand K, Paganga G, *et al.* Oxidisability of low density lipoproteins in patients with carotid or femoral artery atherosclerosis. *Atherosclerosis* 1995; **112**:77–84.

8. Bergmark C, Wu R, de Faire U, *et al.* Patients with early-onset peripheral vascular disease have increased levels of autoantibodies against oxidised LDL. *Arteriosclerosis Thromb Vasc Biol* 1995; **15**:441–5.

9. Molgaard J, Klausen IC, Lassvik C, *et al.* Significant association between low-molecular weight apolipoprotein(a) isoforms and intermittent claudication. *Arteriosclerosis Thromb Vasc Biol* 1992; **12**:895–901.

10. Valentine RJ, Grayhurn PA, Vega GL, Grundy SM. Lp(a) is an independent discriminating risk factor for premature peripheral atherosclerosis among white men. *Arch Intern Med* 1994; **154**:801–6.

11. Cantin B, Moorjani S, Dagenais G, Lupien P-J. Lipoprotein(a) distribution in a French Canadian population and its relation to intermittent claudication (The Quebec Cardiovascular Study). *Am J Cardiol* 1995; **75**:1224–8.

12. Kronenberg F, Kathrein H, Konig P, *et al.* Apolipoprotein(a) phenotypes predict the risk for carotid atherosclerosis in patients with end-stage renal disease. *Arteriosclerosis Thromb* 1994; **14**:1405–11.

13. Baldasarre D, Tremoli E, Franceschini G, *et al.* Plasma lipoprotein(a) is an independent risk factor associated with carotid wall thickening in severely but not moderately hypercholesterolemic patients. *Stroke* 1996; **27**:1044–9.

14. Kannel WB. Risk factors for atherosclerotic cardiovascular outcomes in different arterial territories. *J Cardiovasc Risk* 1994; **1**:333–40.

15. Criqui MH, Langer RD, Fronek A, *et al.* Mortality over a period of ten years in patients with peripheral arterial disease. *N Engl J Med* 1992; **326**:381–6.

16. Fowkes FGR, Housley E, Riemersma RA, *et al.* Smoking, lipids, glucose intolerance, and blood pressure as risk factors for peripheral atherosclerosis compared with ischemic heart disease in the Edinburgh artery study. *Am J Epidemiol* 1992; **135**:331–40.

17. Leng GC, Lee AJ, Fowkes FG, *et al.* Incidence, natural history and cardiovascular events in symptomatic and asymptomatic peripheral arterial disease in the general population. *Int J Epidemiol* 1996; **25**:1172–81.

18. Leng GC, Fowkes, FGR. The Edinburgh claudication questionnaire: an improved version of the WHO/Rose questionnaire for use in epidemiological surveys. *J Clin Epidemiol* 1992; **45**:1101–9.

19. Lee AJ, Fowkes FG, Carson MN, *et al.* Smoking, atherosclerosis and risk of abdominal aortic aneurysm. *Eur Heart J* 1997; **18**:671–6.

20. Price JF, Lee AJ, Fowkes FG. Hyperinsulinaemia: a risk factor for peripheral arterial disease in the non-diabetic population. *J Cardiovasc Risk* 1996; **3**:501–5.

21. Leng GC, Price JF, Jepson RG. Lipid-lowering therapy for lower limb atherosclerosis (Cochrane Review). In: *The Cochrane Library.* Oxford: Update Software; 1999: issue 1.

22. Duffield RG, Lewis B, Miller NE, *et al.* Treatment of hyperlipidaemia retards progression of symptomatic femoral atherosclerosis. A randomised controlled trial. *Lancet* 1983; ii:639–42.

23. Blankenhorn DH, Azen SP, Crawford DW, *et al.* Effects of colestipol-niacin therapy on human femoral atherosclerosis. *Circulation* 1991; **83**:438–47.

24. Buchwald H, Varco RL, Matts JP, *et al.* Effect of partial ileal bypass on mortality and morbidity from coronary heart disease in patients with hypercholesterolemia. *N Engl J Med* 1990; **323**:946–55.

25. Walldius G, Erikson U, Olsson AG, *et al.* The effect of probucol on femoral atherosclerosis: the Probucol Quantitative Regression Swedish Trial (PQRST). *Am J Cardiol* 1994; **74**: 875–83.

26. Pedersen TR, Kjekshus J, Pyorälä K, *et al.* Effect of simvastatin on ischemic signs and symptoms in the Scandinavian Simvastatin Survival Study (4S). *Am J Cardiol* 1998; **81**: 333–5.

27. Wendelhag I, Wiklund O, Wikstrand WJ. Atherosclerotic changes in femoral and carotid arteries in familial hypercholesterolemia. Ultrasonographic assessment of intima-media thickness and plaque occurrence. *Arteriosclerosis Thromb Vasc Biol* 1993; **13**:1404–11.

28. Salonen R, Nyyssonen K, Porkkala E, *et al.* Kuopio Atherosclerosis Prevention Study (KAPS). A population-based primary preventive trial of the effect of LDL lowering on atherosclerotic progression in carotid and femoral arteries. *Circulation* 1995; **92**:1758–64.

29. Crouse JR, Byington RP, Bond MG, *et al.* Pravastatin, lipids and atherosclerosis in the carotid arteries (PLAC-II). *Am J Cardiol* 1995; **75**:455–9.

30. Probstfield JL, Margitic SE, Byington RP, *et al.* Results of the primary outcome measure and clinical events from the Asymptomatic Carotid Artery Progression Study. *Am J Cardiol* 1995; **76**:47C–53C.

31. Wilt TJ, Davis BR, Meyers DG, *et al.* Prevalence and correlates of symptomatic peripheral atherosclerosis in individuals with coronary heart disease and cholesterol levels less than 240 mg/dL: baseline results from the Cholesterol and Recurrent Events (CARE) Study. *Angiology* 1996; **47**:533–41.

32. Jukema JW, Brushke AVG, van Boven AJ, *et al.* Effects of lipid lowering by pravastatin on progression and regression of coronary artery disease in symptomatic men with normal to moderately elevated serum cholesterol levels. The Regression Growth Evaluation Statin Study (REGRESS). *Circulation* 1995; **91**: 2528–40.

33. West of Scotland Coronary Prevention group. Influence of Pravastatin and plasma lipids on clinical events in the West of Scotland Coronary Prevention Study (WOSCOPS). *Circulation* 1998; **97**:1440–5.

34. The LIPID Study Group. Prevention of cardiovascular events and death with pravastatin in patients with coronary heart disease and a broad range of initial cholesterol levels. *N Engl J Med* 1998; **339**:1349–57.

35. Herd JA, Ballantyne CM, Farmer JA, *et al.* Effects of fluvastatin on coronary atherosclerosis in patients with mild to moderate cholesterol elevations (Lipoprotein and Coronary Atherosclerosis Study [LCAS]). *Am J Cardiol* 1997; **80**:278–86.

36. WHO European Collaboration Group. European collaborative trial of multifactorial prevention of coronary heart disease: final report on the 6-year results. *Lancet* 1986; i:869–72.

37. Manttari M, Elo O, Frick MH, *et al.* The Helsinki Heart Study: basic design and randomisation procedure. *Eur Heart J* 1987; **8(suppl. I)**:1–29.

38. Vigna GB, Bolzan M, Romagnoni F, *et al.* Lipids and other risk factors selected by discriminant analysis in symptomatic patients with supra-aortic and peripheral atherosclerosis. *Circulation* 1992; **85**:2205–11.

39. Powell JT, Franks PJ, Poulter NR. Does nibbling or grazing protect the peripheral arteries from atherosclerosis? *J Cardiovasc Risk* 1999; **6**:19–22.

40. Iso H, Jacobs DR, Wentworth D, *et al.* Serum cholesterol and six-year mortality from stroke in 350 977 men screened for the Multiple Risk Factor Intervention Trial. *N Engl J Med* 1989; **320**:904–10.

41. Herbert PR, Gaziano JM, Chan KS, Hennekens CH. Cholesterol lowering with drugs, risk of stroke, and total mortality. *JAMA* 1997; **278**:313–21.

42. Papadakis JA, Mikhailidis DP, Winder AF. Lipids and stroke: neglect of a useful preventive measure? *Cardiovasc Res* 1998; **40**: 265–71.

43. Reed DM. The paradox of high risk of stroke in population with low risk of coronary heart disease. *Am J Epidemiol* 1990; **131**:579–88.

44. Hart CL, Davey Smith G, Hole DJ, Hawthorne VM. Alcohol consumption and mortality from all causes, coronary heart disease, and stroke: results from a prospective cohort study of Scottish men with 21 years of follow-up. *Br Med J* 1999; **318**:1725–9.

45. Sempere AP, Duarte J, Cabezas C, Claveria LE. Etiopathogenesis of transient ischemic attacks and minor ischemic strokes: a community-based study in Segovia, Spain. *Stroke* 1998; **29**:40–5.

46. Schreiner PJ, Chambless LE, Brown SA, *et al.* Lipoprotein(a) as a correlate of stroke and transient ischaemic attack prevalence in a biracial cohort: the ARIC Study. Atherosclerosis

Risk in Communities. *Ann Epidemiol* 1994; **4**:351–9.

47. Criqui MH, Denenburg JO, Langer RD, Fronek A. The epidemiology of peripheral arterial disease: importance of identifying the population at risk. *Vascular Medicine* 1997; **2**: 221–6.

48. McDermott MM, Mehta S, Ahn H, Greenland P. Atherosclerotic risk factors are less intensively treated in patients with peripheral arterial disease than in patients with coronary artery disease. *J Gen Int Med* 1997; **12**: 209–15.

49. Von Kemp K, van den Brande P, Peterson T, *et al*. Screening for concomitant disease in peripheral vascular patients. *Int Angiol* 1997; **16**:114–22.

50. Gimbrone MA, Nagel T, Topper J. Biomechanical activation: an emerging paradigm in endothelial adhesion biology. *J Clin Invest* 1997; **100(suppl. 11)**:S61–S65.

51. Gimbrone MA, Reznick N, Nagel T, *et al*. Hemodynamics, endothelial gene expression, and atherogenesis. *Ann NY Acad Sci* 1997; **811**:1–11.

52. Ishida T, Takahashi M, Corson MA, Berk BC. Fluid shear-stress mediated signal transduction: how do endothelial cells transduce mechanical force into biological responses? *Ann NY Acad Sci* 1997; **811**:12–24.

53. Resnick N, Yahav V, Khachigian LM, *et al*. Endothelial gene regulation by shear stress. *Adv Exp Biol Med* 1997; **430**:155–64.

11

Implications of high lipid levels in the hypertensive patient

Brian Tomlinson

Introduction

Hypertension and hyperlipidaemia occur together more often than would be expected by chance. They are both features of underlying insulin resistance and obesity but there is some evidence that hyperlipidaemia itself may predispose to hypertension and that lipid-lowering interventions may have a beneficial effect on blood pressure, or at least on vascular reactivity. Hypertension and hyperlipidaemia have a more than additive effect on cardiovascular risk and it is important to consider them both along with other risk factors before embarking on drug therapy. Some antihypertensive treatments may have an adverse effect on plasma lipid levels and an inappropriate choice of therapy could worsen the overall cardiovascular risk profile in some individuals. The large trials with statins have shown that these lipid-lowering agents are just as effective in reducing cardiovascular events in patients with hypertension as in those without. Lipid-lowering drugs are generally safe and well tolerated in hypertensives but there may be a slight risk of drug interactions between them and some of the antihypertensive agents.

Association between hypertension and hyperlipidaemia

It has been found repeatedly in epidemiological studies that hypertension is often associated with lipid abnormalities as well as with type 2 diabetes, insulin resistance and obesity.[1,2] The combination of these conditions is called the 'metabolic syndrome' or 'insulin-resistance syndrome' and it is associated also with increased coagulation factors and hyperuricaemia.[3] Dyslipidaemia, with low HDL-cholesterol and raised triglyceride levels is more prevailing in the syndrome than raised LDL-cholesterol levels. In patients with type 2 diabetes the prevalence of hypertension is extremely high.[4] For instance in the Rancho Bernardo Study, over 40% of the diabetic subjects were taking antihypertensive drugs, which was nearly twice the rate of that in the non-diabetic population.[5]

Hypertension and dyslipidaemia can occur together in the absence of diabetes but insulin resistance may still be the underlying link. Modan *et al.* found that in a large Israeli cohort, fasting and postload insulin levels were significantly elevated in the hypertensive group independent of obesity, glucose intolerance, age, and antihypertensive medications. They concluded that insulin resistance and/or hyperinsulinaemia were present in the majority of hypertensives in their population.[6] In the study in Tecumseh, Michigan, elevated plasma cholesterol, triglycerides and insulin levels and low HDL-cholesterol levels were found in young subjects with borderline and white-coat hypertension.[7] The relationship between blood pressure and these metabolic risk factors was linear and even extended into the normotensive range.

It has been shown in other studies that evidence of a relationship between serum lipids and blood pressure can be found even after adjusting for confounding variables such as age and body mass index. A review of seven studies including over 41 000 subjects showed that significant correlations existed between blood pressure and measurements of total cholesterol, LDL-cholesterol and triglycerides.[8]

The term familial dyslipidaemic hypertension (FDH) was used by the late Roger Williams to describe some cohorts of patients in Utah.[9] A diagnosis of FDH was considered if two or more siblings had both hypertension and abnormal lipids before the age of 60 years and they were found to have an increased risk for CHD. Concordant abnormalities in fasting serum lipid concentrations were observed in two or more siblings in 48% of the hypertensive sibships and at least one lipid level was abnormal in almost all concordant sibships. This suggested an association between hypertension and a syndrome of mixed lipid abnormalities, probably familial combined hyperlipidaemia or dyslipidaemia as a low HDL-cholesterol level was the most common abnormality. This condition was found in about 1% of the general population and 12% of the hypertensive subjects in the Utah studies. The lipid abnormalities occurred 10–20 years before hypertension developed and CHD developed another 10 years after the onset of hypertension. Some of the relatives had lipid abnormalities without hypertension. The

pathophysiology was thought to involve insulin resistance and central obesity.[10]

Not surprisingly, insulin resistance and the resulting hyperinsulinaemia are the factors linking hypertension and metabolic changes that have received the most attention. Insulin resistance may occur predominantly in skeletal muscle,[11] whereas other tissues may remain sensitive to insulin and show an exaggerated physiological response to the high circulating insulin levels. The order of events in the development of the metabolic syndrome has not been established clearly, despite extensive study. The pathophysiology leading to the typical dyslipidaemia of the metabolic syndrome is quite well understood but whether dyslipidaemia more commonly precedes, follows or occurs simultaneously with the development of hypertension remains unclear. Increased release of free fatty acids from adipose tissue, particularly from visceral fat into the portal veins, stimulates the production of triglyceride-rich lipoproteins in the liver with release of more and larger VLDL particles. This in turn has effects on other lipoprotein particles resulting in reduced levels of HDL-cholesterol and LDL particles developing a predominant small dense pattern.[12] Increased activity of hepatic lipase and decreased activity of lipoprotein lipase contribute to these changes. Increased postprandial lipaemia also occurs.

Hyperinsulinaemia may result in hypertension because insulin can increase the sympathetic drive, promote sodium retention, alter membrane ion transport and stimulate vascular hypertrophy.[12] An alternative scenario, which has been suggested by Julius[13] and others, is that the haemodynamic changes in hypertension are the forerunners of insulin resistance. Reduced nutritional blood flow to skeletal muscles from the vascular changes resulting from hypertension may cause insulin resistance in these tissues. Insulin resistance is associated with increased peripheral vascular resistance and rarefaction of blood vessels in skeletal muscle. This decreased capillarisation correlates with reduced activity of lipoprotein lipase in skeletal muscle. Thus, overactivity of the sympathetic nervous system might induce the metabolic syndrome in individuals with a genetic predisposition to decreased capillarisation.[14]

Whatever the precise mechanism of the underlying pathophysiology, it is generally thought to be a combination of genetic and environmental factors. Changes in the environment of modern society have allowed the expression of genetic proclivities for physical inactivity and weight gain. Genetic traits will play a permissive role in some individuals, allowing sedentary behaviours and dietary excesses to result in obesity and insulin resistance. The genetic causes of insulin resistance have not been identified so far. Recent studies in the spontaneously hypertensive rat, which is an insulin-resistant model, have detected a defective gene known as Cd36, which encodes a fatty acid translocase and this may prove to be relevant to insulin resistance in humans.[15] An alternative theory for the cause of the metabolic syndrome is the fetal origin hypothesis which considers that CHD, stroke, type 2 diabetes and hypertension originate from adaptations that the fetus makes to malnutrition, which result in permanent changes in the body's structure and physiology.[16]

Whatever the cause of the link between hypertension and hyperlipidaemia, the combined occurrence of these or other risk factors increases CHD risk exponentially[17] and lowers the threshold for intervention. The Multiple Risk Factor Intervention Trial (MRFIT), which involved over 300 000 men, showed that each risk factor alone had a relatively weak effect on CHD risk but in combination the risk increased more than additively. Sub-jects in the highest quintiles for serum cholesterol and systolic or diastolic blood pressure had about 10 times the CHD death rate of those in the lowest quintiles. Those who were smokers with high serum cholesterol and systolic blood pressure levels had approximately 20 times the death rate from CHD compared with those without these three risk factors (Figure 11.1).[18]

Most of the epidemiological data came from studies of middle-aged Caucasian men and risk profiles may not be the same in other ethnic groups. A recent study in eastern Asian populations, where stroke is still more common than CHD, showed a stronger association between blood pressure and stroke than in western populations, possibly because haemorrhagic stroke was more frequent than in Caucasians.[19] Cholesterol levels affected the proportions of stroke subtypes more than the overall stroke numbers. Rapid economic developments in Asian countries have brought about changes in diet and lifestyle which are likely to result in a greater prevalence of CHD.[20] This has already been seen in Singapore, where CHD rates increased to levels seen in western countries along with increases in plasma cholesterol levels. Studies of Indian migrants and native residents show that they have a higher risk of CHD at lower levels of plasma cholesterol than Caucasians, probably related to a high prevalence of diabetes, obesity, sedentary lifestyle and hypertension[21] and this may be the case with other ethnic groups.

Choice of antihypertensive drug
Guidelines

Guidelines from expert bodies on the management of hypertension have been divided on whether diuretics and beta-blockers should be

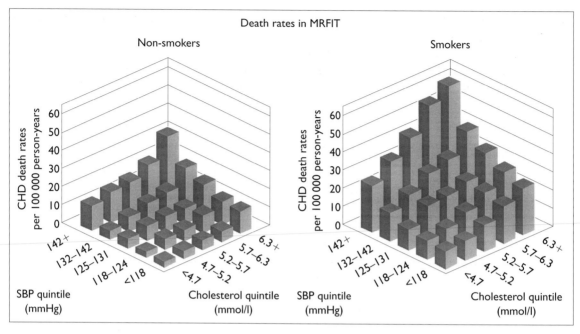

Fig. 11.1

Combined influence of systolic blood pressure (SBP) and serum cholesterol on age-adjusted death rates from coronary heart disease (CHD) in cigarette smokers and non-smokers for 316 099 men screened for the Multiple Risk Factor Intervention Trial (MRFIT).
Adapted from Neaton et al., 1992.[18]

the preferred first-line pharmacological treatment for hypertension or whether other classes of drug are equally appropriate. It has been suggested that adverse metabolic effects may reduce the benefit of blood pressure reduction with some agents. In a meta-analysis of 13 interventional trials in hypertensive patients, predominantly with diuretics and beta-blockers, the average reduction in diastolic blood pressure was 5–6 mmHg over 5 years. Stroke was reduced by 42%, suggesting that virtually all of the epidemiologically expected reduction in stroke appears rapidly: CHD was reduced by only 14%, suggesting that just over half of

the epidemiologically expected CHD reduction of 20–25% appears rapidly.[22,23] Furthermore, the reduction in stroke in these early trials could have been a reduction in predominantly haemorrhagic stroke as it was not possible to distinguish this from thrombotic stroke in these studies. Thus some of the risks from hypertension would appear to persist despite pharmacological treatment.

All of the most recent guidelines for the management of hypertension stress the multiple risk factor approach. The World Health Organisation–International Society of Hypertension (WHO–ISH) guidelines[24] consider that all available drug classes are suitable for the initiation and maintenance of antihypertensive therapy, but the choice of drugs is influenced by many factors. Dyslipidaemia is considered a possible contraindication for diuretics and beta-blockers but a possible indication for alpha-blockers.[24] Because of the weight of evidence from clinical trials that supports their effectiveness, diuretics and beta-blockers have always been favoured as first-line agents in the American guidelines unless contraindicated, unacceptable, or not tolerated. The latest guidelines from the Joint National Committee on the Prevention, Evaluation, and Treatment of High Blood Pressure[25] consider the problem of hypertensive patients with dyslipidaemia and discuss the adverse effects of beta-blockers and high-dose diuretics on lipid levels. They conclude that low-dose thiazide diuretics do not have adverse effects and that beta-blockers have advantages because of their benefits in secondary prevention. Recent recommendations from the Joint European Societies[26] are reviewed in a later chapter. These emphasise the importance of reducing blood pressure and point out that the benefits of regimens based on diuretic, beta-blocker and some calcium channel blockers are well established.

The pros and cons of different classes of antihypertensives

Thiazides

As the thiazides have shown more protection against stroke than against CHD events in long-term controlled trials and adverse metabolic effects may occur with high doses, the use of small doses for treating hypertension seems prudent. In some recent trials using low doses of thiazides plus potassium-sparing diuretics, the number of sudden deaths was reduced more than in other trials that used high doses of diuretics alone: this suggests that

small doses or these combinations may be more effective in reducing cardiac events.[27] Another analysis showed that the risk of primary cardiac arrest was increased with high doses of diuretic but actually decreased with low doses of diuretic.[28] However, these data cannot be regarded as conclusive and a randomised double-blind trial comparing outcome with low and high doses of thiazide diuretics and potassium-sparing drugs should be performed but probably never will be.

Beta-blockers

Not all trials of beta-blockers in hypertension have shown favourable results. A meta-analysis of the effects of beta-blockers compared with diuretics in elderly hypertensive patients showed that both regimens reduced cerebrovascular events and stroke mortality, but only diuretics reduced the incidence of nonfatal CHD events, CHD mortality and all-cause mortality.[29] In the MRC trial in the elderly, only the diuretic-treated group showed benefit; the atenolol-treated group had the same cumulative incidence of coronary events as those patients who received placebo.[30] In the earlier MRC trial, the benefits of propranolol on stoke incidence were negated in subjects who smoked.[31] In the study in elderly patients, the ineffectiveness of beta-blockers may have been related to their weak antihypertensive efficacy as only one-third of the patients studied had their blood pressure controlled by beta-blocker monotherapy whilst two-thirds achieved control by diuretic alone. However, beta-blockers have been shown to have a clear benefit in secondary prevention of myocardial infarction,[32] which may be attributed to fewer arrhythmias, reduced infarction size, and a lower rate of re-infarction. None the less, this benefit has not been shown definitively in primary prevention studies in hypertension, although the recent United Kingdom Prospective Diabetes Study Group (UKPDS) found that tight blood pressure control with the beta-blocker atenolol was just as effective as that with captopril in reducing macrovascular and microvascular events in diabetic patients with hypertension.[33]

Angiotensin-converting enzyme (ACE) inhibitors

ACE inhibitors are advocated for hypertensive patients with cardiac failure or left ventricular dysfunction and for diabetics with evidence of nephropathy.[24] They may also be more effective than some of the other antihypertensive agents in reducing left ventricular and vascular hypertrophy and have favourable effects on other surrogate endpoints. However, the first outcome study using an ACE inhibitor for primary prevention in hypertension was somewhat disappointing. The Captopril Prevention Project (CAPPP) trial compared the effects of ACE inhibition using captopril with conventional therapy on cardiovascular morbidity and mortality in patients with hypertension. The investigators found that the two regimens did not differ in efficacy in preventing cardiovascular morbidity and mortality but fatal and non-fatal stroke were more common with captopril.[34] This unexpected finding may be explained by differences in the baseline risk factors in the two treatment groups, but further studies will be needed to provide more conclusive data.

Angiotensin II receptor antagonists

Angiotensin II receptor antagonists may provide similar benefits to the ACE inhibitors but without the side-effect of cough, which appears to be more frequent in some Asian countries.[35] They have a favourable tolerability profile but as yet no data are available from outcome trials in hypertensive subjects.

Calcium channel blockers

Calcium channel blockers gained great popularity for the treatment of hypertension before any long-term clinical trial data were available. They are effective in reducing blood pressure in most patients, particularly in blacks and Asians.[36] They have few contraindications and are often recommended as first-line treatment in patients with diabetes or dyslipidaemia. Doubts about their safety were raised when high doses of short-acting calcium channel blockers were found to be associated with an increased risk of myocardial infarction in an observational study[37] and a meta-analysis of secondary prevention trials.[38] It was suggested that these adverse events could occur due to negative inotropic effects, proarrhythmic effects, prohaemorrhagic effects, proischaemic effects from the coronary steal phenomenon and a reflex increase in sympathetic activity, which could theoretically produce plaque rupture. The multiple-day dosing required of short-acting agents may also lead to poorer compliance and blood pressure control. There has been much debate of the merits and potential dangers of calcium antagonists but recent trials have shown a beneficial outcome, at least for stroke. The nondihydropyridine calcium antagonists, verapamil and diltiazem, have been shown to improve prognosis after myocardial infarction so they may be preferred in patients at high risk for CHD.[39] Further information is awaited from ongoing trials such as the ALLHAT study which will compare the effects of a diuretic, a calcium channel blocker and an ACE inhibitor on cardiovascular outcomes in hypertensive patients.[40]

Alpha-blockers

Alpha-blockers have not achieved the acceptance they deserve from their beneficial metabolic effects and lack of contraindications. The problem is that a low starting dose is required to avoid first dose hypotension and then a protracted period of titration is often needed to overcome the counter-regulatory responses that occur and to achieve adequate blood pressure control. This proves too tedious for many clinicians and patients alike; in addition high doses of alpha-blockers may cause orthostatic symptoms, drowsiness or other side-effects. Newer formulations may overcome some of these problems but there are no outcome trials to demonstrate long-term benefits with this class of drugs.

Metabolic effects of antihypertensive treatment

The effects of antihypertensive agents on serum lipid levels in different patient populations were reviewed in a meta-analysis of 474 controlled and uncontrolled clinical trials involving over 65 000 patients.[41] The results were similar to those reported in earlier reviews.[42–44] On average, diuretics caused small increases in total cholesterol (5.03 mg/dl, 95% CI = 3.48–6.96; or 0.13 mmol/l, 95% CI = 0.09–0.18). With higher doses these changes almost doubled and significant increases in LDL-cholesterol levels were also seen. The effects on total and LDL-cholesterol levels were more pronounced in black than in non-black patients. Diuretics also increased triglyceride levels slightly (8.85 mg/dl, CI = 2.65–15.93; or 0.10 mmol/l, 95% CI = 0.03–0.18) in short-term studies and the changes were greater in men than in women. HDL-cholesterol was reduced significantly by diuretics only in patients with diabetes. It has been disputed whether the effects of diuretic therapy on lipid levels decrease with duration of therapy.[27] Kasiske et al.[41] found that cholesterol levels tended to decrease with time in both diuretic-treated and untreated groups, indicating that the relative effects were independent of study duration, but the effects on triglyceride levels decreased over time.

On average, beta-blockers had little effect on total and LDL-cholesterol but caused substantial increases in triglyceride levels (30.97 mg/dl, CI = 27.44–34.52; or 0.35 mmol/l, CI = 0.31–0.39) and reductions in HDL-cholesterol levels (−3.87 mg/dl, CI = −4.64 to −3.09; or −0.10 mmol/l, CI = −0.12 to −0.08), which were less for agents with intrinsic sympathomimetic activity (ISA) such as pindolol.[41] The increase in triglyceride levels was greater in patients with higher baseline levels but less with cardioselective agents and in patients with diabetes. Drugs combining ISA with cardioselectivity reduced total cholesterol and LDL-cholesterol levels. When the 56 trials comparing monotherapy with a placebo control group were analysed separately, similar results were obtained (Figure 11.2). In this meta-analysis, insufficient data were available to comment on the third generation beta-blockers, such as celiprolol or carvedilol, which have additional vasodilating effects through α_1-blockade, β_2-partial agonist effects or other mechanisms. In some studies they have shown neutral or beneficial effects upon plasma lipids,[45,46] presumably because the vasodilating mechanisms counteract any tendency for the beta-blockade to worsen lipid levels.

In the overall analysis, alpha-blockers reduced levels of total cholesterol (−8.89 mg/dl, CI = −10.83 to −6.96; or −0.23 mmol/l, CI = −0.28 to −0.18), LDL-cholesterol (−7.73 mg/dl, CI = −9.67 to −5.8; or −0.20 mmol/l, CI = −0.25 to −0.15) and triglycerides (−6.20 mg/dl, CI = −9.74 to −2.66; or −0.07 mmol/l, CI = −0.11 to −0.03), the effects being greater in persons with higher baseline levels.[41] Alpha-

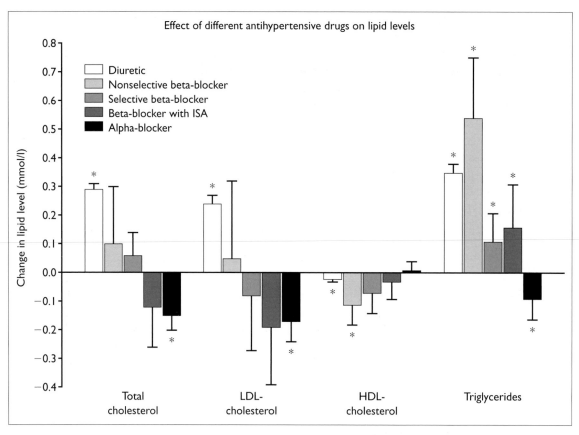

Fig. 11.2
Effects of different antihypertensive drugs on lipid levels in meta-analysis of 56 randomised controlled clinical trials. ACE inhibitors, dihydropyridine calcium antagonists, nondihydropyridine calcium antagonists and sympatholytic drugs had no significant effect in this analysis. Values are means with 95% confidence intervals. *, Significant changes exceeding 95% CI. Adapted from Kasiske et al., 1995.[41]

blockers also increased HDL-cholesterol levels (0.77 mg/dl, CI = 0.38–1.55; or 0.02 mmol/l, CI = 0.01–0.04) but to a lesser extent in older patients. ACE inhibitors reduced triglyceride levels slightly, especially in patients with higher baseline levels but less so in older persons. In diabetics they caused a reduction in total cholesterol levels but there was no effect on HDL-cholesterol levels. The limited data available for angiotensin II antagonists suggest they have no major effects on lipids. Central sympatholytic agents reduced total cholesterol and slightly decreased HDL-cholesterol levels. These effects resulted mostly from studies with guanfacine and guanabenz: the other central sympatholytics appeared to have no significant effect on lipid levels. Vasodilators reduced total and LDL-cholesterol and increased HDL-cholesterol levels. Calcium antagonists were the only group that had no overall effects on lipid levels or insulin resistance.[41]

There were significant correlations between changes in levels of fasting blood glucose and total cholesterol, LDL-cholesterol, triglycerides and HDL-cholesterol during treatment with diuretics, beta-blockers, alpha-blockers and ACE inhibitors. Changes in glycosylated haemoglobin levels also correlated with changes in total cholesterol, LDL-cholesterol and triglyceride levels. Adverse effects on lipid levels, particularly triglycerides, seem to match the effects on insulin sensitivity. Insulin resistance is increased during treatment with most beta-blockers and diuretics but calcium antagonists are neutral. Some ACE inhibitors improve insulin sensitivity, whereas others are neutral or may even lead to slight impairment. Alpha$_1$-blockers generally improve insulin sensitivity.[47]

Many of the metabolic effects of antihypertensive drugs can be attributed to their adverse effects on insulin sensitivity. Likewise, many patients with newly diagnosed type 2 diabetes are already taking antihypertensive drugs and the development of diabetes could be attributed to the long-term use of these medications.[4] One explanation for the effects of different antihypertensive drugs on insulin resistance is their haemodynamic action. Beta-blockers, apart from those with ISA, tend to vasoconstrict and these aggravate insulin resistance, whereas drugs with vasodilating effects, such as ACE inhibitors, angiotensin II antagonists and alpha-blockers, improve insulin resistance.[13] The long-term antihypertensive effects of diuretics are thought to involve a direct vasodilatory action, which one might assume would improve insulin resistance. In this context, the diuretic-induced worsening of insulin resistance is surprising and the underlying mechanisms are not certain but it is thought that potassium depletion may be a mediating factor.

Diuretics and beta-blockers are generally not recommended as first-line therapy for diabetic patients. Diuretics have been associated with increased mortality in some studies of diabetic patients,[48] and in one study beta-blockers and non-potassium-sparing diuretics were associated with an increased risk for sudden cardiac death.[49] However, beta-blockers have been shown to decrease mortality in patients with type 2 diabetes who have CHD[50] and, as mentioned above, atenolol was equally as effective as captopril in preventing cardiovascular events in diabetic subjects in the UKPDS.[33]

Some of the effects of beta-blockers are probably mediated directly through lipoprotein lipase (LPL), but a major effect may be through insulin sensitivity. Insulin release from the pancreas is modulated by beta$_2$-adrenergic activity.[51] The mechanism by which beta-blockers inhibit LPL is not clear. Different types of beta-blockers may have different effects on human LPL *in vitro*. One study showed that propranolol had the strongest inhibitory effect and metoprolol had a moderate inhibitory effect, whereas nadolol, at low concentrations, stimulated LPL activity.[52] *In vitro* studies have used generally non-pharmacological doses of beta-blockers and assays of LPL activity in postheparin plasma may not be optimal for detecting beta-blocker effects. Another study showed that high doses of beta-blockers inhibited LPL activity *in vitro* but this did not appear to be due to altered LPL gene transcription and/or translation of LPL mRNA,[53] but there could have been an effect at the protein level. Interestingly, carriers of the Ser447Stop allele of LPL have been shown to escape the negative effects of beta-blockers on HDL-cholesterol levels, which may be because the drugs are less effective in lowering the activity of the mutated LPL variant.[54]

Use of statins in hypertensive patients

Subgroup analyses of the large clinical trials — the Scandinavian Simvastatin Survival Study (4S),[55] the Cholesterol and Recurrent Events Trial (CARE),[56] the Long-Term Intervention with Pravastatin in Ischaemic Disease (LIPID),[57] the Air Force/Texas Coronary Atherosclerosis Prevention Study (AFCAPS/Tex-CAPS)[58] and the Pooled analysis of clinical events of the Pravastatin Atherosclerosis Inter- vention Program[59] — have demonstrated bene- ficial effects in patients with hypertension which were similar and in some cases greater than in non-hypertensive patients (Table 11.1). Examination of pooled data from multi- ple trials with fluvastatin suggested that the efficacy and safety profile of this agent was also similar in patients with and without con- comitant hypertension[60] and that the use of antihypertensive drugs had no obvious effect on the response.[61] The ALLHAT study will examine whether lowering LDL-cholesterol

| Trial | Events/no. of patients | | Risk reduction (%) |
	Placebo	Active treatment	(95% CI)
4S		Simvastatin	
Hypertension	191/589 (32%)	122/573 (21%)	37 (21–50)
No hypertension	431/1634 (26%)	309/1648 (19%)	32 (21–41)
PAIP		Pravastatin	
Hypertension	17/224 (7.6%)	7/292 (2.4%)	69 (25–92)
No hypertension	29/500 (5.8%)	14/560 (2.5%)	57 (20–81)
CARE		Pravastatin	
Hypertension	263/899 (29%)	200/875 (23%)	23 (8–36)
No hypertension	286/1179 (24%)	230/1206 (19%)	24 (9–36)
LIPID		Pravastatin	
Hypertension	314/1891 (17%)	266/1867 (14%)	15 (0–28)
No hypertension	400/2609 (15%)	291/2644 (11%)	30 (19–40)
AFCAPS/TexCAPS		Lovastatin	
Hypertension	62/729 (9%)	38/719 (5%)	NA
No hypertension	121/2572 (5%)	78/2585 (3%)	NA

4S = Scandinavian Simvastatin Survival Study.[55] PAIP = Pooled analysis of clinical events of the Pravastatin Atherosclerosis Intervention Program.[59] CARE = Cholesterol and Recurrent Events Trial.[56] LIPID = Long-Term Intervention with Pravastatin in Ischaemic Disease.[57] AFCAPS/TexCAPS = Air Force/Texas Coronary Atherosclerosis Prevention Study.[58] NA = not available.

Table 11.1
Effects of lipid-lowering treatment on major cardiac events in patients with and without hypertension in the major trials using statins.

levels with pravastatin in moderately hyper-cholesterolaemic patients taking various anti-hypertensive agents will reduce all-cause mortality.[40]

Effects of lipid lowering on blood pressure

Reductions in lipid levels may be associated with a small reduction in blood pressure although most of the available data were obtained from trials that were not intended to look at this effect. Similarly, the more recent large, lipid-lowering trials with statins were not designed to address this issue. A review of eight lipid-lowering studies including over 17 000 patients found that falls in blood pressure occurred, even though the reduction in cholesterol was quite modest in many studies.[8] The WHO study examined the effect of clofi-brate in 5000 men with hypercholesterolaemia and found a 25% reduction in the incidence of hypertension in the men treated with clofibrate compared with those given placebo.[62] Other studies found that patients with hypercholes-terolaemia showed an increased blood pressure response to both mental stress and exercise, even when resting blood pressure was normal. Reductions in the increased blood pressure response to various stimuli or the basal blood pressure have also been described after cholesterol-lowering treatments.[63]

Alteration in vascular responsiveness with lipid-lowering treatments may be due to increased vasodilation or decreased vasocon-striction. Many studies in animals and humans have shown that oxidised LDL-cholesterol can impair endothelial-dependent vasodilation in both coronary and peripheral arteries.[64] It had been suggested that outside the coronary cir-culation, hypercholesterolaemia results in a functional abnormality of vascular smooth muscle rather than in endothelial dysfunction. One study compared the vasodilator responses to acetylcholine, methacholine and sodium nitroprusside (an endothelium-independent vasodilator) in the forearm resistance vessels of men with primary hypercholesterolaemia com-pared with normocholesterolaemic controls. The results showed impaired vasodilation in response to acetylcholine, but not methacholine or sodium nitroprusside, in hypercholesterol-aemic patients, suggesting that endothelial dys-function in hypercholesterolaemic subjects is generalised and extends to vascular beds other than the coronary circulation.[65] Therefore, reduction of plasma LDL-cholesterol levels in hypercholesterolaemic patients should improve nitric oxide-mediated vasodilator responses. It was shown that endothelial function improves during statin treatment by a mechanism that involves increased bioavailability of nitric oxide.[66] LDL-cholesterol also potentiates the responses to vasoconstrictors such as noradren-aline and endothelin-1 in the absence of endothelium, possibly by enhancing calcium influx into vascular smooth muscle cells. Cho-lesterol reduction with pravastatin treatment over 3 weeks in mildly hypertensive patients reduced the diastolic but not the systolic pres-sor responses to noradrenaline and angiotensin II infusions, but there was no change in the response to the physical stressors of cold pres-sor testing and isometric exercise.[67]

Low-density lipoprotein was reported to increase intracellular free calcium in vascular smooth muscle cells and to cause vasoconstric-tion of rat aortic rings.[68] However, the relative contribution of changes in endothelial-depen-dent vasodilation and vasoconstrictor or inotropic responses remains to be established. The excessive pressor responses in hyperlipi-daemic subjects could be attributed to increases in sympathetic nerve activity linked to the metabolic syndrome,[69] although there was no evidence of increased baseline sympa-thetic activity in one study which measured plasma catecholamines.[63] However this may not have been adequate to assess sympathetic tone.

The effects of statin therapy on glycaemia or insulin resistance have been inconsistent and probably vary with the type of patient studied. One study showed that pravastatin treatment improved fasting hyperinsulinaemia in elderly hypercholesterolaemic hypertensive subjects despite the continued use of beta-blockers and diuretics.[70] It is possible that short-term changes in LDL-cholesterol levels produce favourable changes in cardiovascular responsiveness that may influence the development of ischaemic events, giving rise to some of the early benefits seen in the large statin studies.

Interaction of lipid-lowering treatments with antihypertensive therapy

Most of the large studies and reviews of trial data have found that lipid-lowering treatments are just as effective and safe in patients undergoing treatment for hypertension as in those not receiving other treatments.[61] Nevertheless, the statins do have some potential for interaction with other drugs. They are metabolised predominantly by the cytochrome P450 enzyme, CYP3A4. Exceptions are fluvastatin which is metabolised mainly by CYP2C9, cerivastatin which is eliminated through the duel metabolic pathways of CYP3A4 and CYP2C8, and pravastatin which is excreted mainly unchanged. Other drugs that inhibit CYP3A4 will increase the plasma concentration of lovastatin, simvastatin and atorvastatin, which may predispose to the development of myopathy or, in the most severe cases, rhabdomyolysis and acute renal failure. This was a problem with the T-type calcium channel blocking agent mibefradil,

which is a potent inhibitor of CYP3A4: its interaction with statins was one of the reasons for its withdrawal.[71]

The L-type calcium channel blocking drugs, diltiazem and verapamil, also produce some inhibition of CYP3A4 and could potentially cause interactions with statins that could be important when higher doses of either type of drug are employed. In a pharmacokinetic interaction study, Azie et al. found that diltiazem given as 120 mg twice daily for two weeks increased the area under the curve of single doses of 20 mg lovastatin by 1.5–9-fold (mean 3.6-fold) but had no effect on the area under the curve for pravastatin.[72] Other drugs that might result in interactions through inhibition of CYP3A4 include cyclosporine, macrolide antibiotics such as erythromycin, azole antifungal agents such as ketoconazle, protease inhibitors such as ritonavir[73] and possibly cimetidine, but the use of these drugs is not peculiar to hypertensive patients.

Practical approach to treating hypertensive patients with dyslipidaemia

A global risk factor reduction approach should always be taken. Hypertensive patients should have their plasma lipid and glucose levels checked during the initial assessment. The lipid profile should include HDL-cholesterol and fasting triglycerides as these are more often abnormal than LDL-cholesterol in this group. The opportunity should be taken to measure fasting plasma glucose to detect impaired fasting glucose (IFG) or diabetes. Appropriate dietary and lifestyle advice should be given, including advising smokers to give up the habit. The thresholds for starting therapy will be lower for the hypertension or hyperlipidaemia in patients with both problems. If LDL-cholesterol levels remain high despite dietary measures, treatment with a statin should be commenced. A fibrate may be more appropriate if there is predominant and marked elevation of triglycerides but the response should be monitored to ensure that LDL-cholesterol does not rise above threshold values; this would require the addition of, or change to, a statin.

If specific lipid-lowering therapy is given it may not matter which antihypertensive therapy is chosen. Other factors can be given more weight in determination of the first-line treatment as the small adverse effects on lipids produced by beta-blockers and diuretics will be swamped by the effects of hypolipidaemic agents. Diltiazem and verapamil should be avoided if high doses of statins are to be used, for example in familial hypercholesterolaemia; however with moderate doses of statins, the possible interaction could be seen as an advantage. Adverse effects on insulin sensitivity might still occur with beta-blockers and diuretics, but as long as hyperglycaemia does not occur, there is no clear evidence that this is detrimental. Patients with borderline abnormalities of lipids present a greater challenge as they may be more susceptible than those with normal levels to the adverse effects of beta-blockers and diuretics, and increases in LDL-cholesterol or triglycerides may push them to a level requiring drug therapy. An alpha-blocker may be a good choice in this situation but if this produces side-effects or the response is inadequate, despite titration of the dose, it would be reasonable to switch to a calcium channel blocker, an ACE inhibitor or an angiotensin II receptor antagonist.

An analysis of the effects of antihypertensive therapy and blood pressure control in dyslipidaemic men in the placebo arm of the Helsinki Heart Study showed that the relative risk of CHD and total mortality were similar in adequately treated hypertensives and those with normal blood pressure at study entry, whereas those with untreated or inadequately controlled hypertension had higher relative risks (Table 11.2).[74] The benefits of satisfactory blood pressure control were seen despite the use of mainly diuretics and beta-blockers and lower levels of HDL-cholesterol and higher triglycerides at the start of the study. Adequate blood pressure control is therefore probably more important than slight changes in lipid levels and an effort should be made to reach a target of less than 140/90 mmHg, or even lower in diabetics. The recent Hypertension Optimal Treatment (HOT) trial showed the benefit of lowering the diastolic blood pressure down to about 82 mmHg.[75] This study also demonstrated that the majority of hypertensive patients would require combination therapy to achieve adequate blood pressure targets. Issues of drug tolerability and compliance become extremely important in long-term blood pressure control but they are often neglected. Angiotensin II receptor antagonists have potential advantages in this context as they can be given once daily, are relatively free of side-effects and can be combined effectively with a low-dose diuretic or a calcium channel blocker.

Conclusions

Dyslipidaemia is common in hypertensive patients and should be identified and treated aggressively as the two problems magnify the risk of CHD. Insulin resistance and hyperinsulinaemia frequently underlie these conditions and impaired fasting glucose, glucose intolerance or diabetes may be present and will require attention. Beta-blockers can be predicted to increase triglycerides and decrease HDL-cholesterol levels to an extent, depending upon the baseline levels and the type of

Category	n	HDL-C	Triglycerides	RR CHD	RR death
I	1254	1.27 (0.29)	1.9 (1.1)	1	1
II	540	1.25 (0.28)	2.2 (1.8)	2.1 (1.3–3.3)	1.9 (0.9–3.9)
III	76	1.20 (0.25)	2.4 (1.2)	0.9 (0.2–3.8)	1.0 (0.1–7.3)
IV	165	1.18 (0.29)	2.5 (1.7)	2.0 (1.0–4.1)	4.4 (2.0–9.6)

Categories: I = normal blood pressure at study entry, no antihypertensive treatment; II = untreated hypertensives; III = successful antihypertensive treatment; IV = remained hypertensive despite drug treatment. HDL-C = high-density lipoprotein cholesterol. Values are mean (SD) for this and triglycerides. RR = relative risk (95% CI) using a Cox proportional hazards model with category I as the reference group. Adapted from Mänttäri *et al.* 1995.[74]

Table 11.2
Effects of antihypertensive therapy and blood pressure control on relative risk of CHD and total mortality in dyslipidaemic men in the placebo arm of the Helsinki Heart Study.

drug used. Diuretics are likely to increase total and LDL-cholesterol levels slightly and both groups of drug will aggravate insulin resistance. These drugs may convert a borderline lipid abnormality into one where drug therapy is indicated, which will worsen the problems of compliance and cost, so other choices may be better in these circumstances. In patients who require lipid-lowering treatment, the main considerations should be that the antihypertensive drugs chosen will reduce blood pressure effectively and are well tolerated to maximise compliance.

Acknowledgements

The author gratefully acknowledges support for research on hyperlipidaemia and hypertension provided by a grant from the Strategic Research Programme (SRP9702) of The Chinese University of Hong Kong.

References

1. Stamler J, Wentworth D, Neaton JD. Prevalence and prognostic significance of hypercholesterolemia in men with hypertension. Prospective data on the primary screenees of the Multiple Risk Factor Intervention Trial. *Am J Med* 1986; **80**:33–9.

2. Laurenzi M, Mancini M, Menotti A, *et al.* Multiple risk factors in hypertension: results from the Gubbio study. *J Hypertens* 1990; **8**:S7–S12.

3. Reaven GM, Banting Lecture 1988. Role of insulin resistance in human disease. *Diabetes* 1988; **37**:1595–607.

4. Jarrett RJ, Fitzgerald AP. Non-insulin-dependent diabetes mellitus, glucose intolerance, blood pressure, hypertension, and antihypertensive drugs. *Diabetic Med* 1994; **11**:646–9.

5. Reaven PD, Barrett-Connor EL, Browner DK. Abnormal glucose tolerance and hypertension. *Diabetes Care* 1990; **13**:119–25.

6. Modan M, Halkin H, Almog S, *et al.* Hyperinsulinemia. A link between hypertension obesity and glucose intolerance. *J Clin Invest* 1985; **75**:809–17.

7. Julius S, Jamerson K, Mejia A, *et al*. The association of borderline hypertension with target organ changes and higher coronary risk. Tecumseh Blood Pressure study. *JAMA* 1990; **264**:354–8.

8. Goode GK, Miller JP, Heagerty AM. Hyperlipidaemia, hypertension, and coronary heart disease, *Lancet* 1995; **345**:362–4.

9. Williams RR, Hunt SC, Hopkins PN, *et al*. Familial dyslipidemic hypertension. Evidence from 58 Utah families for a syndrome present in approximately 12% of patients with essential hypertension. *JAMA* 1988; **259**:3579–86.

10. Williams RR, Hopkins PN, Hunt SC, *et al*. Population-based frequency of dyslipidemia syndromes in coronary-prone families in Utah. *Arch Intern Med* 1990; **150**:582–8.

11. Natali A, Santoro D, Palombo C, *et al*. Impaired insulin action on skeletal muscle metabolism in essential hypertension. *Hypertension* 1991; **17**:170–8.

12. DeFronzo RA, Ferrannini E. Insulin resistance. A multifaceted syndrome responsible for NIDDM, obesity, hypertension, dyslipidemia, and atherosclerotic cardiovascular disease. *Diabetes Care* 1991; **14**:173–94.

13. Julius S. Coronary disease in hypertension: a new mosaic. *J Hypertens* 1997; **15**:S3–S10.

14. Lind L, Lithell H. Decreased peripheral blood flow in the pathogenesis of the metabolic syndrome comprising hypertension, hyperlipidemia, and hyperinsulinemia. *Am Heart J* 1993; **125**:1494–7.

15. Aitman TJ, Glazier AM, Wallace CA, *et al*. Identification of Cd36 (Fat) as an insulin-resistance gene causing defective fatty acid and glucose metabolism in hypertensive rats. *Nat Genet* 1999; **21**:76–83.

16. Barker DJ. Fetal origins of coronary heart disease. *Br Med J* 1995; **311**:171–4.

17. Wilson PW. Established risk factors and coronary artery disease: the Framingham Study. *Am J Hypertens* 1994; **7**:7S–12S.

18. Neaton JD, Wentworth D, for the Multiple Risk Factor Intervention Trial Research Group. Serum cholesterol, blood pressure, cigarette smoking, and death from coronary heart disease. Overall findings and differences by age for 316 099 white men. *Arch Intern Med* 1992; **152**:56–64.

19. Eastern Stroke and Coronary Heart Disease Collaborative Research Group. Blood pressure, cholesterol, and stroke in eastern Asia. *Lancet* 1998; **352**:1801–7.

20. Janus ED, Postiglione A, Singh RB, Lewis B. The modernization of Asia. Implications for coronary heart disease. Council on Arteriosclerosis of the International Society and Federation of Cardiology. *Circulation* 1996; **94**:2671–3.

21. Singh RB, Rastogi V, Niaz MA, *et al*. Serum cholesterol and coronary artery disease in populations with low cholesterol levels: the Indian paradox. *Int J Cardiol* 1998; **65**:81–90.

22. Collins R, Peto R, MacMahon S, *et al*. Blood pressure, stroke, and coronary heart disease. Part 2, Short-term reductions in blood pressure: overview of randomised drug trials in their epidemiological context. *Lancet* 1990; **335**:827–38.

23. MacMahon S, Peto R, Cutler J, *et al*. Blood pressure, stroke, and coronary heart disease. Part 1, Prolonged differences in blood pressure: prospective observational studies corrected for the regression dilution bias. *Lancet* 1990; **335**:765–74.

24. Guidelines Subcommittee. 1999 World Health Organization–International Society of Hypertension Guidelines for the Management of Hypertension. *J Hypertens* 1999; **17**:151–83.

25. Joint National Committee on Prevention, Evaluation, and Treatment of high blood pressure. The sixth report of the Joint National Committee on prevention, detection, evaluation, and treatment of high blood pressure. *Arch Intern Med* 1997; **157**:2413–46.

26. Wood D, de Backer G, Faergeman O, *et al*. Prevention of coronary heart disease in clinical practice. Summary of recommendations of the Second Joint Task Force of European and other Societies on Coronary Prevention. *J Hypertens* 1998; **16**: 1407–14.

27. Freis ED. The efficacy and safety of diuretics in treating hypertension. *Ann Intern Med* 1995; **122**:223–6.

28. Siscovick DS, Raghunathan TE, Psaty BM, *et al*. Diuretic therapy for hypertension and the risk of primary cardiac arrest. *N Engl J Med* 1994; **330**:1852–7.

29. Messerli FH, Grossman E, Goldbourt U. Are beta-blockers efficacious as first-line therapy for hypertension in the elderly? A systematic review. *JAMA* 1998; **279**:1903–7.

30. MRC Working Party. Medical Research Council trial of treatment of hypertension in older adults: principal results. *Br Med J* 1992; **304**:405–12.

31. Medical Research Council Working Party. MRC trial of treatment of mild hypertension: principal results. *Br Med J* 1985; **291**:97–104.

32. Yusuf S, Lessem J, Jha P, Lonn E. Primary and secondary prevention of myocardial infarction and strokes: an update of randomly allocated, controlled trials. *J Hypertens* 1993; **11**: S61–S73.

33. UK Prospective Diabetes Study Group. Efficacy of atenolol and captopril in reducing risk of macrovascular and microvascular complications in type 2 diabetes: UKPDS 39. *Br Med J* 1998; **317**:713–20.

34. Hansson L, Lindholm LH, Niskanen L, *et al*. Effect of angiotensin-converting-enzyme inhibition compared with conventional therapy on cardiovascular morbidity and mortality in hypertension: the Captopril Prevention Project (CAPPP) randomised trial [see comments]. *Lancet* 1999; **353**:611–6.

35. Tomlinson B, Young RP, Chan JC, *et al*. Pharmacoepidemiology of ACE inhibitor-induced cough [letter]. *Drug Safety* 1997; **16**:150–1.

36. Tomlinson B. Pharmacokinetic and pharmacodynamic responses to cardiovascular drugs in Asians. *Acta Pharm Sinica* 1998; **19(suppl.)**: 12–13.

37. Psaty BM, Heckbert SR, Koepsell TD, *et al*. The risk of myocardial infarction associated with antihypertensive drug therapies. *JAMA* 1995; **274**:620–5.

38. Furberg CD, Psaty BM, Meyer JV. Nifedipine. Dose-related increase in mortality in patients with coronary heart disease. *Circulation* 1995; **92**:1326–31.

39. Gibson RS, Boden WE. Calcium channel antagonists: friend or foe in postinfarction patients? *Am J Hypertens* 1996; **9**:172S–176S.

40. Davis BR, Cutler JA, Gordon DJ, *et al*. Rationale and design for the Antihypertensive and Lipid Lowering Treatment to Prevent Heart Attack Trial (ALLHAT). *Am J Hypertens* 1996; **9**:342–60.

41. Kasiske BL, Ma JZ, Kalil RS, Louis TA. Effects of antihypertensive therapy on serum lipids. *Ann Intern Med* 1995; **122**:133–41.

42. Ames RP. Antihypertensive drugs and lipid profiles. *Am J Hypertens* 1988; **1**:421–7.

43. Weidmann P, Ferrier C, Saxenhofer H, *et al*. Serum lipoproteins during treatment with antihypertensive drugs. *Drugs* 1988; **35**: 118–34.

44. Chait A. Effects of antihypertensive agents on serum lipids and lipoproteins. *Am J Med* 1989; **86**:5–7.

45. Herrmann JM, Bischof F, von Heymann F, *et al*. Effects of celiprolol on serum lipids in systemic hypertension. *Am J Cardiol* 1988; **61**:41C–44C.

46. Tomlinson B, Prichard BN, Graham BR, Walden RJ. Clinical pharmacology of carvedilol. *Clinical Investigator* 1992; **70**:S27–S36.

47. Lithell H. Hypertension and hyperlipidemia. A review. *Am J Hypertens* 1993; **6**:303S–308S.

48. Parving HH. Excess mortality associated with diuretic therapy in diabetes mellitus [letter]. *Arch Intern Med* 1992; **152**:1093–4, 1097.

49. Hoes AW, Grobbee DE, Lubsen J, *et al*. Diuretics, beta-blockers, and the risk for sudden cardiac death in hypertensive patients. *Ann Intern Med* 1995; **123**:481–7.

50. Jonas M, Reicher-Reiss H, Boyko V, *et al*. Usefulness of beta-blocker therapy in patients with non-insulin-dependent diabetes mellitus and coronary artery disease. Bezafibrate Infarction Prevention (BIP) Study Group. *Am J Cardiol* 1996; **77**:1273–7.

51. Day JL, Simpson N, Metcalfe J, Page RL. Metabolic consequences of atenolol and propranolol in treatment of essential hypertension. *Br Med J* 1979; **1**:77–80.

52. Kihara S, Kubo M, Ikeda N, *et al*. Inhibition of purified human postheparin lipoprotein lipase by beta-adrenergic blockers in vitro. *Biochem Pharmacol* 1989; **38**:407–11.

53. Raynolds MV, Awald PD, Gordon DF, *et al*. Lipoprotein lipase gene expression in rat adipocytes is regulated by isoproterenol and insulin through different mechanisms. *Mol Endocrinol* 1990; **4**:1416–22.

54. Groenemeijer BE, Hallman MD, Reymer PW, *et al*. Genetic variant showing a positive interaction with beta-blocking agents with a beneficial influence on lipoprotein lipase activity, HDL cholesterol, and triglyceride levels in coronary artery disease patients. The Ser447-stop substitution in the lipoprotein lipase gene. REGRESS Study Group. *Circulation* 1997; **95**:2628–35.

55. The Scandinavian Simvastatin Survival Study Group. Randomised trial of cholesterol lowering in 4444 patients with coronary heart disease: the Scandinavian Simvastatin Survival Study (4S). *Lancet* 1994; **344**:1383–9.

56. Sacks FM, Pfeffer MA, Moye LA, *et al*. The effect of pravastatin on coronary events after myocardial infarction in patients with average cholesterol levels. Cholesterol and Recurrent Events Trial investigators. *N Engl J Med* 1996; **335**:1001–9.

57. The Long-Term Intervention with Pravastatin in Ischaemic Disease (LIPID) Study Group. Prevention of cardiovascular events and death with pravastatin in patients with coronary heart disease and a broad range of initial cholesterol levels. *N Engl J Med* 1998; **339**: 1349–57.

58. Downs JR, Clearfield M, Weis S, *et al*. Primary prevention of acute coronary events with lovastatin in men and women with average cholesterol levels: results of AFCAPS/TexCAPS. Air Force/Texas Coronary Atherosclerosis Prevention Study. *JAMA* 1998; **279**: 1615–22.

59. Byington RP, Jukema JW, Salonen JT, *et al*. Reduction in cardiovascular events during pravastatin therapy. Pooled analysis of clinical events of the Pravastatin Atherosclerosis Intervention Program. *Circulation* 1995; **92**: 2419–25.

60. Peters TK, Mehra M, Muratti EN. Efficacy and safety of fluvastatin in hypertensive patients. An analysis of a clinical trial database. *Am J Hypertens* 1993; **6**:340S–345S.

61. Peters TK, Jewitt-Harris J, Mehra M, Muratti EN. Safety and tolerability of fluvastatin with concomitant use of antihypertensive agents. An analysis of a clinical trial database. *Am J Hypertens* 1993; **6**:346S–352S.

62. Committee of Principal Investigators. A cooperative trial in the primary prevention of ischaemic heart disease using clofibrate. *Br Heart J* 1978; **40**:1069–118.

63. Minami M, Atarashi K, Ishiyama A, *et al*. Pressor hyperreactivity to mental and hand-grip stresses in patients with hypercholesterolemia. *J Hypertens* 1999; **17**: 185–92.

64. Howes LG, Abbott D, Straznicky NE. Lipoproteins and cardiovascular reactivity. *Br J Clin Pharmacol* 1997; **44**:319–24.

65. Chowienczyk PJ, Watts GF, Cockcroft JR, Ritter JM. Impaired endothelium-dependent vasodilation of forearm resistance vessels in hypercholesterolaemia. *Lancet* 1992; **340**: 1430–2.

66. John S, Schlaich M, Langenfeld M, *et al*. Increased bioavailability of nitric oxide after lipid-lowering therapy in hypercholesterolemic patients: a randomized, placebo-controlled, double-blind study. *Circulation* 1998; **98**: 211–16.

67. Straznicky NE, Howes LG, Lam W, Louis WJ. Effects of pravastatin on cardiovascular reactivity to norepinephrine and angiotensin II in patients with hypercholesterolemia and systemic hypertension. *Am J Cardiol* 1995; **75**: 582–6.

68. Sachinidis A, Mengden T, Locher R, *et al*. Novel cellular activities for low density lipoprotein in vascular smooth muscle cells. *Hypertension* 1990; **15**:704–11.

69. Julius S, Gudbrandsson T, Jamerson K, *et al*. The hemodynamic link between insulin resistance and hypertension. *J Hypertens* 1991; **9**:983–6.

70. Chan P, Tomlinson B, Lee CB, *et al*. Beneficial effects of pravastatin on fasting hyperinsulinemia in elderly hypertensive hypercholesterolemic subjects. *Hypertension* 1996; **28**:647–51.

71. Schmassmann-Suhijar D, Bullingham R, Gasser R, *et al*. Rhabdomyolysis due to interaction of simvastatin with mibefradil [letter]. *Lancet* 1998; **351**:1929–30.

72. Azie NE, Brater DC, Becker PA, *et al*. The interaction of diltiazem with lovastatin and pravastatin. *Clin Pharmacol Ther* 1998; **64**:369–77.

73. Von Moltke LL, Greenblatt DJ, Grassi JM, *et al*. Protease inhibitors as inhibitors of human

cytochromes P450: high risk associated with ritonavir. *J Clin Pharmacol* 1998; 38:106–11.

74. Mänttäri M, Tenkanen L, Manninen V, *et al*. Antihypertensive therapy in dyslipidemic men. Effects on coronary heart disease incidence and total mortality. *Hypertension* 1995; 25:47–52.

75. Hansson L, Zanchetti A, Carruthers SG, *et al*. Effects of intensive blood-pressure lowering and low-dose aspirin in patients with hypertension: principal results of the Hypertension Optimal Treatment (HOT) randomised trial. HOT Study Group. *Lancet* 1998; 351: 1755–62.

12

Lipids in heart transplant patients

Mahmud Barbir, Fawzi Lazem and Magdi Yacoub

Introduction

Heart transplantation is the optimal treatment for end-stage heart failure, of which ischaemic heart disease constitutes the commonest indication in most centres. More than 30 000 heart transplantations have been performed worldwide, and improved management strategies have led to a dramatic reduction in early post-transplant morbidity and mortality. Allograft coronary vasculopathy (ACV), an accelerated form of atherosclerotic vascular disease, is considered to be due to chronic rejection[1] and is the most serious medium- and long-term complication of transplantation. The incidence of ACV increases progressively to 20–45% by 3 years.[2,3] The disease causes episodic and sustained myocardial ischaemia and may progress rapidly. ACV presents a major clinical problem for the foreseeable future. The aetiology of the disease appears to be multifactorial; both immunological[4,5] and non-immunological[6–8] factors have been implicated in the pathogenesis. There is smooth muscle proliferation and later development of lesions similar but not identical to those associated with non-transplant atherosclerosis. Hyperlipidaemia is common and contributes to the development of ACV. In this chapter we review the prevalence, mechanisms, clinical implication and management of hyperlipidaemia in heart transplant patients.

Prevalence

Many studies have documented that lipid abnormalities are common after heart transplantation.[9,10] In one series, up to 80% of recipients developed a total cholesterol level greater than 220 mg/dl (5.7 mmol/l).[11] Several studies have evaluated the changes in lipid levels that occur after transplantation. Most of the series have shown uniformly that increases in total cholesterol, LDL-cholesterol, triglycerides and apolipoprotein B levels develop at between 3 to 18 months after heart transplantation.[12,13] HDL-cholesterol levels are more variable, with some studies showing no change,[14] some showing an increase[15] and others showing an increase early after transplantation with subsequent return to normal levels.[16] Interestingly, in one study lipoprotein(a) [Lp(a)] levels were found to decrease by 40% after heart transplantation.[17]

Aetiology

Cardiac transplant recipients are a fairly heterogeneous population and are subject to many influential factors in the early postoperative period. Diabetes mellitus, obesity, medication with immunosuppressants (such as cyclosporin and prednisolone) and with diuretics are all common in transplant recipients and can adversely affect lipid metabolism.

In addition genetic predisposition (for example towards familial hyperlipidaemia) is common, especially in patients with preoperative diagnosis of ischaemic heart disease.[18] In one study, patients with pretransplant diagnosis of ischaemic heart disease had significantly higher post-transplant total cholesterol levels of 282.3 mg/dl (7.3 mmol/l) compared with 224.3 mg/dl (5.8 mmol/l) in those with diagnosis of dilated cardiomyopathy.[19]

Heart transplant recipients usually receive a triple drug immunosuppressive regime with cyclosporin A, azathioprine and oral prednisolone to prevent allograft rejection during the first 12 months. Thereafter prednisolone is gradually withdrawn to avoid long-term problems such as obesity, osteoporosis, diabetes and hypertension.

Numerous studies in transplant patients receiving long-term prednisolone therapy have found increases in total cholesterol, LDL-cholesterol and serum triglyceride levels.[20] Interestingly, it has been reported that prednisolone has induced an increase in HDL-cholesterol levels. This increase may not be beneficial, since it reflects increases in HDL3 at the expense of HDL2, which is regarded the protective subfraction of HDL.[18]

In patients who show evidence of acute cardiac rejection, the standard management is high-dose intravenous methyl prednisolone for 48–72 hours followed by tapering course of oral prednisolone. Recently we have shown that pulsed prednisolone therapy significantly increase total cholesterol, triglyceride and apolipoprotein A-1 levels as well as mevalonic acid. This may suggest that prednisolone increases cholesterol synthesis even after short-term administration (unpublished data). Prednisolone also enhances the activity of acetyl-coenzyme A carboxylase and free fatty acid synthesis and it inhibits lipoprotein lipase. This results in an increase in plasma concentration of very low density lipoprotein (VLDL), total cholesterol and triglycerides. Another important pathway leading to hyperlipidaemia is insulin resistance induced by prednisolone. Kemma *et al.* reported a high prevalence of severe glucose intolerance, hyperinsulinism, hypertriglyceridaemia and hypercholesterolaemia in heart transplant recipients.[21]

Frequently, cyclosporin A and prednisolone have been reported to cause hyperlipidaemia.[21-23] Cyclosporin A inhibits 26-hydroxylase, a key enzyme in the bile acid synthetic pathway. Furthermore cyclosporin A has been shown to increase hepatic lipase activity and decrease lipoprotein lipase activity, resulting in impaired clearance of VLDL and LDL. In addition, cyclosporin A is reported to bind to LDL receptors, which resulted in increased levels of LDL-cholesterol.

Hyperlipidaemia as a risk factor in allograft coronary vasculopathy

Several studies have shown a link between ACV and high levels of total cholesterol, LDL-cholesterol, triglycerides, lipoprotein (a) and, more recently, oxidised LDL.[9,16,23-25] In a study of 120 heart transplant recipients from Harefield Hospital, increased levels of total cholesterol and LDL-cholesterol were significantly higher in patients who developed ACV compared with a similar group of patients who remained disease free. There was striking increase in Lp(a) levels in patients who developed ACV. Furthermore, hyperlipidaemia appears to be predictive of future ACV (Table 12.1).

In another study from Harefield Hospital of 207 heart transplant recipients, the cumulative probability of ACV in those with a total cho-

Variable	No ACV (n = 97)	ACV (n = 33)	P*
Total cholesterol (mmol/l)	6.3 (1.7)	7.1 (2)	0.02
LDL-cholesterol (mmol/l)	4.4 (1.0)	4.9 (1.6)	0.03
Triglycerides (mmol/l)	2.0 (1.0)	2.3 (1.3)	0.54
HDL-cholesterol (mmol/l)	1.15 (0.3)	1.4 (0.9)	0.68
Lipoprotein(a) (mg/dl)	22 (1–170)	71 (3–193)	0.0006

ACV = allograft coronary vasculopathy. Results as mean (SD) except for Lp(a), which is given as median (range). *P value calculated using Mann-Whitney test. From Barbir *et al.* with permission.

Table 12.1
Fasting serum lipid and lipoprotein values.

lesterol level greater than 224 mg/dl (5.8 mmol/l) was 9.3% at 2 years, 24.4% at 3 years and 45% at 4 years compared with 4.3% at 2 years, 7.4% at 3 years and 14% at 4 years in those with a total cholesterol level less than 224 mg/dl (5.8 mmol/l) (Figures 12.1 and 12.2).[23] Similarly the incidence of ACV was increased in patients with serum triglyceride levels greater than 54.14 mg/dl (1.4 mmol/l). The same authors reported in a subsequent study that circulating Lp(a) also has a strong predictive value for ACV (Figure 12.3).

The exact mechanism by which dyslipidaemia contributes to ACV is not fully elucidated. It has been suggested that ACV results from a response to injury of the endothelium.[26] This injury may be induced by a number of factors which include oxidised LDL-cholesterol, CMV infection, cellular immune responses and cyclosporin, all of which may act on the coronary endothelium. In an autopsy study, McManus *et al.*[27] found that mean total cholesterol, esterfied cholesterol, and free cholesterol content in trans-

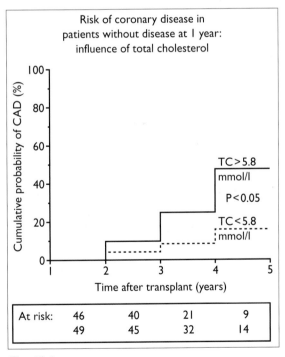

Fig. 12.1
Influence of total cholesterol on risk of coronary artery disease in patients without disease at 1 year. From Barbir et al. with kind permission of the authors and publishers, Elsevier Science Publishers.[9]

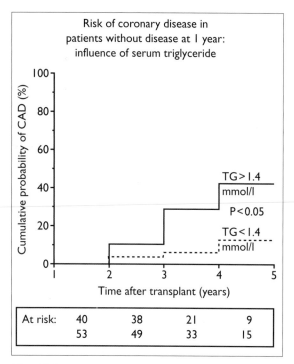

Fig. 12.2
Influence of serum triglyceride on risk of coronary arterial disease in patients without disease at 1 year. From Barbir et al. with kind permission of the authors and publishers, Elsevier Science Publishers.[9]

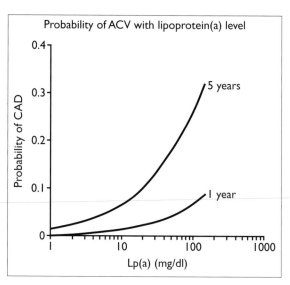

Fig. 12.3
Predicted probability of allograft coronary vasculopathy (ACV) versus lipoprotein(a) level for men without hypertension, 1 and 5 years after transplantation. From Barbir et al. with kind permission of the authors and Lancet.[23]

planted arteriopathic coronaries were 10-fold higher than in comparable native coronary segments. The amount of lipids in the arterial wall was correlated strongly with digitised per cent luminal narrowing, suggesting that lipid accumulation is an important early and persistent phenomenon in the development of this disease.

Management of hyperlipidaemia in heart transplant recipients

We have discussed the importance of hyperlipidaemia in the development of ACV, and it is apparent that its management might be significant in the prevention of ACV. In contrast to the wealth of data on the management of hyperlipidaemia for both primary and secondary prevention in the non-transplant population, there are only a few trials that investigated the risks and benefits of lipid-lowering therapy after heart transplantation. Dietary modification and optimisation of medical management are the safest forms of treatment of hyperlipidaemia, but this is usually inadequate and lipid-lowering drugs are necessary. The bile acid sequestrants, fibric acid derivatives and nicotinic acids are usually not recommended due to the lack of efficacy and frequent adverse effects. In an open randomised study comparing the efficacy and safety of eicosapeutaenoic acid plus docosohexaenoic (Maxepa™) with bezafibrate in 87 heart transplant recipients, bezafibrate had better lipid, apolipoprotein and haemostatic modifying properties but it had an adverse effect on renal function.[28]

Inhibitors of 3-hydroxy-3-methylglutaryl coenzyme A (HMG-CoA) reductase lower blood cholesterol levels and have been associated with regression of atherosclerotic lesions in non-transplant patients with CAD.[30]

There are few published studies using lovastatin, simvastatin and pravastatin and ongoing studies using fluvastatin, cerivastatin and atorvastatin in the management of hyperlipidaemia in heart transplant recipients. In one study simvastatin at a dose of 10 mg was well tolerated and had favourable modifying properties, resulting in a decrease in levels of total cholesterol, LDL-cholesterol and triglycerides by 38, 42 and 25%, respectively.[30] Furthermore in a 4-year prospective randomised study, Wenke *et al.* found that in comparison with dietary measures alone, the combination of a low-cholesterol diet and low-dose simvastatin after heart transplantation led to a significant reduction in cholesterol levels, a significantly higher long-term survival rate and a low incidence of ACV.[31]

In a primary prevention study, 97 heart transplant recipients were randomly assigned within 2 weeks after heart transplantation to receive either pravastatin (20 or 40 mg per day) or placebo. At 1-year follow-up in this non-blinded, single-centre trial, patients treated with pravastatin showed a significant reduction in mortality rate as well as a significantly lower incidence of ACV. The pravastatin-treated group also had significant reductions in haemodynamically significant rejection and in natural killer cytotoxicity.[32]

At Harefield, a series of 244 heart transplant recipients with hyperlipidaemia were given various statin therapies, simvastatin,

pravastatin or fluvastatin, and followed for a mean period of 10 years. The recent, yet to be published, data from this study showed that those who had responded well to treatment (more than 77 mg/dl or 2 mmol/l reduction in total cholesterol) tended to survive longer.

There are several potential mechanisms whereby statins may have improved the clinical outcome. Statins have been shown to decrease antibody dependent cellular cytotoxicity and natural killer cell function.[33] Statins may also have a direct vascular effect on intimal proliferation. Simvastatin has been shown to reduce ACV without significant changes in lipoprotein concentration in a rat model of heart transplantation on FK506 immunosuppressive therapy.[31,34] In addition marked reduction in plasma lipoprotein concentration may influence cyclosporin activity, as the majority of cyclosporin in plasma is bound, exclusively, to lipoproteins. A marked decrease in lipoprotein concentration would lead to an increased proportion of free cyclosporin in plasma, and this might lead to significant increases in the biological activity of cyclosporin even with a similar whole blood trough level.[35]

Rhabdomyolysis is a potentially serious complication of statin therapy.[36] The results of 11 post-transplantation series that used lovastatin, simvastatin, or pravastatin as monotherapy[37-40] have shown a low incidence of rhabdomyolysis (defined as creatinine kinase more than 10 times the upper limit of normal with muscle symptoms): lovastatin = 1.1% (2/186), simvastatin = 1.4% (1/71), and pravastatin = 0% (0/47), or 1.01% (3/304) overall. The incidence of rhabdomyolysis was dose dependent. Interaction with other drugs such as gemfibrozil, nicotinic acid, erythromycin, or itraconozole also increases the risk of rhabdomyolysis. Other drugs metabolised by the cytochrome P450 system, for example macrolides and calcium channel blockers, also increase the risk of this complication. It is advisable that patients on statin therapy should be informed about the potential side-effect of muscular ache and their creatinine kinase levels should be measured on a regular basis. Statins differ in their pharmacokinetic profiles with respect to hydrophilicity, first-pass extraction by the liver, plasma half-life and protein binding. Pharmacokinetic studies have shown that cyclosporin interacts with simvastatin which is lipophilic[39] and also with pravastatin, which is more hydrophilic. In heart transplant recipients co-administration of cyclosporin alters the disposition of pravastatin, producing a 20-fold increase in the area under the curve and a seven-fold increase in maximum plasma concentration (Cmax).[39]

It is generally accepted that low doses of HMG-CoA reductase inhibitors can be used safely in heart transplant recipients. However in some patients who are resistant to lipid-lowering drugs or unable to tolerate statins, LDL apheresis may have a therapeutic benefit. In a pilot study at Harefield Hospital, six heart transplant recipients with refractory hyperlipidaemia and angiographic evidence of ACV had bi-weekly LDL apheresis for a period of 12 months. LDL apheresis was well tolerated and effective in reducing LDL-cholesterol, triglyceride and Lp(a) levels without interfering with plasma cyclosporin level. Others have shown that LDL apheresis with heparin-induced LDL precipitation (HELP system) is effective in reducing LDL-cholesterol, fibrinogen and Lp(a) levels by about 55%, 50% and 60%, respectively. Furthermore the weekly LDL apheresis (HELP system) led to ACV regression.[41] Further large controlled studies are needed to substantiate these findings.

Conclusions

Hyperlipidaemia is common after heart transplantation, with up to 80% of recipients developing a total cholesterol level greater than 220 mg/dl (5.7 mmol/l). The aetiology appears to be multifactorial. Pretransplant diagnosis of ischaemic heart disease and the use of immunosuppressive drugs such as corticosteroids and cyclosporin are contributors to the development of hyperlipidaemia following transplantation. Higher concentrations of serum total cholesterol, triglycerides and Lp(a) are strongly associated with, and predictive of, an increased risk of ACV after heart transplantation.

Hypercholesterolaemia, in particular the oxidised forms of LDL, have been shown to alter the composition of endothelial cell membranes and cause endothelial dysfunction. Recently, an association between the plasma level of oxidised LDL and the extent of transplant ACV has been demonstrated. This association was independent of other possible inducers of endothelial injury.

The management of hyperlipidaemia may have important implications in the prevention of ACV. Dietary modification and optimisation of medical management are the safest forms of treatment of hyperlipidaemia. However these are usually inadequate and lipid-lowering drugs are necessary. Bile acid sequestrants, fibric acid derivatives and nicotinic acid are not recommended due to lack of efficacy and frequent adverse effects. When given in low doses the statins, particularly simvastatin and pravastatin, are well tolerated and highly effective in reducing LDL-cholesterol levels. Recent studies suggest that statin therapy may improve long-term survival.

References

1. Hosenpud JD, Novick RJ, Breen TJ, *et al*. The Registry of the International Society for Heart and Lung Transplantation: twelfth official report — 1995. *J Heart Lung Transplant* 1995; **15**(5):805–15.

2. Reid C, Banner N, O'Brien C, *et al*. Prevalence and significance of coronary artery disease after heart transplantation in patients receiving cyclosporin and azathioprine. *Br Heart J* 1988; **59**:116–20.

3. Fragomeni LS, Kaye MP. The registry of the international society for heart transplantation. Fifth official reports 1988. *J Heart Transplant* 1988; **7**:249–53.

4. Hruban RH, Beschorner WE, Baumgartner WA, *et al*. Accelerated arteriosclerosis in heart transplant recipients is associated with a T-lymphocyte-mediated endothelialitis. *Am J Pathol* 1990; **137**(4):871–82.

5. Salomon RN, Hughes CC, Schoen FJ, *et al*. Human coronary transplantation-associated arteriosclerosis. Evidence for a chronic immune reaction to activated graft endothelial cells. *Am J Pathol* 1991; **138**(4):791–8.

6. Taylor PM, Rose ML, Yacoub MH. Coronary artery immunogenicity: a comparison between explanted recipient or donor hearts and transplanted hearts. *Transplant Immunol* 1993; **1**(4): 294–301.

7. Johnson MR. Transplant coronary disease: nonimmunologic risk factors. *J Heart Lung Transplant* 1992; **11**:S124–S132.

8. Loebe M, Schiller S, Zaus O, *et al*. Role of cytomegalovirus in the development of coronary artery disease in transplanted heart. *J Heart Lung Transplant* 1990; **9**:707–11.

9. Barbir M, Banner N, Thompson GR, *et al*. Relationship of immunosuppression and serum lipids to the development of coronary arterial disease in the transplanted heart. *Int J Cardiol* 1991; **32**(1):51–56.

10. Stamler JS, Vaughan DE, Rudd MA, *et al*. Frequency of hypercholesterolemia after cardiac transplantation. *Am J Cardiol* 1988; **62**: 1268–72.

11. Miller LW, Schlant RC, Kobashigawa J, *et al*. 24th Bethesda conference: Cardiac transplantation Task Force 5: Complications. *J Am Coll Cardiol* 1993; **22**(1):41–54.

12. Ballantyne CM, Jones PH, Payton-Ross C, *et al*. Hyperlipidemia following heart transplantation: natural history and intervention with mevinolin (lovastatin). *Transplant Proc* 1987; **19**(5):60–2.

13. Kirk JK, Dupuis RE. Approaches to the treatment of hyperlipidemia in the solid organ transplant recipient. *Ann Pharmacother* 1995; **29**(9):879–91.

14. Grady LK, Costanzo-Nordin MR, Herold LS, *et al*. Obesity and hyperlipidemia after heart transplantation. *J Heart Lung Transplant* 1991; **10**:449–54.

15. Bilodea M, Fitchett DH, Guerraty A, Sniderman AD. Dyslipidemia after heart and heart–lung transplantation: Potential relations to accelerated graft arteriosclerosis. *J Heart Lung Transplant* 1989; **8**:454–9.

16. Keogh A, Simons L, Spratt P, *et al*. Hyperlipidemia after heart transplantation. *J Heart Transplant* 1988; **7**(3):171–5.

17. Farmer JA, Ballantyne CM, Frazier OH, *et al*. Lipoprotein(a) and apolipoprotein changes after cardiac transplantation. *J Am Coll Cardiol* 1991; **18**:926–30.

18. Taylor DO, Thompson JA, Hastillo A, *et al*. Hyperlipidemia after clinical heart transplantation. *J Heart Transplant* 1989; **8**:209–13.

19. Barbir M, Banner NR, Trayner I, *et al*. High prevalence of lipid and apolipoprotein abnormalities in heart transplant recipients. *European Heart J* 1989; **10**:188 [abstract].

20. Becker DM, Chamberlain B, Swank R. Relationship between corticosteroid exposure and plasma lipid levels in heart transplant recipients. *Am J Med* 1988; **85**(5):632–8.

21. Kemma MS, Valantine HA, Hunt SA, *et al*. Metabolic risk factors for atherosclerosis in heart transplant recipients. *Am Heart J* 1994; **128**:68–72.

22. De Groen PC. Cyclosporine, low density lipoprotein, and cholesterol. *Mayo Clin Proc* 1988; **63**:1012–21.

23. Barbir M, Kushwaha S, Hunt B, *et al*. Lipoprotein(a) and accelerated coronary artery disease in cardiac transplant recipients. *Lancet* 1992; **340**(8834–8835):1500–2.

24. Mehra MR, Ventura HO, Chambers R, *et al*. Predictive model to assess risk for cardiac allo-

graft vasculopathy: an intravascular ultrasound study. *J Am Coll Cardiol* 1995; **26(6)**: 1537–44.

25. Holvoet P, Stassen JM, van Cleemput J, *et al*. Oxidized low density lipoproteins in patients with transplant-associated coronary artery disease. *Arteriosclerosis Thromb Vasc Biol* 1998; **18(1)**:100–7. *Am J Surg Pathol* 1994 **18(4)**:338–46.

26. Gaudin PB, Rayburn BK, Hutchins GM, *et al*. Peritransplant injury to the myocardium associated with the development of accelerated arteriosclerosis in heart transplant recipients. *Am J Surg Pathol* 1994; **18(4)**:338–46.

27. McManus BM, Horley KJ, Wilson JE, *et al*. Prominence of coronary arterial wall lipids in human heart allografts. Implications for pathogenesis of allograft arteriopathy. *Am J Pathol* 1995; **147(2)**:293–308.

28. Barbir M, Hunt B, Kushwaha S, *et al*. Maxepa versus bezafibrate in hyperlipidemic cardiac transplant recipients. *Am J Cardiol* 1992; **70(20)**:1596–601.

29. Summary of the Second Report of the National Cholesterol Education Program (NCEP) Expert Panel on Detection, Evaluation, and Treatment of High Blood Cholesterol in Adults. *JAMA* 1993; **269(23)**:3015–23.

30. Barbir M, Rose M, Kushwaha S, *et al*. Low-dose simvastatin for the treatment of hypercholesterolaemia in recipients of cardiac transplantation. *Int J Cardiol* 1991; **33(2)**: 241–6.

31. Wenke K, Meiser B, Thiery J, *et al*. Simvastatin reduces graft vessel disease and mortality after heart transplantation: a four-year randomized trial. *Circulation* 1997; **96(5)**:1398–402.

32. Kobashigawa JA, Katznelson S, Laks H, *et al*. Effect of pravastatin on outcomes after cardiac transplantation. *N Engl J Med* 1995; **333(10)**:621–7.

33. Cutts JL, Bankhurst AD. Reversal of lovastatin-mediated inhibition of natural killer cell cytotoxicity by interleukin 2. *J Cell Physiol* 1990; **145(2)**:244–52.

34. Meiser BM, Wenke K, Thiery J, *et al*. Simvastatin decreases accelerated graft vessel disease after heart transplantation in an animal model. *Transplant Proc* 1993; **25(2)**:2077–9.

35. Awni WM, Heim-Duthoy K, Kasiske BL. Impact of lipoproteins on cyclosporine pharmacokinetics and biological activity in transplant patients. *Transplant Proc* 1990; **22(3)**:1193–6.

36. Ballantyne CM, Jones PH, Payton-Ross C, *et al*. Hyperlipidemia following heart transplantation: natural history and intervention with mevinolin (lovastatin). *Transplant Proc* 1987; **19(4 suppl. 5)**:60–2.

37. Kuo PC, Kirshenbaum JM, Gordon J, *et al*. Lovastatin therapy for hypercholesterolemia in cardiac transplant recipients. *Am J Cardiol* 1989; **64(10)**:631–65.

38. Pflugfelder PW, Huff M, Oskalns R, *et al*. Cholesterol-lowering therapy after heart transplantation: A 12-month randomized trial. *J Heart Lung Transplant* 1995; **14(4)**: 613–22.

39. Regazzi MB, Iacona I, Campana C, *et al*. Clinical efficacy and pharmacokinetics of HMG-CoA reductase inhibitors in heart transplant patients treated with cyclosporin A. *Transplant Proc* 1994; **26(5)**:2644–5.

40. Kabashikawa JA, Murphy FL, Stevenson LW, *et al*. Low dose lovastatin safely lowers cholesterol after heart transplantation. *Circulation* 1990; **82**:IV281–IV283.

41. Park JW, Merz M, Braun P. Regression of transplant coronary artery disease during chronic low-density lipoprotein-apheresis. *J Heart Lung Transplant* 1997; **16(3)**:290–7.

13

Diabetes, lipids and coronary heart disease: what have we learnt from lipid lowering trials?

George Steiner

The problem of atherosclerosis in diabetes

Atherosclerosis is the most common complication of diabetes.[1] In virtually every population, the risk of atherosclerotic cardiovascular disease in those with diabetes is two to four times greater than it is in those without.[1-5] It is responsible for the death of approximately 75% of those with diabetes, the deaths occurring primarily because of coronary artery disease. Several factors contribute to this increased mortality. The incidence of myocardial infarction is greatly increased in diabetes. Furthermore, the morbidity and case fatality for heart attacks in those who have diabetes is much greater than in those who do not.[6-10] This is both immediately and over the longer period after the heart attack. Because so many who suffer heart attacks die even before reaching adequate medical care, the most effective way to reduce coronary mortality in the general population, as well as in those with diabetes, is to prevent the heart attack from occurring. This chapter will describe the current information available and that being obtained with respect to the effectiveness of intervening in dyslipoproteinemias as a method of coronary risk reduction.

Coronary risk and dyslipoproteinemias

Hyperglycemia is the feature common to both type 1 and type 2 diabetes. However, there is ongoing uncertainty about the role of hyperglycemia itself as a coronary risk factor.[11-15] Both the Diabetes Control and Complications Trial (DCCT)[16] and the United Kingdom Prospective Diabetes Study (UKPDS)[17] found that improved glycemic control had a minor effect on coronary artery disease. Thus, in attempting to reduce atherosclerosis in diabetes, one must pay more attention to other factors. There are many that could lead to the massive increase in atherosclerotic cardiovascular disease in diabetes. Among them are alterations in lipoproteins, which will be covered in this chapter. Other atherogenic factors in diabetes include alterations in coagulation factors,[18-20] nonenzymatic glycation of tissue proteins and of lipoproteins,[21,22] accumulation of advanced glycation endproducts,[23,24] hypertension,[25-28] microalbuminuria and proteinuria,[29,30] possibly insulin resistance and hyperinsulinemia.[31-37]

The lipoproteins in diabetes may be altered both in quantity and in quality. The quantitative changes most commonly seen are an increase in the TG-rich lipoproteins and a decrease in HDL.[38-42] These changes can be seen at[43,44] and even before the diagnosis of diabetes. In general it is agreed that LDL concentrations in diabetes are similar to those in the general population.[45] However, there is some suggestion that with improved control, a person's LDL levels may be somewhat decreased.[45] In the case of LDL, the qualitative changes seen in diabetes are probably more important than are quantitative changes. These qualitative changes include changes in the size and density of LDL,[46–49] glycation of the lipoprotein,[22,50] and its oxidation.[51–53] All of these changes can make lipoproteins more atherogenic.

The term 'dyslipoproteinemias' will be used to describe that group of lipoprotein changes that are present in diabetes. This is because the lipoprotein changes are qualitative as well as quantitative. Furthermore, as triglyceride rich lipoproteins are increased and HDL levels are decreased in diabetes, it would be incorrect to use the term '*hyper*lipoproteinemia'. This chapter will not deal with the causes or nature of the dyslipoproteinemias seen in diabetes. Rather, it will be concerned with the clinical trials of lipoprotein intervention that have been, or are being, conducted in those with diabetes. However, before discussing these trials, one must consider whether the dyslipoproteinemias do increase the risk of coronary artery disease in diabetes.

Although the prevalence of hypercholesterolemia is not increased in diabetes, it still does confer a risk of coronary artery disease. This was clearly demonstrated by the Multiple Risk Factor Intervention Trial.[54] Furthermore, it found that the shape of the curve relating increasing cholesterol levels to an increasing incidence of coronary artery disease in those with diabetes is similar to that in those without diabetes. However, the coronary artery disease risk at any given cholesterol level is two to four times greater in those with diabetes than it is in the general population. One possible reason for this could be that any

given amount of LDL might be more atherogenic in those with diabetes, because of the qualitative changes noted earlier. It is also possible that other factors in diabetes make the artery more susceptible to the atherogenic effects of a given amount of LDL.

The risk impact of hypertriglyceridemia in diabetes has not been so clearly established. The first study to point out a link was the WHO Multinational Study.[55] This was a cross-sectional study of people with diabetes that showed an association between hypertriglyceridemia and ischemic ECG changes. Subsequently, the Paris Prospective Study demonstrated a positive relation between hypertriglyceridemia and coronary artery disease mortality in men with impaired glucose tolerance or diabetes.[56] Unfortunately, that study did not assess HDL levels. It is generally recognized that triglyceride and HDL cholesterol concentrations are inversely related to each other. HDL is generally recognized to be lipoprotein that is associated with a reduced risk of coronary artery disease.[41,57–61] Thus, the risk associated with hypertriglyceridemia might also reflect an increase in coronary disease because of a low concentration of HDL. A more recent prospective study was conducted in Finland. That study demonstrated that both high triglyceride rich lipoprotein and low HDL levels were predictive of CAD in type 2 diabetes.[42,46]

We have examined the relation between coronary disease and the numbers of triglyceride rich lipoprotein particles, not just the concentration of their major lipid triglyceride. Three-quarters of the triglyceride rich lipoproteins are found in the smaller, denser subfraction.[63,64] In a group of people with plasma triglycerides ranging up to approximately 8 mmol/l (309 mg/dl), 70–80% of the difference in plasma triglyceride levels between individuals can be accounted for by an increase in the numbers of particles and only

20–30% by an increase in their size.[63,64] This pattern is similar in diabetes and in the general population. In diabetes the angiographic severity of coronary artery disease is positively related to the numbers of triglyceride rich lipoprotein particles in the plasma.[65] Interestingly, the relationship between the severity of coronary artery disease and triglyceride rich lipoproteins appears to be present in those with mild to moderate coronary disease. However, it disappears as one progresses from moderate to severe disease. This raises the intriguing possibility that other factors become more important in the later occlusive stages of the disorder.

Intervention trials
Rationale

As dyslipoproteinemias are risk factors for atherosclerotic cardiovascular disease in diabetes, one might postulate that correcting them would prevent this major complication. However, it should be recognized that identifying something as a risk factor does not mean that it is a causative factor. It is possible that the dyslipoproteinemia serves only to mark an individual who has other atherogenic factors such as hypertension or a coagulopathy. Furthermore, other atherogenic factors may be so strong in the person with diabetes that they minimize the effects of the dyslipoproteinemias. Finally, perhaps by the time that treatment is initiated in those with diabetes, it may be too late to be of benefit. Therefore, it is vital to examine the postulate that correcting the dyslipoproteinemias in diabetes will reduce the risk of coronary artery disease.

Lipid intervention trials in the general population

Almost all 'lipid intervention studies' reported to date have been undertaken in general populations, not in specific subpopulations such as those with diabetes. Recommendations for those in the special subpopulations by and large have been based on extrapolation from these studies. A large number of studies have consistently demonstrated that reducing LDL-cholesterol levels results in decreased coronary risk. These studies have used both angiographic[66,67] and clinical events as primary endpoints. The latter group have been conducted both as primary intervention trials (that is, in people with no prior clinical coronary artery disease)[68–73] and as secondary intervention trials (that is, in people with prior clinical coronary artery disease).[74,76] They have used many different approaches to lower cholesterol. Many different methods have been used to reduce plasma cholesterol. Early studies used bile acid binding resins,[68,69] and nicotinic acid.[72] Later studies have used a variety of HMG CoA reductase inhibitors,[70,73] partial ileal bypass surgery[71] or lifestyle modification.[77] Regardless of the treatment approach or the endpoint chosen, they have consistently shown a decrease in coronary artery disease. From this, one can conclude that the benefit is not the specific effect of one treatment, but a general effect of the LDL-cholesterol reduction.

The data on triglyceride and HDL levels are fewer. Such as they are, they indicate that intervening in hypertriglyceridemia, possibly with an accompanying increase in HDL, will reduce the risk of coronary artery disease in those who already have it. These observations were made in the Stockholm Ischemic Heart Disease Secondary Intervention Study[78] and in the BECAIT Study.[79] The former was a study using clofibrate and niacin and demonstrated a reduction in reinfarction. The latter used bezafibrate and, although designed as an angiographic study in a small population of men, also found a reduction in clinical events.

The Helsinki Heart Study[80–82] was a primary intervention study that observed a reduction in coronary events in men who were treated with gemfibrozil. This could only partially be explained by the reduction in their LDL levels and also reflected an increase in their HDL levels. Furthermore, while the Helsinki Heart Study was primarily aimed at HDL, the greatest benefit was found in those who had a combination of low HDL and high triglyceride levels.[82] Finally, the very recently concluded Veterans Administration HDL Intervention Trial (VA-HIT) was a secondary intervention study which demonstrated that increasing levels of HDL-cholesterol and reducing levels of plasma triglyceride with gemfibrozil, even in the presence of normal LDL levels, reduces coronary artery disease in a group of men with known coronary disease.[83] There is a general consensus that those at highest risk for coronary artery disease benefit the most from cholesterol reduction. Thus, secondary intervention is more generally accepted as being beneficial than is primary intervention. Against that background, it is important to note that Haffner et al. have reported that the risk of infarction occurring in those with diabetes and no prior infarct is equal to that seen in those who do not have diabetes but have had a prior infarct.[84] Thus, if there is an argument for intervention, some may feel that it is stronger in those with diabetes than it is in those without.

Lipid intervention trials in the diabetic population: post-hoc subgroup analysis

At present, most of the clinical trial information with respect to diabetes comes from studies of large populations, among which a subpopulation had diabetes. That diabetic subgroup was then examined post hoc. This has certain obvious limitations. These include the fact that at randomization the participants were not stratified according to the presence or absence of diabetes. The five that have been published will be reviewed briefly.

The Helsinki Heart Study

As mentioned earlier, a large group of men were treated with gemfibrozil and found to have a significant reduction in their coronary events. This was related not only to the reduction in their LDL-cholesterol levels but also to the increase in their HDL-cholesterol levels. A small number of participants in that study had diabetes. When they were analyzed as a separate subgroup, those treated with gemfibrozil were found to have fewer coronary events.[85] However, the numbers of participants with diabetes and the number of events in that group were far too few to make this significant.

The Veterans Administration HDL Intervention Trial (VA-HIT)

As noted earlier, this study tested the hypothesis that 'raising HDL-cholesterol levels and lowering levels of triglycerides would reduce death from coronary heart disease and nonfatal myocardial infarction in men with coronary heart disease who had low levels of both HDL-cholesterol and LDL-cholesterol'.[83] One-quarter of the population had diabetes, presumably type 2 diabetes. When the study endpoints were expanded to include confirmed stroke, those with diabetes who were treated with active gemfibrozil had a 24% risk reduction, with a significance equal to 0.05 but a 95% confidence interval that went from −0.1 to 43% reduction. Thus, the study provides very suggestive information in those men with diabetes who have existing coronary artery disease. However, it is still limited by the general confines of post-hoc analyses, by the lack of stratification for diabetes at the time of randomization and by its borderline significance.

The Air Force/Texas Coronary Atherosclerosis Prevention Study (AFCAPS/TexCAPS)

This was a large study of healthy middle-aged men and women with average total and LDL-cholesterol levels and below average HDL-cholesterol levels. They were treated with lovastatin or placebo. Among the 6605 participants, 155 had diabetes. During the follow-up period of at least 5 years, six of those with diabetes who were treated with placebo had a coronary event, while this happened in only four of those treated with active drug. Although the trend would appear to be in the right direction and the per cent reduction would appear to be great, the numbers of events and the differences are too small to make even this post-hoc analysis significant.[73]

Scandinavian Simvastatin Survival Study (4S)

In the 4S study, 4444 hypercholesterolemic men and women with preexisting coronary artery disease were treated with simvastatin. There was a significant reduction in coronary and in overall mortality among those in the active treatment group.[74] Of these people, 202 had diabetes. This represented 5% of the 4S population, a prevalence that is much lower than that of diabetes in Scandinavians of similar age. This was because the participants legitimately were selected to fit the primary intent of the study. One of the exclusion criteria was plasma triglyceride levels exceeding 2.5 mmol/l (96.7 mg/dl). Thus, the most frequent form of hyperlipoproteinemia in diabetes, hypertriglyceridemia and low HDL-cholesterol levels, was excluded. Post-

hoc analysis of the data from this subgroup revealed that those who were treated with the active drug had a significant reduction in coronary events.[86] There was no reduction in mortality. However, the numbers of individuals were too few to demonstrate this. It is interesting that there was a tendency toward a greater treatment effect in those who had entry triglyceride levels over 1.7 mmol/l (65.7 mg/dl) than in those whose triglyceride levels were below this.

Cholesterol and Recurrent Events (CARE) Trial

This subgroup analysis examined data from 586 people with diabetes who were part of a total population of 4159 individuals treated with pravastatin or placebo. The mean triglyceride level for the group was 1.85 mmol/l (71.5 mg/dl) and individuals with levels exceeding 2.82 mmol/l (109 mg/dl) were excluded. The risk of coronary events was reduced by 25% in those treated with the active drug.[87]

Long-term Intervention with Pravastatin in Ischemic Disease (LIPID) Trial

Yet another secondary intervention study with pravastatin, the LIPID study, was conducted in Australia. Although the direction of change in coronary events was toward a benefit in the actively treated group, LIPID contrasted to the two other statin studies, in that the reduction in coronary events in the subgroup with diabetes was not significant.[88]

Hence, these three studies have raised very interesting suggestions that treating hypercholesterolemia in diabetes will reduce CAD. However, they are not uniform in their observations and they have their limitations.

Lipid intervention trials designed to examine arteries other than native coronary vessels in the diabetic population

Two studies have been conducted with the primary aim of intervening on plasma lipids in people with diabetes. However, they were not designed to examine the effects of such intervention on native coronary arteries.

The Post Coronary Artery Bypass Graft Study

The Post CABG study used a two-by-two factorial design to examine the effect of warfarin and of intensive versus moderate control of cholesterol on saphenous vein grafts and on clinical events in people who had undergone CABG. Two groups were studied: those with type 2 diabetes and those without. Warfarin had no effect on the outcome of the study subjects. The intensive versus moderate cholesterol reduction was achieved by using a statin alone or in combination with a bile acid binding resin. Intensive cholesterol reduction had the same effect in those with diabetes as it did in those without. There was a risk reduction in both groups. This was noted both as a better angiographic status of the grafted saphenous veins and as a reduction in clinical events. However, the statistical significance of this was low as the 95% confidence intervals all crossed a relative risk of one.[89]

The St Mary's, Ealing, Northwick Park Diabetes Cardiovascular Disease Prevention (SENDCAP) Study

The SENDCAP study, conducted in a group of London hospitals, was designed to determine whether the treatment of dyslipoproteinemias in type 2 diabetes with bezafibrate would affect the intimal medial thickening of the carotid arteries. It did not. However, along with a reduction in triglycerides and an increase in HDL-cholesterol levels, the investigators found that there was a decrease in ischemic heart disease, defined very broadly as MI or ischemic ECG changes.[90]

Lipid intervention trials designed specifically to examine coronary artery disease in the diabetic population

At the time of writing, no study has been completed and reported that has been specifically designed to examine whether correcting dyslipoproteinemias in those with diabetes will reduce the risk of coronary artery disease. Four studies are now underway that are exclusively examining those with diabetes. A fifth has included those with diabetes in its study population. They will be reviewed below and are summarized in Table 13.1.

The Diabetes Atherosclerosis Intervention Study (DAIS)

This is the first of these studies that will be completed. It was started in 1993, at the request of the World Health Organization. DAIS is an angiographic study involving 418 people (305 men and 113 women) with type 2 diabetes, 200 of whom have had previously known coronary disease and 218 of whom have not. It is a double-blind randomized placebo-controlled trial in which the active drug used to treat the dyslipoproteinemias is micronized fenofibrate (200 mg/day). The lipid entry criteria for DAIS are a total cholesterol/HDL-cholesterol ratio greater than or equal to 4 and either an LDL-cholesterol level of 3.5–4.5 mmol/l (135–174 mg/dl) and a triglyceride level less than or equal to 5.2 mmol/l (201 mg/dl) *or* a triglyceride level of 1.7–5.2 mmol/l (65.7–210 mg/dl) and an LDL-cholesterol level less than or equal to 4.5 mmol/l (174 mg/dl). The study is being conducted in 11 clinics located in Canada, Finland, France and Sweden. The details of the DAIS protocol,[91] the population's baseline characteristics,[92] and the angiographic methods[93] have been published. The treatment period, which is between 3 and 5 years, has been completed and the repeat angiograms performed. It is expected that data analysis will be completed and the study results will be reported in the summer of 2000.

It is interesting that 27% of the population in DIAS are women. This figure compares very closely to the 24.7% reported in the MRC/BHF Heart Protection Study (see below). Both of these populations contrast with the gender distribution reported for diabetes in the USA.[94] In the general US population, the rate of diabetes in women is slightly higher than that in men. In the age group 45–65 years, it is equal. The reasons for the lower representation of women in DAIS and in the MRC/BHF Heart Protection Study are not clear. In DIAS, it was noted that once women volunteered and were identified as being potentially eligible for entry, the percentage who were excluded was the same as that for men.[92] This suggested that whatever the reason for the smaller percentage of women, it was something that occurred before the stages of volunteering and identification.

The Fenofibrate Intervention and Event Lowering in Diabetes (FIELD) Trial

The FIELD trial is a second study using micronized fenofibrate (200 mg/day) as its active lipid lowering drug. The endpoints for this study are coronary mortality and coronary events. This study is being conducted in Australia, Finland and New Zealand. It is currently in its active recruitment phase and plans to recruit 8000 men and women with type 2 diabetes: 2000 with and 6000 without prior coronary artery disease. The lipid eligibility

criteria are a total cholesterol/HDL-cholesterol ratio greater than or equal to 4.0 or a fasting triglyceride level greater than or equal to 1.0 mmol/l (38.7 mg/dl) and less than 5.0 mmol/l (193.3 mg/dl). Those with a total cholesterol less than 3.0 mmol/l (116 mg/dl) or greater than 6.5 mmol/l (251.4 mg/dl) (in Finland the upper value is greater than 5.5 mmol/l, or 212.7 mg/dl) are excluded. It is a clinical event study that plans a treatment period of 5–7 years and should report after 2004 (Keech A, personal communication).

The Lipids in Diabetes Study (LDS)

The Lipids in Diabetes Study is also a randomized primary prevention clinical outcome study. The study population will consist of men and women between 40 and 75 years with type 2 diabetes who are not thought to have clinically significant cardiovascular disease. They should have an LDL-cholesterol level less than 4.1 mmol/l (158.5 mg/dl) and triglyceride levels less than 4.5 mmol/l (174 mg/dl). Its unique feature is that it examines the effects of both fenofibrate (200 mg/day) and cerivastatin (0.4 mg/day), using two-by-two factorial design. The study is being conducted in 30 clinics in the United Kingdom and is recruiting 5000 people, 1250 in each treatment cell. It is presently in its active recruitment phase. The treatment period will be at least 5 years and not more than 6.5 years. The planned completion date for this study is 2006.[95]

The Collaborative Atorvastatin Diabetes Study (CARDS)

CARDS is studying the effects of atorvastatin (10 mg/day) in a population of 2120 men and women with type 2 diabetes who have at least one other major coronary risk factor but have no known previous coronary artery disease. The lipid entry criteria for entry are LDL-

	DAIS	FIELD	LDS	CARDS	MTC/BHF HPS
DIABETES	Type 2	Type 2	Type 2	Type 2	Not specified
POPULATION Gender	Men & women	Men & women	Men & women	Men & women	Men & women
Age (years)	40–65	50–75	40–75	40–75	40–80
Numbers	418 recruited	8000 planned	5000 planned	2120 planned	5963 with diabetes of a total population 20 536
Prior clinical CAD (+ve/−ve)	200/218	2000/6000 planned	0/5000	0/2120 but must have ≥1 other risk factor	1978/3985
LIPIDS Plasma triglyceride (mmol/l)	1.7–5.2 if LDL ≤4.5	1.0–5.0 or total/HDL cholesterol as below	<4.5	≤6.78	Not specified
Cholesterol (mmol/l)	LDL 3.5–4.5 if TG ≤5.2	Total 3.0–6.5	LDL <4.1	LDL ≤4.14	Total >3.5
Total/HDL cholesterol	Either of above plus total/HDL cholesterol ≥4.0	Triglyceride as above or total/HDL cholesterol ≥4.0	Not specified	Not specified	Not specified
LIPID INTERVENTION	Micronized fenofibrate	Micronized fenofibrate	Micronized fenofibrate &/or cerivastatin in 2 × 2 design	Atorvastatin	Simvastatin &/or antioxidants in 2 × 2 design
ENDPOINT	Coronary angiographic changes	Coronary mortality and total coronary events	Coronary death & nonfatal MI or revascularization	Coronary death & nonfatal MI or revascularization	Mortality (all-cause & cause-specific)
ANTICIPATED REPORTING	2000	2004	2006	2002	2002

Table 13.1
Summary of lipid intervention trials being undertaken specifically to examine CHD in diabetes

cholesterol levels less than or equal to 4.14 mmol/l (160 mg/dl) and triglyceride levels less than or equal to 6.78 mmol/l (262.2 mg/dl). It is looking for an effect on clinical endpoints and is planned to be completed in 2002 (Betteridge DJ, personal communication).

The MRC/BHF Heart Protection Study

The Heart Protection Study[96] is not confined to those with diabetes. It has a broad population of 20 536 men and women with a prior atherosclerotic cardiovascular disease or diabetes or hypertension and a total blood cholesterol level greater than 3.5 mmol/l (135.3 mg/dl). It uses a two-by-two factorial design to examine the effects of antioxidant vitamins (vitamin E, 600 mg/day plus vitamin C, 250 mg/day plus β-carotene, 20 mg/day) and of simvastatin (40 mg/day). Of the study population, 5963 have known preexisting type 1 or type 2 diabetes. This population was 24.7% female, a figure very similar to that in DAIS: 3985 had known prior coronary disease; 1978 did not. The primary endpoint is all-cause and cause-specific mortality. Once again, it should be completed some time after 2003.

Conclusions

It is clear that the biggest problem confronting the person with diabetes is coronary artery disease. Although improvement in the management of those who have had an infarct is reducing the rate of death from this disease, a much bigger impact will be made when it can be prevented. This will not only cut down coronary mortality. It will greatly reduce the morbidity associated with chronic ischemic heart disease. Although a number of risk factors that contribute to coronary disease in diabetes have been identified, information about

the effects of reversing them is limited at best. Most information that is available relates to the dyslipoproteinemias, and among them to hypercholesterolemia. This information is based largely on extrapolation from intervention trials in general populations. Those few studies that have included people with diabetes have, on post-hoc subgroup analysis, suggested that similar benefits will be obtained. However, these studies are secondary intervention studies, have the limitations of post-hoc subgroup analyses, and in some cases are of marginal or no significance. Currently there are some studies underway that are specifically designed to examine whether correcting the dyslipoproteinemias occurring in diabetes will reduce the risk of coronary artery disease. Thus, over the next few years there should be a more definitive answer to this question.

References

1. Steiner G. Atherosclerosis, the major complication of diabetes. In: Vranic M, Hollenberg CH, Steiner G, eds. *Comparison of Type I and Type II Diabetes: Similarities and Dissimilarities in Etiology, Pathogenesis and Complications.* New York: Plenum Press, 1985: 277–97.
2. Steiner G. Diabetes and atherosclerosis—a lipoprotein perspective. *Diabetic Med* 1997; **14**:S38–S44.
3. Keen H, Jarrett RJ. The WHO multinational study of vascular disease in diabetes: 2. Macrovascular disease prevalence. *Diabetes Care* 1979; **2**:187–95.
4. Burchfiel CM, Reed DM, Marcus EB, *et al.* Association of diabetes mellitus with coronary atherosclerosis and myocardial lesions. An autopsy study from the Honolulu Heart program. *Am J Epidemiol* 1993; **137**:1328–40.
5. Howard BV, Lee ET, Cowan LD, *et al.* Coronary heart disease prevalence and its relation to risk factors in American Indians. The Strong Heart Study. *Am J Epidemiol* 1995; **142**:254–68.
6. Miettinen H, Lehto S, Salomaa V, *et al.* Impact

of diabetes on mortality after the first myocardial infarction. The FINMONICA Myocardial Infarction Register Study group. *Diabetes Care* 1998; **21**:69–75.

7. Maher M, Singh HP, Dias S, *et al*. Coronary artery bypass surgery in the diabetic patient. *Ir J Med Sci* 1995; **164**:136–38.

8. Jaffe AS, Spadaro JJ, Schechtman K, *et al*. Increased congestive heart failure after myocardial infarction of modest extent in patients with diabetes mellitus. *Am Heart J* 1984; **108**:31–37.

9. Lehto S, Pyorala K, Miettinen H, *et al*. Myocardial infarct size and mortality in patients with non-insulin-dependent diabetes mellitus. *J Intern Med* 1994; **236**:291–97.

10. Gwilt DJ, Petri M, Lewis PW, *et al*. Myocardial infarct size and mortality in diabetic patients. *Br Heart J* 1985; **54**:466–72.

11. Folsom AR, Eckfeldt JH, Weitzman S, *et al*. Relation of carotid artery wall thickness to diabetes mellitus, fasting glucose and insulin, body size, and physical activity. Atherosclerosis Risk in Communities (ARIC) Study Investigators. *Stroke* 1994; **25**:66–73.

12. Behar S, Boyko V, Benderly M, *et al*. Asymptomatic hyperglycemia in coronary heart disease: frequency and associated lipid and lipoprotein levels in the bezafibrate infarction prevention (BIP) register. The BIP Study Group. *J Cardiovasc Risk* 1995; **2**:241–46.

13. Lehto S, Ronnemaa T, Haffner SM, *et al*. Dyslipidemia and hyperglycemia predict coronary heart disease events in middle-aged patients with NIDDM. *Diabetes* 1997; **46**:1354–59.

14. Fuller JH, McCartney P, Jarrett RJ, *et al*. Hyperglycemia and coronary heart disease: the Whitehall Study. *J Chronic Dis* 1979; **32**:721–28.

15. Barrett-Connor E, Ferrara A. Isolated postchallenge hyperglycemia and the risk of fatal cardiovascular disease in older women and men. The Rancho Bernardo Study. *Diabetes Care* 1998; **21**:1236–39.

16. Anonymous. Effect of intensive diabetes management on macrovascular events and risk factors in the Diabetes Control and Complications Trial. *Am J Cardiol* 1995; **75**:894–903.

17. Anonymous. Intensive blood-glucose control with sulphonylureas or insulin compared with conventional treated and risk of complications in patients with type 2 diabetes (UKPDS 33). UK Prospective Diabetes Study (UKPDS) Group. *Lancet* 1998; **352**:837–53.

18. Colwell JA. Pathophysiology of vascular disease in diabetes: effects of gliclazide. *Am J Med* 1991; **90**:S50–S54.

19. Kelleher CC. Plasma fibrinogen and factor VII as risk factors for cardiovascular disease. *Eur J Epidemiol* 1992; **8**:79–82.

20. Kannel WB, D'Agostino RB, Wilson PW, *et al*. Diabetes, fibrinogen, and risk of cardiovascular disease: the Framingham experience. *Am Heart J* 1990; **120**:672–76.

21. Lyons TJ, Lopes-Virella MF. Glycation related mechanisms. In: Draznin B, Eckel RH, eds. *Diabetes and Atherosclerosis*. Amsterdam: Elsevier; 1993: 169–90.

22. Lyons TJ. Lipoprotein glycation and its metabolic consequences. *Diabetes* 1992; **41**: S67–S73.

23. Bucala R, Vlassara H. Advanced glycosylation end products in diabetic renal and vascular disease. *Am J Kidney Dis* 1995; **26**:875–88.

24. Nakamura Y, Horii Y, Nishino T, *et al*. Immunohistochemical localization of advanced glycosylation end products in coronary atheroma and cardiac tissue in diabetes mellitus. *Am J Pathol* 1993; **143**:1649–56.

25. Hsueh WA, Anderson PW. Systemic hypertension and the renin–angiotensin system in diabetic vascular complications. *Am J Cardiol* 1993; **72**:H14–H21.

26. Giugliano D, Ceriello A, Paolisso G. Diabetes mellitus, hypertension, and cardiovascular disease: which role for oxidative stress? *Metabolism* 1995; **44**:363–68.

27. Ferrannini E, Santoro D, Manicardi V. The association of essential hypertension and diabetes. *Compr Ther* 1989; **15**:51–58.

28. Davis BR, Cutler JA, Gordon DJ, *et al*. Rationale and design for the Antihypertensive and Lipid Lowering Treatment to Prevent Heart Attack Trial (ALLHAT). ALLHAT Research Group. *Am J Hypertens* 1996; **9**:342–60.

29. Kuusisto J, Mykkanen L, Pyorala K, Laakso M. Hyperinsulinemic microalbuminuria. A new risk indicator for coronary heart disease. *Circulation* 1995; **91**:831–37.

30. Lanfredini M, Fiorina P, Peca MG, *et al.* Fasting and post-methionine load homocyst(e)ine values are correlated with microalbuminuria and could contribute to worsening vascular damage in non-insulin-dependent diabetes mellitus patients. *Metab Clin Exper* 1998; **47**:915–21.

31. Barakat HA, Carpenter JW, McLendon VD, *et al.* Influence of obesity, impaired glucose tolerance, and NIDDM on LDL structure and composition. Possible link between hyperinsulinemia and atherosclerosis. *Diabetes* 1990; **39**:1527–33.

32. Bavenholm P, Proudler A, Tornvall P, *et al.* Insulin, intact and split proinsulin, and coronary artery disease in young men. *Circulation* 1995; **92**: 1422–29.

33. Katz RJ, Ratner RE, Cohen RM, *et al.* Are insulin and proinsulin independent risk markers for premature coronary artery disease? *Diabetes* 1996; **45**:736–41.

34. Laakso M. Insulin resistance and coronary heart disease. *Curr Opin Lipidol* 1996; **7**: 217–26.

35. Modan M, Or J, Karasik A, *et al.* Hyperinsulinemia, sex, and risk of atherosclerotic cardiovascular disease. *Circulation* 1991; **84**: 1165–75.

36. Fontbonne AM, Eschwege EM. Insulin and cardiovascular disease. Paris Prospective Study. *Diabetes Care* 1991; **14**:461–69.

37. Despres JP, Lamarche B, Mauriege P, *et al.* Hyperinsulinemia as an independent risk factor for ischemic heart disease. *N Engl J Med* 1996; **334**:952–57.

38. Steiner G. Diabetes mellitus, dyslipoproteinaemias and atherosclerosis. *Diabetologia* 1997; **40**:S147–S148.

39. Steiner G, Dyslipoproteinemias in diabetes. *Med Clin Exp* 1995; **18**:282–87.

40. Laakso M, Pyörälä K. Lipid and lipoprotein abnormalities in diabetic patients with peripheral vascular disease. *Atherosclerosis* 1988; **74**:55–63.

41. Laakso M. Lipids and lipoproteins as risk factors for coronary heart disease in non-insulin-dependent diabetes mellitus. *Ann Med* 1996; **28**:341–45.

42. Laakso M., Dyslipidemia, morbidity, and mortality in non-insulin-dependent diabetes mellitus. Lipoproteins and coronary heart disease in non-insulin-dependent diabetes mellitus. *J Diabetes Complications* 1997; **11**:137–41.

43. Anonymous. UK Prospective Diabetes Study 27. Plasma lipids and lipoproteins at diagnosis of NIDDM by age and sex. *Diabetes Care* 1997; **20**:1683–87.

44. Mykkanen L, Kuusisto J, Haffner SM, *et al.* Hyperinsulinemia predicts multiple atherogenic changes in lipoproteins in elderly subjects. *Arterioscler Thromb* 1994; **14**:518–26.

45. Reaven PD, Picard S, Witztum J. Low-density lipoprotein metabolism in diabetes. In: Draznin B, Eckel RH, eds. *Diabetes and Atherosclerosis. Molecular Basis and Clinical Aspects.* New York: Elsevier, 1993: 17–38.

46. Gray RS, Robbins DC, Wang W, *et al.* Relation of LDL size to the insulin resistance syndrome and coronary heart disease in American Indians. The Strong Heart Study. *Arterioscler Thromb Vasc Biol* 1997; **17**:2713–20.

47. Lahdenpera S, Tilly-Kiesi M, Vuorinen-Markkola H, *et al.* Effects of gemfibrozil on low-density lipoprotein particle size, density, distribution, and composition in patients with type II diabetes. *Diabetes Care* 1993; **16**:584–92.

48. Lahdenpera S, Sane T, Vuorinen-Markkola H, *et al.* LDL particle size in mildly hypertriglyceridemic subjects: no relation to insulin resistance or diabetes. *Atherosclerosis* 1995; **113**:227–36.

49. Austin MA, Hokanson JE, Brunzell JD. Characterization of low-density lipoprotein subclasses: methodologic approaches and clinical relevance. *Curr Opin Lipidol* 1994; **5**: 395–403.

50. Austin MA. Small dense low-density lipoprotein as a risk factor for coronary heart disease. *Int J Clin Lab Res* 1994; **24**:187–92.

51. Kawamura M, Heinecke JW, Chait A. Pathophysiological concentrations of glucose promote oxidative modification of low density lipoprotein by a superoxide-dependent pathway. *J Clin Invest* 1994; **94**:771–78.

52. Chait A, Brazg RL, Tribble DL, Krauss RM. Susceptibility of small, dense, low-density lipoproteins to oxidative modification in subjects with the atherogenic lipoprotein phenotype, pattern B. *Am J Med* 1993; **94**:350–56.

53. Grundy SM. Oxidized LDL and atherogenesis: relation to risk factors for coronary heart disease. *Clin Cardiol* 1993; **16**:13–15.

54. Stamler J, Vaccaro O, Neaton JD, Wentworth D. Diabetes, other risk factors, and 12-yr cardiovascular mortality for men screened in the Multiple Risk Factor Intervention Trial. *Diabetes Care* 1993; **16**:434–44.

55. West KM, Ahuja MM, Bennett PH, *et al*. The role of circulating glucose and triglyceride concentrations and their interactions with other 'risk factors' as determinants of arterial disease in nine diabetic population samples from the WHO multinational study. *Diabetes Care* 1983; **6**:361–69.

56. Fontbonne A, Eschwege E, Cambien F, *et al*. Hypertriglyceridaemia as a risk factor of coronary heart disease mortality in subjects with impaired glucose tolerance or diabetes. Results from the 11-year follow-up of the Paris Prospective Study. *Diabetologia* 1989; **32**: 300–4.

57. Drexel H, Amann FW, Rentsch K, *et al*. Relation of the level of high-density lipoprotein subfractions to the presence and extent of coronary artery disease. *Am J Cardiol* 1992; **70**:436–40.

58. Hamsten A, Walldius G, Szamosi A, *et al*. Relationship of angiographically defined coronary artery disease to serum lipoproteins and apolipoproteins in young survivors of myocardial infarction. *Circulation* 1986; **73**:1097–110.

59. Corti MC, Guralnik JM, Salive ME, *et al*. HDL cholesterol predicts coronary heart disease mortality in older persons [see comments]. *JAMA* 1995; **274**:539–44.

60. Frick MH, Syvanne M, Nieminen MS, *et al*. Prevention of the angiographic progression of coronary and vein-graft atherosclerosis by gemfibrozil after coronary bypass surgery in men with low levels of HDL cholesterol. Lipid Coronary Angiography Trial (LOCAT) Study Group. *Circulation* 1997; **96**:2137–43.

61. Streja D, Steiner G, Kwiterovich PO Jr. Plasma high-density lipoproteins and ischemic heart disease: studies in a large kindred with familial hypercholesterolemia. *Ann Intern Med* 1978; **89**:871–80.

62. Laakso M, Lehto S, Penttila I, Pyorälä K. Lipids and lipoproteins predicting coronary heart disease mortality and morbidity in patients with non-insulin-dependent diabetes. *Circulation* 1993; **88**:1421–30.

63. Poapst M, Reardon M, Steiner G. Relative contribution of triglyceride-rich lipoprotein particle size and number to plasma triglyceride concentration. *Arteriosclerosis* 1985; **5**:381–90.

64. Steiner G, Tkac I, Uffelman KD, Lewis GF. Important contribution of lipoprotein particle number to plasma triglyceride concentration in type 2 diabetes. *Atherosclerosis* 1998; **137**:211–14.

65. Tkac I, Kimball BP, Lewis G, *et al*. The severity of coronary atherosclerosis in type 2 diabetes mellitus is related to the number of circulating triglyceride-rich lipoprotein particles. *Arterioscler Thromb Vasc Biol* 1997; **17**:3633–38.

66. Brown G, Albers JJ, Fisher LD, *et al*. Regression of coronary artery disease as a result of intensive lipid-lowering therapy in men with high levels of apolipoprotein B. *N Engl J Med* 1990; **323**:1289–98.

67. Blankenhorn DH, Azen SP, Kramsch DM, *et al*. Coronary angiographic changes with lovastatin therapy. The monitored atherosclerosis regression study (MARS). *Ann Intern Med* 1993; **119**:969–76.

68. Anonymous. The Lipid Research Clinics Coronary Primary Prevention Trial results I. Reduction in the incidence of coronary heart disease. *JAMA* 1984; **251**:351–64.

69. Anonymous. The Lipid Research Clinics Coronary Primary Prevention Trial results. II. The relationship of reduction in incidence of coronary heart disease to cholesterol lowering. *JAMA* 1984; **251**:365–74.

70. Anonymous. Influence of pravastatin on plasma lipids on clinical events in the West of Scotland Coronary Prevention Study (WOSCOPS). *Circulation* 1998; **97**:1440–45.

71. Buchwald H, Varco RL, Boen JE, *et al*. Effective lipid modification by partial ileal bypass reduced long-term coronary heart disease mortality and morbidity: five-year posttrial follow-up report from the POSCH. Program on the Surgical Control of the Hyperlipidemias. *Arch Intern Med* 1998; **158**:1253–61.

72. Canner PL, Berge KG, Wenger NK, *et al*. Fif-

teen year mortality in Coronary Drug Project patients: long-term benefit with niacin. *J Am Coll Cardiol* 1986; **8**:1245–55.

73. Downs JR, Clearfield M, Weis S, *et al*. Primary prevention of acute coronary events with lovastatin in men and women with average cholesterol levels: results of AFCAPS/Tex-CAPS. Air Force/Texas Coronary Atherosclerosis Prevention Study. *JAMA* 1998; **279**: 1615–22.

74. Anonymous. Randomised trial of cholesterol lowering in 4444 patients with coronary heart disease: the Scandinavian Simvastatin Survival Study (4S). *Lancet* 1994; **344**:1383–89.

75. Anonymous. Design, rational, and baseline characteristics of the Prospective Pravastatin Pooling (PPP) project – a combined analysis of three large-scale randomized trials: Long-term Intervention with Pravastatin in Ischemic Disease (LIPID), Cholesterol and Recurrent Events (CARE), and West of Scotland Coronary Prevention Study (WOSCOPS). *Am J Cardiol* 1995; **76**:899–905.

76. Sacks FM, Pfeffer MA, Moye LA, *et al*. The effect of pravastatin on coronary events after myocardial infarction in patients with average cholesterol levels. Cholesterol and recurrent Events Trial investigators. *N Engl J Med* 1996; **335**:1001–9.

77. Ornish D, Scherwitz LW, Billings JH, *et al*. Intensive lifestyle changes for reversal of coronary heart disease. *JAMA* 1998; **280**:2001–7.

78. Carlson LA, Rosenhamer G. Reduction of mortality in the Stockholm Ischaemic Heart Disease Secondary Prevention Study by combined treatment with clofibrate and nicotinic acid. *Acta Med Scand* 1988; **223**:405–18.

79. Ericsson CG. Results of the Bezafibrate Coronary Atherosclerosis Intervention Trial (BECAIT) and an update on trials now in progress. *Eur Heart J* 1998; **19**:37H–41H.

80. Manninen V, Elo MO, Frick MH, *et al*. Lipid alterations and decline in the incidence of coronary heart disease in the Helsinki Heart Study. *JAMA* 1988; **260**:641–51.

81. Frick MH, Elo O, Haapa K, Heinonen OP, *et al*. Helsinki Heart Study: primary-prevention trial with gemfibrozil in middle-aged men with dyslipidemia. Safety of treatment, changes in risk factors, and incidence of coronary heart disease. *N Engl J Med* 1987; **317**:1237–45.

82. Manninen V, Tenkanen L, Koskinen P, *et al*. Joint effects of serum triglyceride and LDL cholesterol and HDL cholesterol concentrations on coronary heart disease risk in the Helsinki Heart Study. Implications for treatment. *Circulation* 1992; **85**:37–45.

83. Bloomfield Rubins H, Robins SJ, Collins D, *et al*. Gemfibrozil for the secondary prevention of coronary heart disease in men with low levels of high-density lipoprotein cholesterol. *N Engl J Med* 1999; **341**:410–18.

84. Haffner SM, Lehto S, Ronnemaa T, *et al*. Mortality from coronary heart disease in subjects with type 2 diabetes and in nondiabetic subjects with and without prior myocardial infarction. *N Engl J Med* 1998; **339**:229–34.

85. Koskinen P, Manttari M, Manninen V, *et al*. Coronary heart disease incidence in NIDDM patients in the Helsinki Heart Study. *Diabetes Care* 1992; **15**:820–25.

86. Pyorälä K, Pedersen TR, Kjekshus J, *et al*. Cholesterol lowering with simvastatin improves prognosis of diabetic patients with coronary heart disease. A subgroup analysis of the Scandinavian Simvastatin Survival Study (4S). *Diabetes Care* 1997; **20**:614–20.

87. Goldberg RB, Mellies MJ, Sacks FM, *et al*. Cardiovascular events and their reduction with pravastatin in diabetic and glucose-intolerant myocardial infarction survivors with average cholesterol levels: subgroup analyses in the cholesterol and recurrent events (CARE) trial. The Care Investigators. *Circulation* 1998; **98**:2513–19.

88. Anonymous. Prevention of cardiovascular events and death with pravastatin in patients with coronary heart disease and a broad range of initial cholesterol levels. The Long-Term Intervention with Pravastatin in Ischaemic Disease (LIPID) Study Group. *N Engl J Med* 1998; **339**:1349–57.

89. Hoogwerf BJ, Waness A, Cressman M, *et al*. Effects of aggressive cholesterol lowering and low-dose anticoagulation on clinical and angiographic outcomes in patients with diabetes: the Post Coronary Artery Bypass Graft Trial. *Diabetes* 1999; **48**:1289–94.

90. Elkeles RS, Diamond JR, Poulter C, *et al*. Cardiovascular outcomes in type 2 diabetes. A

double-blind placebo-controlled study of bezafibrate: the St. Mary's, Ealing, Northwick Park Diabetes Cardiovascular Disease Prevention (SENDCAP) Study. *Diabetes Care* 1998; **21**:641–48.

91. Steiner G. The Diabetes Atherosclerosis Intervention Study (DAIS): a study conducted in cooperation with the World Health Organization. The DAIS Project Group. *Diabetologia* 1996; **39**:1655–61.

92. Steiner G, Stewart D, Hosking JD. Baseline characteristics of the study population in the Diabetes Atherosclerosis Intervention Study (DAIS). *Am J Cardiol* 1999; **84**:1004–10.

93. McLaughlin PR, Gladstone P. Diabetes Atherosclerosis Intervention Study (DAIS): quantitative coronary angiographic analysis of coronary artery atherosclerosis. *Cathet Cardiovasc Diag* 1998; **44**:249–56.

94. Kenny SJ, Aubert RE, Geiss LS. National Diabetes Data Group. eds. NIH Publication No. 95-1468. 47–68. 1995. In: *Diabetes in America*, 2nd edn. National Institutes of Health, National Institutes of Diabetes and Digestive and Kidney Diseases; 1995: 47–68.

95. Holman RR. Lipids in Diabetes Study. *Diabetes* 1999; **48**:A362.

96. Anonymous. MRC/BHF Heart Protection Study of cholesterol-lowering therapy and of antioxidant vitamin supplementation in a wide range of patients at increased risk of coronary heart disease death: early safety and efficacy experience. *Eur Heart J* 1999; **20**:725–41.

14

Lowering cardiovascular risk by cholesterol reduction: evidence from observational studies and randomised trials

Malcolm Law

Introduction

After decades of controversy, there is no longer serious dissent from the fact that increasing serum cholesterol is an important cause of cardiovascular disease and that lowering serum cholesterol reduces risk. Indeed the high fat diet typical of many Western countries over the greater part of the 20th century is the major underlying factor in the epidemic of ischaemic heart disease. Modern cholesterol lowering drugs, used in adequate dosages, can substantially reduce mortality.[1]

Serum total and LDL-cholesterol

The high saturated fat content of the diet in Western countries means that the entire distribution of serum total and low density lipoprotein- (LDL-) cholesterol is high in relation to those in other communities. Table 14.1 illustrates this for total serum cholesterol, by showing average levels in contrasting populations.[2] These data question the use of the term 'normal' in reference to average Western cholesterol levels: subsistence farming and hunter–gatherer societies have serum choles-

This chapter is adapted, with permission, from Law M. Lipids and cardiovascular disease. In: Yusuf S, Camm J, Cairns J, *et al.*, eds. *Evidence Based Cardiology*. London: BMJ Books; 1998: 191–205.

terol levels of about 3.5 mmol/l (130 mg/dl). Since these are likely to be typical of those in human populations throughout almost all of mankind's time on Earth, the level of about 3.5 mmol/l may be the best definition of 'normal'. The term hypercholesterolaemia could be applied to average Western levels.

Of the average total serum cholesterol of 6.0 to 6.4 mmol/l (230 to 250 mg/dl) in middle-aged and older adults in Western populations, two-thirds is low density lipoprotein- (LDL-) cholesterol and one-quarter is high density lipoprotein- (HDL-) cholesterol. Many of the large epidemiological studies and randomised trials measured only total serum cholesterol, and results based on total serum cholesterol have been taken to estimate effects of LDL-cholesterol. Fortuitously the approximation is a good one. The absolute reduction in total serum cholesterol produced by diet and by most drugs is similar to the reduction in LDL-cholesterol (simvastatin for example reduced total and LDL-cholesterol by 1.8 mmol/l (70 mg/dl).[1] Observational differences between individuals in total cholesterol are close to the corresponding differences in LDL-cholesterol, because HDL-cholesterol is independent of total serum cholesterol.[3,4] This arises because the tendency for HDL-cholesterol to be positively associated with total cholesterol, because HDL-cholesterol is part of the total, is offset by the small inverse association

Population	Cholesterol (mmol/l)
Hunter–gatherer societies	3.0–3.5
Rural China	3.5
Japan: rural	4.5
urban	5.0
Mediterranean areas	5.2–5.6
USA	5.7
Northern Europe	6.0–6.4
Finland (20 years ago)	7.0

Levels of low density lipoprotein- (LDL-) cholesterol are about 2 mmol/l lower in each population.[2]

Table 14.1
Typical total serum cholesterol values in men aged 45 to 64 years in different populations

between HDL and LDL-cholesterol.[3] Much epidemiological and clinical trial data are therefore available in estimating quantitatively the effect of lowering serum LDL-cholesterol on the risk of ischaemic heart disease.

Serum cholesterol and ischaemic heart disease

Three important practical questions arise — the nature of the dose–response relationship, the size of the effect and the speed of the reversal of risk. To answer these questions, data from both observational epidemiology (cohort or prospective studies) and from randomised controlled trials are necessary. The two are complementary, examining trial data alone is misleading. Table 14.2 summarises the advantages of each. In cohort studies there is no intervention; serum cholesterol is measured in a large number of individuals and subsequent heart disease mortality (or incidence of myocardial infarction) is recorded. Cohort studies are therefore easier to conduct than trials and can be much larger with a longer follow-up period. Accordingly their statistical

power is greater, and they can examine the association across a wider range of serum cholesterol values and a wider range of ages than the trials have done. Cohort studies are thus the more informative on the nature of the dose–response relationship and the size of the effect at different ages. Differences between individuals in total and LDL-cholesterol that are observed in cohort studies will have been present for many years before the time of recruitment, so cohort studies, in contrast to trials, show the effects of long-term cholesterol differences. Trials show the effect of short-term differences — how rapidly risk can be reversed.

Most of the cohort studies and trials of cholesterol and ischaemic heart disease recruited men — for reasons of economy as ischaemic heart disease is more common in men. The limited data from women indicate a similar effect as that found in men.[1,5]

The nature of the dose–response relationship: is there a threshold?

Figure 14.1 shows mortality from ischaemic heart disease in a large cohort study of serum cholesterol and ischaemic heart disease

Objective	Advantage (comment)
Statistical power	Cohort studies (recorded about three times more ischaemic heart disease events than the trials)
Dose–response relationship	Cohort studies (observation across wider range of cholesterol levels)
Wide age range	Cohort studies (ischaemic heart disease events occurred at age 35–85, mostly 55–65 in trials)
Long-term effects of cholesterol differences	Cohort studies (on recruitment the serum cholesterol differences between persons had been present for many years beforehand)
Short-term effects of cholesterol differences	Randomised trials (on recruitment serum cholesterol was the same in intervention and control groups)
Avoid bias	Randomised trials (not a major advantage — bias in cohort studies can be allowed for)

Table 14.2
Relative advantages of cohort studies and randomised trials in assessing the relationship between serum cholesterol and ischaemic heart disease

Fig. 14.1
Mortality from ischaemic heart disease (with 95% confidence intervals) according to serum cholesterol in a large cohort study.[6]

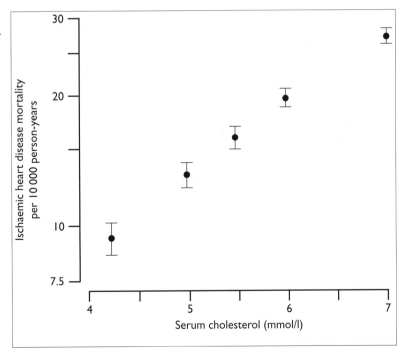

(MRFIT Screenees).[6] The subjects are divided into fifths of the ranked serum cholesterol measurements. With ischaemic heart disease plotted on a logarithmic scale the relationship is described almost perfectly by a straight line linking the proportional change in ischaemic heart disease to the absolute difference in serum cholesterol ($r = 0.997$). Other cohort studies show the same relationship.[5] The 95% confidence limits of the risk estimates in each sub-group do not overlap, establishing that there is no threshold below which a further decrease in serum cholesterol is not associated with a further decrease in risk of ischaemic heart disease. The exponential relationship indicated by the straight line means that a given absolute difference in serum cholesterol concentration from any point on the cholesterol distribution is associated with a constant percentage difference in the incidence of ischaemic heart disease.

This absence of a threshold has been contentious; many published guidelines on lowering cholesterol invoke one. Yet the evidence is firmly against any threshold. The data in Figure 14.1 (which alone are conclusive) are supported by data from other large cohort studies,[5] including one from China which shows that the continuous relationship extends below serum cholesterol levels of 4 mmol/l (160 mg/dl).[7] In the '4S' trial serum cholesterol was lowered to about 4 mmol/l in the quarter of the patients with lowest total or LDL-cholesterol on entry, and the proportionate reduction in myocardial infarction and heart disease death in these patients was similar to that in patients with higher serum cholesterol on entry,[8] again excluding a threshold above 4 mmol/l. Experimental data on the transfer of cholesterol from the blood into atheromatous lesions exclude a threshold as low as 1 mmol/l (40 mg/dl).[9]

The size of the long-term effect

As above, cohort studies estimate the long-term effect because the serum cholesterol differences between individuals recorded on entry to a cohort study will have been present for decades beforehand. Trials, on the other hand, show the effect of short-term differences. Cohort studies are subject to bias but this can be corrected. The major bias is the so-called 'regression dilution bias',[3] which effects not only serum cholesterol but non-interventional studies of all associations in which the explanatory (horizontal axis) variable is, like serum cholesterol, subject to random fluctuation over time in an individual. For example, in a group of men all selected because a single serum cholesterol reading was relatively high (say about 7 mmol/l (270 mg/dl)), the true (long-term average) level will be closer to 6 mmol/l (230 mg/dl) in some of the men (in whom the single reading of 7 mmol/l was unusually high), and closer to 8 mmol/l (310 mg/dl) in others (in whom the single reading of 7 mmol/l was unusually low). A long-term average serum cholesterol of 6 mmol/l is common, however, and one of 8 mmol/l uncommon, so in the group as a whole the long-term average serum cholesterol will be lower than 7 mmol/l. Correspondingly in a group of men selected because a single cholesterol measurement was relatively low (say about 5 mmol/l (190 mg/dl)) the long-term average will be greater than this. The effect is that random error introduces bias. The range of serum cholesterol concentrations based on single measurements will be wider than that based on long-term average levels. Both are associated with the same range of heart disease death rates, so a plot of heart disease mortality against serum cholesterol concentration will be steeper (by about 50%)[3] if based on long-term average levels.

| Age (years) | Estimated percentage decrease in risk for a serum cholesterol reduction (mmol/l) of: | | | |
	0.3 (5%)	0.6 (10%)	1.2 (20%)	1.8 (30%)
40	32	54	79	90
50	22	39	63	77
60	15	27	47	61
70	11	20	36	49
80	10	19	34	47

From 10 cohort studies.[5]

Table 14.3
Estimates of the percentage decrease in risk of ischaemic heart disease according to extent of serum cholesterol reduction and age

Table 14.3 shows estimates of the long-term percentage decrease in the risk of ischaemic heart disease according to the decrease in serum cholesterol concentration and age at death. The estimates are taken from an analysis of the 10 largest cohort studies, corrected for the regression dilution bias and for the minor distinction between differences in total and in LDL-cholesterol discussed above.[3,5] A cholesterol reduction of 0.6 mmol/l (23 mg/dl) (about 10%) is associated with a decrease in risk of ischaemic heart disease of about 50% at age 40, 40% at 50, 30% at 60 and 20% at 70–80. The proportionate decrease in risk decreases with age, but the absolute benefit increases because the disease becomes more common with age. The increasing reduction in risk with greater reduction in serum cholesterol shown in Table 14.3 follows from the continuous relationship described above. For a 0.6 mmol/l cholesterol reduction at age 60, for example, the reduction in risk is 27% and the relative risk is therefore 0.73; with a serum cholesterol reduction three times as great (1.8 mmol/l or 70 mg/dl) the relative risk is 0.73 raised to the third power (0.73^3), which is 0.39 — corresponding to a reduction in risk of 61% as shown in Table 14.3.

Speed of reversal and consistency of observational and trial data

Randomised trials, as discussed above, show how quickly the long-term difference in heart disease risk (from cohort studies) can be attained after a serum cholesterol reduction. Analysis of the older cholesterol lowering trials (testing all interventions except statin drugs), in which the average serum cholesterol reduction was 0.6 mmol/l, showed that in the first two years there was little reduction in risk (in fact none in the first year), but between two and five the average reduction in risk was 22%, and after five years the reduction was 25%.[5] The ischaemic heart disease events in these trials mostly occurred at an average age of about 60, and at this age the estimate of the long-term effect from the cohort studies is 27% (Table 14.3). The similarity of the estimates of effect from the cohort studies and from the trial data from the third year onwards therefore indicate that the reversal of risk is near maximal after two years — a surprisingly rapid effect.

The trial data show that the proportionate reduction in risk from lowering serum cholesterol is similar in persons with and without previous myocardial infarction or other clinical evidence of coronary artery disease.[5]

Six large trials of 'statin' drugs have been published (Table 14.4).[1,10–14] The serum cholesterol reduction attained (1.0–1.8 mmol/l or 40–70 mg/dl), substantially greater than in the older trials) and the reduction in coronary events (also substantial) are shown. Importantly, however, this too depended on duration of follow-up: these recent trials, like the older ones, showed a relatively small proportionate reduction in heart disease in the first two years, but a reduction after two years that is close to the maximum indicated by the cohort studies. The average age for incurring an ischaemic heart disease event was again about 60 years. In one of the trials the average reduction in serum total and LDL-cholesterol was 1.8 mmol/l (70 mg/dl).[1] The expected long-term reduction in ischaemic heart disease mortality (Table 14.3) is 61% and this was close to the observed reduction in the trial from the third year onwards. In the other large statin trials the average serum cholesterol reduction was about 1.0 mmol/l (40 mg/dl), the corresponding expected long-term reduction in ischaemic heart disease mortality from the cohort studies is about 40% and again, this is close to the observed reduction from the third year onwards in these trials. As expected, therefore, the greater the serum cholesterol reduction the greater the reduction in risk.

In prescribing statin drugs, it follows from the above that a drug and a dosage should be chosen that has been demonstrated, in experimental studies correlating dose against cholesterol reduction, to reduce total and LDL-cholesterol on average by about 1.8 mmol/l. Some statin drugs cannot attain this. Also, it is misleading (as is often done) to cite the average reduction in heart disease attained over the typical five-year duration of these statin trials. What is important is that a reduction in risk of 60% can be attained from the third year onwards.

As with the cohort studies and the older trials, these statin trials have shown a similar proportionate reduction in heart disease risk in men and women, and a similar proportionate reduction at different starting levels of total or LDL-cholesterol. They have also confirmed reductions in heart disease in different age groups, but the variation of the size of the effect with age shown in Table 14.3 could not be confirmed independently in the trials — they would need to be unrealistically large to have the statistical power to do this.

Serum cholesterol and stroke

The relationship between serum cholesterol and stroke is a complex one. For thrombotic stroke a continuous dose–response relationship has been shown in a large cohort study,[15] analogous to that shown for ischaemic heart disease (in the same cohort study) in Figure 14.1. The older cholesterol lowering trials were uninformative on stroke because they recorded relatively few deaths and attained relatively small reductions in cholesterol. The large statin trials are more informative because they record non-fatal events (which are far more numerous) and attain larger cholesterol reductions. The results are shown in Table 14.4. A reduction in treated patients is evident. A published metaanalysis that included smaller trials but not the recently published LIPID trial yielded an overall combined estimate of a 26% reduction in risk (95% confidence interval 11%, 38%).[16] The stroke data in the major trials listed in Table 14.4 yield virtually the same estimate. This resolves the uncertainty from the observational studies, supporting the association shown in Table 14.4, of an increasing risk of non-haemorrhagic stroke as serum cholesterol

Trial	Drug	No. of patients		LDL-cholesterol (mmol/l):		No. of coronary events	No. of strokes
		Treated	Placebo	Average level in placebo group	Reduction in treated group	Treated v placebo	Treated v placebo
Patients with known coronary disease							
4S[1,8]	simvastatin	2221	2223	4.9	1.8	431 v 623	70 v 98
CARE[10]	pravastatin	2081	2078	3.6	1.1	212 v 274	54 v 78
Pravastatin Atherosclerosis Intervention programme[11]	pravastatin	995	936	4.4	1.2	29 v 52	5 v 13
LIPID[12]	pravastatin	4512	4502	3.9	1.0	557 v 715	169 v 204
Patients without known coronary disease							
West of Scotland[13]	pravastatin	3302	3293	5.0	1.0	150 v 218	46 v 51
AFCAPS/TexCAPS[14]	lovastatin	3304	3301	4.0	1.1	116 v 183	not yet reported

Table 14.4
Major trials of statin drugs: cholesterol reduction attained, numbers of patients, coronary events (ischaemic heart disease deaths and non-fatal myocardial infarction) and strokes (fatal and non-fatal)

increases above 4 mmol/l (160 mg/dl). As with heart disease it is likely that a greater long-term reduction is diluted by the absence of an early effect.[11]

For haemorrhagic stroke (intracranial and subarachnoid) there is no association with serum cholesterol across the greater part of its distribution.[15] At the lowest serum cholesterol levels found in Western populations, studies recording sufficient numbers of deaths at low levels have tended to show an excess risk — an L-shaped association.[15] Whether the association is due to cause and effect is uncertain. It is more difficult to see how an association with intracranial haemorrhage might arise through the disease (or predisposition to the disease) lowering serum cholesterol than is the case with depression and suicide, or cancer.[17] The cholesterol lowering trials tended not to recruit subjects with relatively low cholesterol, so that the numbers of treated patients with serum cholesterol levels of around 4 mmol/l were too few to enable the trials to test whether the excess risk of haemorrhagic stroke is causal. Even if the association is cause and effect, however, the increased mortality from haemorrhagic stroke at very low cholesterol concentrations is small compared to the lower mortality from ischaemic heart disease and other circulatory diseases. Even at the lowest serum cholesterol concentrations in Western populations, mortality from all circulatory diseases is substantially lower than in the next lowest group.

Safety of cholesterol reduction

The uncertainty concerning the excess mortality from haemorrhagic stroke at very low serum cholesterol concentration is unresolved, as discussed above. This apart, there are no material grounds for concern. The trials of statin drugs, particularly informative on safety because of the large reduction in serum cholesterol that they attain, have resolved the issue of safety because they show no excess mortality from non-circulatory causes. The excess mortality from cancer and accidents and suicide at very low serum cholesterol in observational studies is attributable to cancer or depression lowering serum cholesterol, not the reverse.[17] The excess mortality from accidents and suicide in two of the older cholesterol lowering trials (which was not statistically significant) occurred among men who had not taken the medication, and was therefore attributable to chance.[18] Further reassurance on safety is provided by the condition of heterozygous familial hypobetalipoproteinaemia, in which serum cholesterol levels are as low as 2 to 3 mmol/l (80 to 120 mg/dl). Life expectancy is prolonged because coronary artery disease is avoided, and no adverse effects from the low cholesterol are recognised[19,20] — an important natural experiment.

Policy

In a small proportion of the population (1% or so), notably persons with familial hypercholesterolaemia, the absolute risk of death from ischaemic heart disease at a young age is so great that affected persons should be identified and treated, even though the condition accounts for a fraction of all heart disease deaths in a population. The most appropriate screening strategy has not yet been devised: measuring lipids in first degree relatives of known cases will not identify all cases.

In the general population, measures to reduce dietary fat and serum cholesterol should be directed at the entire population. Serum cholesterol reductions of 0.6 mmol/l (23 mg/dl) (10%) have occurred in entire Western communities,[2] facilitated by health education, the wider availability of healthy food in restaurants and supermarkets and a positive image of healthy eating. A reduction of 0.6 mmol/l (23 mg/dl) is less likely when an individual attempts dietary change in isolation. The most important measures to lower cholesterol in healthy people involve wider public education, adoption of a simple system of labelling of the nutrient content of foods, and widespread availability of palatable low fat foods.

Clinicians direct their activities towards high risk patients, and by far the most important high risk group are survivors of myocardial infarction. Statin drugs are justified because of the high absolute risk of death of these patients — statins can lower serum cholesterol by 1.8 mmol/l (70 mg/dl) (30%)[1] which, as discussed, reduces mortality from heart disease by as much as 60% after two years.

The 'population' and 'high risk' approaches are complementary — the first primarily a public health issue aimed at altering the population diet and hence the incidence of ischaemic heart disease, the second primarily a clinical activity, identifying and treating with statins patients with coronary artery disease.

References

1. Scandinavian Simvastatin Survival Study Group. Randomised trial of cholesterol lowering in 4444 patients with coronary heart disease: the Scandinavian Survival Study (4S). *Lancet* 1994; **344**:1383–9.
2. Law MR, Wald NJ. An ecological study of serum cholesterol and ischaemic heart disease between 1950 and 1990. *Eur J Clin Nutr* 1994; **48**:305–25.
3. Law MR, Wald NJ, Wu T, Hackshaw A, Bailey A. Systematic underestimation of association between serum cholesterol concentration and ischaemic heart disease in observational studies: data from the BUPA study. *BMJ* 1994; **308**:363–6.
4. Pocock SJ, Shaper AG, Phillips AN. Concentrations of high density lipoprotein cholesterol, triglycerides, and total cholesterol in ischaemic heart disease. *BMJ* 1989; **298**:998–1002.
5. Law MR, Wald NJ, Thompson SG. By how much and how quickly does reduction in serum cholesterol concentration lower risk of ischaemic heart disease? *BMJ* 1994; **308**: 367–72.
6. Neaton JD, Wentworth D. Serum cholesterol, blood pressure, cigarette smoking, and death from coronary heart disease. *Arch Intern Med* 1992; **152**:56–64.
7. Chen Z, Peto R, Collins R *et al*. Serum cholesterol concentration and coronary heart disease in a population with low cholesterol concentrations. *BMJ* 1991; **303**:276–82.
8. Scandinavian Simvastatin Survival Study Group. Baseline serum cholesterol and treatment effect in the Scandinavian Simvastatin Survival Study (4S). *Lancet* 1995; **345**:1274–5.
9. Smith EB, Slater RS. Relationship between low-density lipoprotein in aortic intima and serum-lipid levels. *Lancet* 1972; **1**:463–9.
10. Sacks FM, Pfeffer MA, Moye LA *et al*. The effect of pravastatin on coronary events after myocardial infarction in patients with average cholesterol levels. *N Engl J Med* 1996; **335**:1001–9.
11. Byington RP, Juhema JW, Salonen JT *et al*. Reduction in cardiovascular events during pravastatin therapy: pooled analysis of clinical events of the Pravastatin Atherosclerosis Intervention Program. *Circulation* 1995; **92**: 2419–25.
12. The Long-Term Intervention with Pravastatin in Ischaemic Heart Disease (LIPID) Study Group. Prevention of cardiovascular events and death with pravastatin in patients with coronary heart disease and a broad range of initial cholesterol levels. *N Engl J Med* 1998; **339**:1349–57.
13. Shepherd J, Cobbe SM, Ford I *et al*. Prevention of coronary heart disease with pravastatin in men with hypercholesterolemia. *N Engl J Med* 1995; **333**:1301–7.
14. Downs RJ, Clearfield M, Weis S *et al*. Primary prevention of acute coronary events with lovastatin in men and women with average cholesterol levels. *JAMA* 1998; **279**:1615–22.

15. Neaton JD, Blackburn H, Jacobs D *et al.* Serum cholesterol level and mortality findings for men screened in the multiple risk factor intervention trial. *Arch Intern Med* 1992; **152:**1490–500.

16. Crouse JR, Byington RP, Furberg CD. HMG-CoA reductase inhibitor therapy and stroke risk reduction: an analysis of clinical trials data. *Atherosclerosis* 1998; **138:** 11–24.

17. Law MR, Wald NJ, Thompson S. Assessing possible hazards of reducing serum cholesterol.

BMJ 1994; **308:**373–9.

18. Wysowski DK, Gross TP. Deaths due to accidents and violence in two recent trials of cholesterol-lowering drugs. *Arch Intern Med* 1990; **150:**2169–72.

19. Linton MF, Farese RV, Young SG. Familial hypobetalipoproteinemia. *J Lipid Res* 1993; **34:**521–41.

20. Glueck CJ, Gartside P, Fallat RW, Sielski J, Steiner PM. Longevity syndromes: familial hypobeta and familial hyperalpha lipoproteinemia. *J Lab Clin Med* 1976; **88:**941–57.

15

Women and coronary heart disease: lipid risk factors

Jacques E Rossouw

Which lipids are risk factors in women?

Much has been made of the differences between women and men in respect of CHD risk.[1,2] On average, the onset of CHD is delayed by 10–15 years in women compared to men. The delay may be related to lower LDL-cholesterol and higher HDL-cholesterol levels up to middle age in women, which in turn may be related to differing hormonal milieus. Women more often present with angina as the first symptom, while men more often present with acute myocardial infarction. Once women do have an acute myocardial infarction they have a higher mortality rate than men, as shown by the Framingham study where the 12-month mortality was 45% for women and 20% for men.[3] The higher mortality rate may be related to the older age at which women develop CHD, and a greater prevalence of risk factors such as diabetes, hypertension, and dyslipidemia. The lipid risk factors are said to have a different relative impact in women than men, with HDL-cholesterol and triglycerides being more prominent than LDL-cholesterol. None the less, there are more similarities than dissimilarities between the pathogenesis of CHD in women and men, and pathologically the lesions in women and men are indistinguishable. It is the same disease.

The same lipids and lipoproteins that are risk factors in men are also risk factors in women — total cholesterol, LDL-cholesterol, HDL-cholesterol, triglycerides, and Lp(a). In women as in men, LDL-cholesterol (or total cholesterol) and HDL-cholesterol emerge as independent risk factors in multivariate analyses. The data do not support the concept that the relative impact of LDL-cholesterol may be smaller and that of HDL-cholesterol may be greater in women than in men. The best estimate of the overall univariate risk associated with lipids comes from a pooled analysis of 13 cohort studies in women and 25 studies in men.[4] For women aged less than 65 years, a total cholesterol of 240 mg/dl or higher compared to less than 200 mg/dl was associated with a 144% excess risk of CHD, while for men the excess was 73% (Figure 15.1A). LDL-cholesterol levels of more than 160 mg/dl compared to less than 130 mg/dl increased risk by 227% in women, and 92% in men. Triglyceride levels of 130 mg/dl and above compared to less than 100 mg/dl increased risk by 98% and 16% in women and men respectively. Finally, for HDL-cholesterol levels less than 50 mg/dl compared to 60 mg/dl and above, the excess risks were 113% in women and 131% in men. All of these results were statistically significant. Thus, as judged from univariate analyses, the usual lipid risk factors are relevant in middle-aged women and men, and if anything the risks associated with high total cholesterol, LDL-cholesterol, and triglyceride levels are more pronounced in women. The impact of low HDL-cholesterol of levels appears to be about equal in men and women.

In women and men who are 65 years and older, the relative risks associated with lipids on average attenuate in both women and men (Figure 15.1B). In women the 13% excess risk with high LDL-cholesterol levels, and for men the 9% excess risk with low HDL-cholesterol levels is no longer significant in univariate analyses. However, the average obscures the heterogeneity of the older population.[5] To some degree, the decrease in relative risk at older ages results from the selective survival of some individuals who are resistant to high LDL-cholesterol levels, and to some degree it also reflects the increasingly dominant effect of aging as a risk factor. These influences would constitute a real decrease in risk associated with LDL-cholesterol levels. However, the relative risks may also be seriously confounded by intercurrent illness or debility. A relatively large proportion of the older age groups may have a subclinical or overt illness at the time of measuring lipid levels, and such illness may simultaneously depress lipid levels and increase risk for CHD. Low lipid levels in the elderly are associated with markers of ill health such as involuntary weight loss, low activity levels, low levels of hemoglobin and albumin, and the presence of diabetes.[5,6] The result is that in the ill elderly, there may appear to be no relationship, or even an inverse relationship between current lipid levels and CHD. However, the lipid levels anteceding the illness would still have influenced the prevalence and degree of atherosclerosis. In the case of chronic illness, one may have to go back 10 years or more to find the lipid levels that are predictive of CHD.[5]

Importantly, in spite of the survivor and

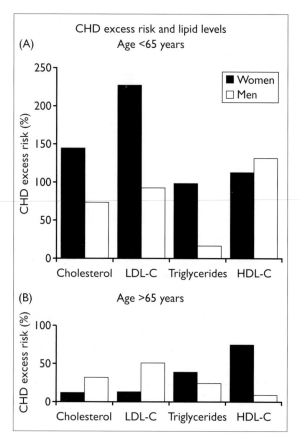

Fig. 15.1
Univariate relative risk of high cholesterol, LDL-cholesterol and triglyceride levels and low HDL-cholesterol levels in (A) middle-aged and (B) older women and men. Adapted from pooled data from 13 cohort studies in women and 25 in men.[4] All results were statistically significant except those for LDL-cholesterol in older women and HDL-cholesterol in older men.

confounding effects noted above, lipid disorders remain predictive of CHD in the healthy elderly. The continued impact of lipids is supported by cross-sectional studies of subclinical atherosclerosis as measured by carotid ultrasonography.[7] Across the age range 45–75 years, LDL-cholesterol and HDL-cholesterol levels were associated with atherosclerosis in both women and men, and the magnitude of the association did not attenuate with age. Lipid-lowering trials have repeatedly shown significant benefit in older women and men.[3,8–12]

Thus, for many older people the risk associated with lipid disorders remains real, and because the population burden of CHD is much higher at older ages, even a small relative risk will translate into a large number of CHD cases associated with the risk factor. From the clinical perspective, the message from these data is that the lipids of relatively healthy older persons should be managed in exactly the same way as in middle-aged persons. Since older women outnumber older men, these considerations are particularly pertinent to women. At these older ages, the absolute risk for CHD in women starts to approximate that of men, and therefore the cost-effectiveness of lipid-lowering treatment is also similar. Cost-effectiveness will eventually diminish at advanced older age, at which point extension of years of life would not be possible.[13]

High Lp(a) levels are associated with a higher risk for CHD in both women and men;[14] however the status of Lp(a) as a risk factor independent of LDL-cholesterol is less certain. In men, more recent prospective studies have been inconsistent, but it is possible that high Lp(a) levels aggravate the deleterious effects of LDL-cholesterol or negate some of the beneficial effects associated with high HDL-cholesterol levels.[15–18] Women in the Framingham Heart Study who had a sinking pre-beta lipoprotein band (a surrogate marker for Lp(a)) were at significantly increased risk for CHD, claudication, and stroke, even after allowing for LDL-cholesterol and HDL-cholesterol levels in a multivariable analysis.[19] In angiographic studies Lp(a) has been strongly

associated with the presence of coronary disease in women, and less so in men.[18,20] It is not clear whether (or why) Lp(a) might have a different import in women than men, and more study of this issue is needed.

For triglycerides, results from observational studies have been mixed. As noted above, univariate analyses generally show an increased risk with higher triglyceride levels, and in a meta-analysis the average excess risk associated with a 38.67 mg/dl (1 mmol/l) increase in triglycerides was 76% in women and 32% in men, both statistically significant (Figure 15.2).[21] When adjusted for HDL-cholesterol levels, the excess risk for high triglycerides was halved, to 37% in women and 14% in men, but was still statistically significant. Unfortunately, in women there were only two studies with data on HDL-cholesterol, therefore further confirmation of the independent status of triglycerides in women is needed. The risk associated with hypertriglyceridemia may be determined by the company it keeps. For some individuals, a high triglyceride level may be a marker of atherogenic triglyceride-rich remnant particles or small dense LDL particles. When triglycerides and LDL particle size are considered together, sometimes triglycerides emerge as an independent factor, and sometimes LDL particle size emerges as an independent factor.[21] The causal factor is more likely to be small dense LDL particles, since these are taken up by the endothelial cell more readily than the large VLDL particles, and are thus able to initiate the processes of atherosclerosis. Isolated hypertriglyceridemia such as is found in familial hypertriglyceridemia (where there is a defect in clearance of VLDL) is not associated with an increased risk for CHD. On the other hand, the overproduction of apoB-containing particles (VLDL and LDL) underlying familial combined hyperlipidemia (FCHL) is commonly associated with CHD. FCHL may

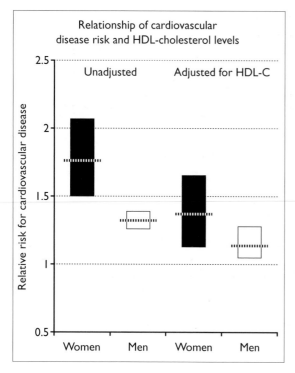

Fig. 15.2
Univariate (unadjusted) and multivariate (adjusted for HDL-cholesterol) relationship of high triglyceride levels to cardiovascular disease risk. Adapted from pooled data from five population-based cohort studies in women and 16 in men.[21] The solid bar represents the typical odds ratio, and the open boxes represent the 95% confidence interval. Values higher than 1.0 indicate increased risk and if the confidence interval does not cross 1.0, the result is statistically significant.

and sympathoadrenal overactivity, and is marked by abdominal obesity, hypertriglyceridemia, small dense LDL particles, low HDL-cholesterol levels, hypertension, abnormal glucose tolerance, and a predisposition to CHD.[22]

Clustering of risk factors is common, whether or not as part of the metabolic syndrome, and this clustering may have a particularly severe impact on women. In the Framingham Offspring Study, clustering of three or more of six metabolically linked risk factors (most adverse quintile of body mass index, total cholesterol, low HDL-cholesterol, triglyceride, systolic blood pressure, and fasting glucose) occurred in 18–19% of women and men, or twice the rate that would be predicted by chance.[23] In women with three or more risk factors, the age-adjusted relative risk for CHD was 4.76 (CI = 1.73–13.13) while in men the risk was 2.68 (CI = 1.63–4.42). Most strikingly, clustering of three or more risk factors accounted for 48% of all CHD in women and 20% of all CHD in men (Table 15.1). Initial obesity level was associated with clustering in women but not in men. Weight gain in both sexes predicted increased clustering, and weight loss predicted decreased clustering. The implications of these findings are that the presence of one risk factor should lead to a search for others so that overall risk can be quantified. Weight management in prevention and treatment may be of particular importance in women.

Trials of lipid lowering

The risk factor concept derives from observational epidemiology, which is focused on identifying exposures or characteristics of individuals that predict higher than average risk for a disease. A biologically plausible, strong, reproducible, dose-dependent associa-

express itself as hypertriglyceridemia, hypercholesterolemia, or both in different family members, and in many the lipid disorder also includes increased numbers of small dense LDL particles and low HDL-cholesterol levels. There is overlap between FCHL and the metabolic syndrome. The metabolic syndrome is postulated to be due to insulin resistance

Risk factor sum	Relative risk (95% confidence interval)	Prevalence (%)	CHD events (number)	Population attributable risk (%)
Women				
0	1 (referent)	32	7	referent
1	1.21 (0.45–3.23)	30	10	6
2	2.89 (1.17–7.13)	19	18	26
3+	5.90 (2.54–13.73)	19	44	48
Men				
0	1 (referent)	33	41	referent
1	1.54 (1.01–2.35)	29	61	14
2	2.02 (1.31–3.12)	19	58	16
3+	2.39 (1.56–3.66)	18	69	20

Table 15.1
Age-adjusted risk factor sum and 16-year coronary heart disease (CHD) risk in persons aged 30–74 years at baseline.[23]

tion of the factor with disease which is statistically independent of other factors lends credence to the risk factor. However for reversible risk factors, final proof of causality rests with randomized controlled clinical trials. For the lipid risk factors it is now abundantly clear from the clinical trials that lowering LDL-cholesterol levels in women is as effective as it is in men, while clinical trial support for the roles of triglycerides, HDL-cholesterol, and Lp(a) remains scanty. In part, this situation has arisen because most of the trials have focused on lowering total cholesterol or LDL-cholesterol and hence persons with high triglyceride levels were often excluded, and in part because it is difficult to design a trial of lipid modification that would lower triglycerides and raise HDL-cholesterol levels without also affecting total cholesterol and LDL-cholesterol levels. None the less, the Helsinki Heart Study in men suggested that gemfibrozil treatment reduced CHD risk in the subset with the combination of high triglycerides and low HDL-cholesterol levels.[24] Angiographic benefit was observed in trials of bezafibrate and gemfibrozil (also in men) which reduced triglycerides and increased HDL-cholesterol levels, but had little effect on LDL-cholesterol levels.[25,26] No trial with clinical outcomes has focused on lowering Lp(a) levels.

Most of the data for women and men derive from trials aimed at lowering total or LDL-cholesterol. Angiographic trials that included women have consistently shown improvement in coronary morphology in women to at least the same degree as in men.[27,28] For clinical outcomes, as recently as 1995 a meta-analysis of clinical trials concluded that there is no evidence from primary prevention trials to suggest that cholesterol lowering affects CHD mortality in healthy women, and limited evidence to suggest that treatment of hypercholesterolemia in women with coronary disease decreases CHD mortality.[29] Since that time, a number of large trials using HMG-CoA reductase inhibitors (statins) have reported their results, and it can now be stated with confidence that cholesterol lowering works as well in women as in men.[8–10,12]

In the arena of primary prevention, data are still sparse. The AFCAPS/TexCAPS trial of lovastatin included women with average cholesterol levels.[9] The reduction in CHD was 46% in women compared with 37% in men, however with only 20 events in women the result was not significant. When added to the existing data from previous primary prevention trials, the meta-analytic odds ratio for CHD in the treatment group was 0.70 (CI = 0.57–0.86) (Table 15.2).[30–32] However, this result is dependent on inclusion of the large Finnish Mental Hospitals diet trial, which was not a true individually randomized trial.[31]

In secondary prevention, the Scandinavian Simvastatin Survival Study (4S) was the first to include relatively large numbers of women (n = 827).[12] Treatment with simvastatin reduced CHD events by one-third, a significant result and similar to that for men. Two subsequent secondary prevention trials have strengthened the evidence of benefit for women with existing heart disease. The Cholesterol and Recurrent Events (CARE) trial included 576 women with existing disease and average lipid levels.[10] Pravastatin reduced recurrent CHD risk by 46% compared with 20% in men (both results were highly significant). In the Long-term Intervention with Pravastatin in Ischaemic Disease (LIPID) trial,

including subjects with a wide range of cholesterol levels, the risk reduction in women (n = 760) was 11% (not significant) versus 26% in men (significant).[8] When added to the data of the three previous secondary prevention trials reporting data in women,[30,33,34] the risk reduction for CHD is overwhelmingly significant, with a meta-analytic odds ratio of 0.65 (CI = 0.53–0.78) (see Table 15.2). Since primary and secondary prevention of CHD simply represent treatment along a different segment of the atherosclerosis continuum, it is reasonable to combine the data from all the trials. This yields a highly significant risk reduction of 33%, identical to the 33% average risk reduction observed in the combined statin trials which included mainly men.[35]

In view of the inconsistent data from observational studies linking lipid levels to CHD risk in older persons, another important finding from the trials is that older persons benefit almost as much as the middle-aged. For example, in the 4S trial the risk reduction in participants aged 60 years and older was 29% while that in younger participants was 39% (both results were significant).[12] Similarly, older participants in the CARE, LIPID, and AFCAPS/TexCAPS trials showed significant benefit from lipid-lowering treatment.[8–10] CARE participants older than 65 years appeared to do even better than younger participants, with a 32% (P = 0.001) reduction in coronary events in older participants compared with 19% reduction (P = 0.005) in younger participants.[11] The older women in CARE showed a 36% risk reduction compared with the 31% reduction in older men, but the result for older women was not significant due to small numbers. The treatment of older participants appeared to be more cost-effective when compared with that of younger participants. Because of the high event rates in older participants, older participants would need to be

	Treatment		Control		Odds ratio (95% confidence interval)
	CHD events (number)	Randomized (number)	CHD events (number)	Randomized (number)	
Primary prevention					
Colestipol[32]	32	601	28	4583	1.11 (0.66–1.87)
Minnesota[30]	62	2344	47	2320	1.31 (0.90–1.92)
Finnish Mental Hospital N[31]	52	2169	107	1773	0.39 (0.28–0.54)
Finnish Mental Hospital K[31]	21	1429	22	1063	0.70 (0.38–1.29)
AFCAPS/TexCAPS[32]	7	499	13	498	0.54 (0.22–1.31)
Subtotal, typical odds ratio	**174**	**7042**	**217**	**6237**	**0.70 (0.57–0.86)**
Secondary prevention					
Newcastle[34]	4	52	13	45	0.23 (0.08–0.67)
Edinburgh[33]	4	57	8	54	0.45 (0.13–1.48)
4S[12]	59	407	91	420	0.62 (0.43–0.88)
CARE[10]	46	286	80	29	0.51 (0.34–0.76)
LIPID[8]	90	756	104	760	0.85 (0.63–1.15)
Subtotal, typical odds ratio	**203**	**1558**	**296**	**1569**	**0.65 (0.53–0.78)**
Grand total, typical odds ratio	**377**	**8600**	**513**	**7806**	**0.67 (0.58–0.77)**

Table 15.2
CHD events in primary and secondary prevention cholesterol-lowering trials in women.

treated for 5 years to prevent one event, compared with 20 younger participants needing to be treated to prevent one event.

Estrogen, lipids, and coronary heart disease

On average, adult women have HDL-cholesterol levels some 10–15 mg/dl higher than men, and this difference is most often cited as the major reason why the onset of CHD is delayed in women. This may be so, but the corollary that the relatively higher HDL-cholesterol levels in women are solely due to endogenous estrogen is questionable. This difference between women and men is initiated during puberty when the HDL-cholesterol levels in young men decline as a result of rising testosterone levels, whereas the HDL-cholesterol levels in women remains fairly constant throughout life (Figure 15.3).[36] The small decrease in HDL-cholesterol levels noted in cohort studies of women passing through the menopause is not sufficient to affect the gap between women and men observed in cross-sectional studies. There are other notable differences in lipids between women and men: up to middle age the average LDL-cholesterol level of women is lower than that of men, whereafter it rises steeply and exceeds that of men. Throughout life women have lower average triglyceride levels than men. These lipid differences are consistent with a delayed onset of CHD in women, and also with the eventual increase in CHD rates in older women, which approximate the rates in males after the age of 75 years. Lp(a) levels are similar in women and men, but some increase occurs in older women.[37,38]

Endogenous sex hormones, both estrogenic and androgenic, are probably key to the explanation of lipid differences between women and men. As noted above, endogenous androgens depress HDL-cholesterol levels in men and are probably a primary determinant of the sex difference in these levels, while estrogens maintain higher levels of HDL-cholesterol throughout life in women.[39–41] Both androgens and estrogens may influence the pattern of LDL-cholesterol by age in opposite directions.[39,40] Endogenous estrogens probably have little effect on triglyceride levels or may even lower them.[39] Estrogens appear to decrease Lp(a) levels but there is little difference in Lp(a) between the sexes.[37] Generally, oophorectomy studies have observed little or no change in triglyceride or HDL-cholesterol levels, while increases in LDL-cholesterol were more consistently observed.[42,43] One recent large study also observed a marked (43–90%) increase in Lp(a) concentrations after oophorectomy.[44]

Trials using transdermal estradiol possibly provide the most reliable indication of the lipid effects of endogenous estrogen. Unlike endogenous estradiol, transdermal estradiol enters the systemic circulation directly, does not undergo first-pass hepatic circulation, and therefore does not stimulate production of apoproteins B and A1 to the same degree as oral estrogens, nor do they stimulate the hepatic production of coagulation proteins.[45] Physiologic doses of transdermal estradiol usually have little effect on HDL-cholesterol, but they do decrease triglyceride levels by about 20% and may modestly decrease LDL-cholesterol levels by up to 10% and Lp(a) levels by 12%.[46–48] The addition of progesterone, whether transvaginal or oral, does not materially change these findings except that some forms of progesterone depress HDL-cholesterol levels. Transdermal estrogens have little or no effect on markers of blood coagulation but retain potentially favorable effects on blood vessel physiology and on the inhibition of LDL oxidation.[45,48–52] The reported increase

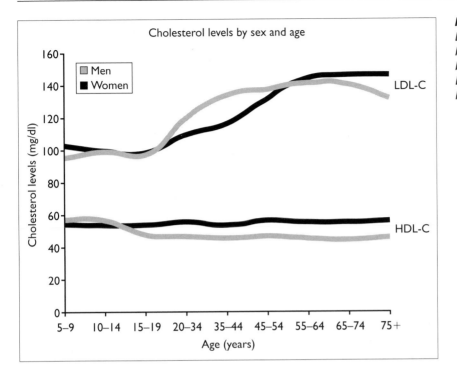

Fig. 15.3
LDL-cholesterol and HDL-cholesterol levels by sex and age in the Lipid Research Clinics Prevalence Study.[36]

in venous thromboembolism in women using transdermal estrogens needs to be confirmed.[53] The biologic importance of the reduction in LDL-cholesterol levels induced by estrogen, whether transdermal or oral, is uncertain because the shift in particle size towards small dense LDL may be countered by a reduced residence time of the particles.[54]

In contrast to transdermal estradiol, the administration of oral estradiol or conjugated equine estrogens (CEE) delivers supraphysiologic concentrations of estrogen to the liver, and this results in a different lipid response.[45] Oral estrogens raise HDL-cholesterol levels by 15–20%, raise triglyceride levels by up to 25%, and induce larger decreases in LDL-cholesterol of about 15% and in Lp(a) levels of about 20%. The effect on HDL-cholesterol appears to be due to increased hepatic production of apoA-1 and inhibition of hepatic lipase activity; the effect on triglycerides is due to increased hepatic production of apoB and VLDL particles; the effect on LDL-cholesterol is due to increased LDL receptor activity, and the effect on Lp(a) is due to reduced production of apo(a).[54–56] Oral progestins blunt the estrogenic effects on HDL-cholesterol and possibly on triglycerides, but do not influence the effects on LDL-cholesterol or Lp(a).[57,58] Oral estrogens with or without progestins produce a multitude of changes in blood clotting proteins, and until recently it was not clear whether these effects were favorable or unfavorable.[48,49,51,56,59] However, recent observational studies and the results of the Heart and Estrogen/Progestin (HERS) trial have clarified that the net effect on blood coagulation is unfavorable, since venous thromboembolism clearly increases in hormone users.[53,60,61]

Some physicians consider estrogen to be a lipid-lowering therapy that can obviate the need for statins or other lipid-lowering drugs, and of course many women are currently on treatment with both estrogen and statins. How does estrogen compare to a statin in respect of lipid lowering, fibrinolysis, and vascular function, and do these classes of drugs have additive or opposing effects on risk factors? These questions have been examined in several studies, and the results indicate that 10 mg of simvastatin is more effective than 0.625 mg of CEE for lowering LDL-cholesterol and apoB levels, while CEE were more effective at raising HDL-cholesterol and apoA-1 levels.[52,54,59] Adding the less effective drug resulted in very modest further change, in other words the drugs were less than fully additive.[59,62] Triglyceride levels were reduced by simvastatin, modestly elevated by CEE, and when the drugs were combined there was little net effect.[59,62,63] Only CEE reduced Lp(a) levels.[59,63] Flow-mediated dilatation was significantly improved by both therapies, with no further improvement on the combination. Concentrations of PAI-1 and of the cell adhesion molecule E-selectin were reduced by CEE but not by simvastatin, with no further change on the combination.[59] Importantly, statins have been proven to prevent CHD and remain the drugs of choice for hypercholesterolemia. The apparent advantages of estrogen in respect of Lp(a), PA-1, and E-selectin relate to risk factors that are less well established than LDL-cholesterol, and treatment of these risk factors has not been demonstrated to result in lowered CHD event rates. Also, estrogen has multiple effects on multiple organ systems, and whether the net effect is beneficial or harmful remains to be established.[64]

The differences in the age of onset of CHD in women and men, together with the gender differences in lipids and the effects of oral estrogens on lipids and on vascular biology, plus consistent observations that hormone users have lower rates of CHD, have led to a widespread assumption that oral estrogens are beneficial. Confirmation from the large randomized controlled clinical trials for primary prevention of CHD is awaited.[65] However, it is worth noting that, to date, the results of randomized controlled clinical trials of secondary prevention in both men and women have been disappointing.

The first randomized controlled clinical trial with CHD as the principal outcome, the Heart and Estrogen/Progestin Replacement Study (HERS) was a landmark study.[61] HERS tested CEE 0.625 mg and medroxyprogesterone (MPA) 2.5 mg daily versus placebo in 2763 postmenopausal women with evidence of CHD. The hormones induced the expected lipid changes, reducing LDL-cholesterol levels by 11%, raising HDL-cholesterol levels by 10%, and raising triglyceride levels by 8% compared with placebo. Over an average study duration of 4.1 years there was no net benefit for the principal outcome of CHD (non-fatal myocardial infarction plus CHD death) with 172 cases in the placebo group and 176 cases in the active treatment group (Table 15.3). However, in the first year there was a nominally significant ($P < 0.05$) excess of CHD events in the treatment group (57) compared with the placebo group (38). In the second year there was no difference in event rates and thereafter there was a trend towards a reduction of CHD events in the treatment group, mainly due to a reduction in non-fatal MI. The trend for CHD over time was significant ($P = 0.009$). There was no benefit for any other cardiovascular outcome, including angina or revascularization procedures. Other

Outcome	Treatment group		Relative hazard (95% CI)	P value
	Estrogen/progestin (n = 1380)	Placebo (n = 1383)		
CHD events	172	176	0.99 (0.80–1.22)	0.91
CHD death	71	58	1.24 (0.87–1.75)	0.23
Non-fatal MI	116	129	0.91 (0.71–1.17)	0.46
Coronary artery bypass surgery	88	101	0.87 (0.66–1.16)	0.36
Percutaneous coronary revascularization	164	175	0.95 (0.77–1.17)	0.62
Stroke/transient ischemic attack	108	96	1.13 (0.85–1.48)	0.40
Venous thromboembolic event	34	12	2.89 (1.50–5.58)	0.002
Cancer	96	87	1.12 (0.84–1.50)	0.44
Breast cancer	32	25	1.30 (0.77–2.19)	0.33
Endometrial cancer	2	4	0.49 (0.09–2.69)	0.41
Fracture	130	138	0.95 (0.75–1.21)	0.70
Hip fracture	12	11	1.10 (0.49–2.50)	0.82
Other fractures	119	129	1.38 (0.73–1.20)	0.50
Gallbladder disease	84	62	1.08 (1.00–1.92)	0.05
All deaths	131	123	1.08 (0.84–1.38)	0.56

Table 15.3
Clinical outcomes in the Heart and Estrogen/Progestin Replacement Study (HERS).[61]

important findings were a significant, almost threefold increase in the risk for venous thromboembolism (34 in the hormone group and 12 in the placebo group, $P = 0.002$) and a marginally significant increase in gallbladder disease (84 in the hormone group and 62 in the placebo group, $P = 0.05$). The excess risk for venous thromboembolism persisted over the duration of the study, but was significant only in the first year. There was no reduction in fractures (130 compared with 138).

Thus, HERS provided some results for HRT that were expected (increased risk for venous thromboembolism and gallbladder disease) and some that were unexpected (no overall reduction in CHD, and no reduction in fractures). The trend over time for CHD was also unexpected. If anything, the immediate effects of HRT on coagulation factors and vascular reactivity reviewed above might have led to an expectation of early benefit, sustained in later years by a benefit from lipid lowering. The early dysbenefit needs to be explained; possibilities include HRT-induced inflammatory changes in unstable plaques, or a procoagulant effect that predominates early on. There is no doubt that HRT is procoagulant, as shown by the excess of venous thromboembolism. The findings may be explained by the existence of a subset of women who are particularly susceptible to one or more of the adverse metabolic changes induced by HRT, and the remaining women are those who survive to reap the later benefit of lipid lowering. The lack of overall benefit for CHD also puts into question the reliability of the observational studies, which indicated likely benefit for both CEE and CEE with MPA.

It is important to keep in mind that oral estrogen is being used as a drug, and is not simply replacing endogenous hormones. The first-pass hepatic circulation of oral estrogen causes metabolic pertubations that are not found with parenteral estrogen or endogenous estrogen. In particular, oral estrogen differs from parenteral estrogen in increasing HDL-cholesterol and triglyceride levels and also markedly changing the levels and activity of a variety of coagulation proteins. It is not known whether the increase in HDL-cholesterol levels is necessary for clinical benefit to the heart, but it is known that the changes in coagulation proteins are responsible for venous thromboembolism. Thus, the clinical effects of oral estrogen on the vascular system may turn out to be quite different from those of parenteral estrogen. Considered as replacement therapy, the apparent optimal dose of estrogen might be one that yields serum levels of estrogen similar to those in premenopausal women, relieves menopausal symptoms, and maintains bone mass. However, because it is a drug undergoing first-pass hepatic circulation, the dose of oral estrogen needed to obtain the desired replacement effect is about 10-fold higher than if used parenterally, the liver is exposed to non-physiologic levels, and this may lead to clinical effects (either harmful or beneficial) that differ from those of parenteral estrogens.

Selective estrogen receptor modulators (SERMs)

Because of the known and putative risks of estrogen, one of the hopes of the future rests with the development of compounds with selective actions on the estrogen receptors in various tissues, so that the potentially beneficial effects on lipids, vascular endothelium, and bone mineral density are retained but the potentially harmful effects on coagulation, the breast, and the endometrium are avoided. Two of these SERMs, raloxifene and tamoxifen, have been examined for their effects on cardiovascular risk factors. A double-blind randomized trial in 390 postmenopausal women examined the effects of two doses of raloxifene, hormone replacement therapy (HRT in the form of CEE 0.625 mg/day and MPA 2.5 mg/day), and placebo on lipids, lipoproteins, and coagulation factors after 3 and 6 months of treatment.[66] Both doses of raloxifene (60 and 120 mg/day) lowered LDL-cholesterol levels by 11%, similar to the 13% reduction seen with HRT. However, raloxifene had less effect on HDL-cholesterol, HDL2-cholesterol, and apoA-1 levels than HRT, and also less effect on Lp(a) levels. Among the coagulation factors tested, raloxifene lowered fibrinogen to a greater extent than HRT, but the reverse was true for PAI-1. Thus, from the combined lipid and coagulation data it is not possible to predict whether raloxifene or HRT is likely to have the more beneficial effect on the vascular tree. The effects of tamoxifen on lipids and coagulation factors are similar to those of raloxifene, except that tamoxifen lowers fibrinogen and PAI-1 levels to a greater extent.

In the absence of clinical outcome data it is not certain that the effect of raloxifene on the heart will be beneficial. Coronary atherosclerosis in ovariectomized monkeys fed an atherogenic diet was not inhibited by low-dose raloxifene (1 mg/kg) or high-dose raloxifene (5 mg/kg), but was reduced by CE 0.04 mg/kg.[67] Also, although the lipid effects of raloxifene are similar to those of tamoxifen, the Breast Cancer Prevention Trial (BCPT) of 13 388 women treated with tamoxifen 20 mg/day or placebo for 5 years did not show a reduction in CHD.[68] The BCPT studied a population at low risk of CHD, none the less it is worth noting that there was no indication of benefit for the cardiovascular system. The numbers of CHD events, angina, and acute ischemic syndrome were virtually identical in the tamoxifen and placebo groups, while strokes tended to be higher (not significant) on tamoxifen. Like HRT, tamoxifen increases the risk for pulmonary embolism about threefold (risk ratio 3.01, CI = 1.15–9.27). Therefore, it can be concluded that tamoxifen is procoagulant in spite of the reductions in fibrinogen and PAI-1 observed in metabolic studies. Thus, proof of whether tamoxifen, raloxifene, or any other SERM is indeed cardioprotective will need to await the results of ongoing large randomized controlled clinical trials.

Are lipids in women being treated?

In the USA, lipid disorders in women have been treated less frequently than those in men because of the perception that women are at lower risk for CHD. It is certainly true that the risk for CHD is considerably lower in younger women, and their lipid profiles are also generally less adverse than those of men. Unless there is a monogenic lipid disorder or a number of other risk factors, it is not cost-effective to treat high blood cholesterol in younger women.[13] This picture changes in older women. After the age of about 55, years LDL-cholesterol levels in women start to rival and eventually exceed those of men, and CHD becomes the most frequent cause of death in women. At about age 75 years, the number of CHD deaths in women equals that in men. Over their lifespan, US women suffer as many CHD deaths as men.[69]

Two recent studies have indicated that lipid disorders in older US women (and men) continue to be undertreated, although progress is being made.[70,71] In a population representative sample of women and men aged 65 years and older surveyed in 1989–1990, 5.1% of women and 3.1% of men without CHD were using cholesterol-lowering drugs, or one-third of the numbers that would have been eligible according to

NCEP guidelines.[70] Only 9.9% of women and 8.2% of men with CHD were using lipid-lowering drugs, or one-tenth of those eligible according to the guidelines. Over the ensuing 6 years to 1995–1996 the percentages using cholesterol-lowering drugs increased to 9.0% of women and 5.7% of men without CHD, and to 15.6% and 16.4% of those with CHD. Thus, by the end of this period half of women and men without CHD, but still only one-quarter of women and one-third of men with CHD who were eligible for treatment were receiving cholesterol-lowering drugs. At the beginning of the period of observation, statins and fibrates were used in equal numbers, but by the end statins were used in four times as many cases as fibrates. The 2763 women (average age 67 years) who volunteered for the HERS trial had to be rigorously documented prior CHD, and might have been expected to be more health conscious than women from the general population.[71] However, although 47% of the women at baseline examination in 1993–1995 were taking a lipid-lowering medication, 91% did not meet the NCEP goal of less than 100 mg/dl. Given the proven effectiveness of lipid lowering, especially in secondary prevention, further efforts need to be made to increase the implementation of diet and drugs and the achievement of optimal lipid levels.

Conclusions

Coronary heart disease is as important to diagnose and treat in women as it is in men; lipid disorders play a similar role as risk factors, and lipid lowering is as effective in women as it is in men. The fact that women develop heart disease at an older age should not be a barrier to treatment since lipid lowering is as effective at older ages as it is in the middle-aged. High-risk women with existing coronary disease or multiple risk factors should be targeted, while drug treatment could be used more cautiously in younger women with isolated lipid disorders only (except for monogenic lipid disorders associated with high risk for CHD). The search for multiple risk factors, especially those associated with obesity and the metabolic syndrome, may be particularly important in women because clustering of risk factors appears to be particularly common in women and diabetes is a major risk factor in women. It is possible but unproven that triglycerides and Lp(a) are more important risk factors in women than in men.

In postmenopausal women oral estrogen reduces Lp(a) and LDL-cholesterol levels, increases HDL-cholesterol and triglyceride levels, and has favorable effects on vascular physiology, but oral estrogen also increases blood coagulation, gallbladder disease, and breast cancer. Based on current knowledge, oral estrogen is not a suitable drug for treatment of lipid disorders or prevention of CHD. Parenteral estrogen retains some of the lipid effects and the vascular effects, and does not affect blood coagulation proteins, but clinical effects on coagulation need to be determined. Unlike oral estrogens, parenteral estrogens do not elevate levels of triglycerides or HDL-cholesterol. For women with high triglyceride levels, transdermal estrogens appear to be safer than oral estrogens.

Currently available selective estrogen receptor modulators (SERMs) have lipid and coagulation effects that differ quantitatively from those of estrogen, but appear to share the clinical effect of increasing venous thromboembolism. The first large randomized controlled clinical trial of hormone replacement therapy (HERS) failed to show the anticipated benefit of reducing CHD. Primary prevention trials are currently being conducted. Preliminary indications are that tamoxifen (one of the

SERMs) will not prevent CHD, but further trials of both tamoxifen and raloxifene are being conducted. A clinical trial of parenteral estrogen is needed, because this route of administration yields metabolic changes that are closer to those of endogenous estrogens.

References

1. Eaker ED, Chesebro JH, Sacks FM, *et al*. Cardiovascular disease in women. *Circulation* 1993; **88**(no. 4, part 1):1999–2009.

2. Mosca L, Manson JE, Sutherland SE, *et al*. Cardiovascular disease in women. A statement for healthcare professionals from the American Heart Association. *Circulation* 1997; **96**: 2468–82.

3. Lerner DJ, Kannel WB. Patterns of coronary heart disease morbidity and mortality in the sexes: A 26-year follow up of the Framingham population. *Am Heart J* 1986; **111**:383–90.

4. Manolio TA, Pearson TA, Wenger NK, *et al*. Cholesterol and heart disease in older persons and women: review of an NHLBI workshop. *Ann Epidemiol* 1992; **2**:161–76.

5. Harris T, Feldman JJ, Kleinman JC, *et al*. The low cholesterol-mortality association in a national cohort. *J Clin Epidemiol* 1992; **45**(6):595–601.

6. Manolio TA, Ettinger WH, Tracy RP, *et al*. Epidemiology of low cholesterol levels in older adults. The Cardiovascular Health Study. *Circulation* 1993; **87**(3):728–37.

7. Howard G, Manolio TA, Burke GL, *et al*. Does the association of risk factors and atherosclerosis change with age? An analysis of the combined ARIC and CHS cohorts. The Atherosclerosis Risk in Communities (ARIC) and Cardiovascular Health Study (CHS) Investigators. *Stroke* 1997; **29**(9): 1693–1701.

8. The Long-Term Intervention with Pravastatin in Ischaemic Disease (LIPID) Study Group. Prevention of cardiovascular events and death with pravastatin in patients with coronary heart disease and a broad range of initial cholesterol levels. *N Engl J Med* 1998; **339**(19):1349–57.

9. Downs JR, Clearfield M, Weis S, *et al*. Primary prevention of acute coronary events with lovastatin in men and women with average cholesterol levels — Results of AFCAPS/TexCAPS. *JAMA* 1998; **279**(20):1615–22.

10. Sacks FM, Pfeffer MA, Moye LA, *et al*. The effect of pravastatin on coronary events after myocardial infarction in patients with average cholesterol levels. *N Engl J Med* 1996; **335**(14):1001–100.

11. Lewis SJ, Moye LA, Sacks FM, *et al*. Effect of pravastatin on cardiovascular events in older patients with myocardial infarction and cholesterol levels in the average range. *Ann Intern Med* 1998; **129**(9):681–9.

12. The Scandinavian Simvastatin Survival Group. Randomized trial of cholesterol lowering in 4444 patients with coronary heart disease: The Scandinavian Simvastatin Survival Study. *Lancet* 1994; **344**(8934):1383–9.

13. Goldman L, Weinstein MC, Goldman PA, Williams LW. Cost-effectiveness of HMB-CoA reductase inhibition for primary and secondary prevention of coronary heart disease. *JAMA* 1991; **265**(9):1145–51.

14. Craig WY, Neveux LM, Palomaki GE, *et al*. Lipoprotein(a) as a risk factor for ischemic heart disease: metaanalysis of prospective studies. *Clin Chem* 1998; **44**(11):2301–6.

15. Klausen IC, Sjol A, Hansen PS, *et al*. Apolipoprotein(a) isoforms and coronary heart disease in men — A nested case-control study. *Atherosclerosis* 1997; **132**:77–84.

16. Cantin B, Gagnon F, Moorjani S, *et al*. Is Lipoprotein(a) an independent risk factor for ischemic heart disease in men? The Quebec Cardiovascular Study. *J Am Coll Cardiol* 1998; **31**:519–25.

17. Bostom AG, Cupples LA, Jenner JL, *et al*. Elevated plasma lipoprotein(a) and coronary heart disease in men aged 55 years and younger. A prospective study. *JAMA* 1996; **276**(7):544–8.

18. Dahlen GH, Stenlund H. Lp(a) lipoprotein is a major risk factor for cardiovascular disease: pathogenic mechanisms and clinical significance. *Clin Genet* 1997; **52**:272–80.

19. Bostom AG, Gagnon DR, Cupples LA, *et al*. A prospective investigation of elevated lipoprotein (a) detected by electrophoresis and cardiovascular disease in women. The Framingham Heart Study. *Circulation* 1994; **90**(4):1688–95.

20. Schwartzman RA, Cox ID, Poloniecki J, *et al*.

Elevated plasma lipoprotein(a) is associated with coronary artery disease in patients with chronic stable angina pectoris. *J Am Coll Cardiol* 1998; **31**(6):1260–6.

21. Austin MA, Hokanson JE, Edwards KL. Hypertriglyceridemia as a cardiovascular risk factor. *Am J Cardiol* 1998; **81**(4A):7B–12B.

22. Reaven GM, Chen YD, Jeppesen J, *et al*. Insulin resistance and hyperinsulinemia in individuals with small, dense low density lipoprotein particles. *J Clin Invest* 1993; **92**(1):141–6.

23. Wilson PWF, Kannel WB, Silbershatz H, D'Agostino RB. Clustering of metabolic factors and coronary heart disease. *Arch Intern Med* 1999; **159**:1104–9.

24. Manninen V, Tenkanen L, Koskinen P, *et al*. Joint effects of serum triglyceride and LD cholesterol and HDL cholesterol concentrations on coronary heart disease risk in the Helsinki heart study: implications for treatment. *Circulation* 1992; **85**(1):37–45.

25. Frick MH, Syvanne M, Nieminen MS, *et al*. Prevention of the angiographic progression of coronary and vein-graft atherosclerosis by gemfibrozil after coronary bypass surgery in men with low levels of HDL cholesterol. Lopid Coronary Angiography Trial (LOCAT) Study Group. *Circulation* 1997; **96**(7):2113–14.

26. Ericsson CG, Hamsten A, Nilsson J, *et al*. Angiographic assessment of effects of bezafibrate on progression of coronary artery disease in young male postinfarction patients. *Lancet* 1996; **347**(9005):849–53.

27. Waters D, Higginson L, Gladstone R, *et al*. Effects of cholesterol lowering on the progression of coronary atherosclerosis in women. A Canadian Coronary Atherosclerosis Intervention Trial (CCAIT) substudy. *Circulation* 1995; **92**(9):2404–10.

28. Haskell WL, Alderman EL, Fair JM, *et al*. Effects of intensive multiple risk factor reduction on coronary atherosclerosis and clinical cardiac events in men and women with coronary artery disease. The Stanford Coronary Risk Intervention Project (SCRIP). *Circulation* 1994; **89**(3):975–90.

29. Walsh JME, Grady D. Treatment of hyperlipidemia in women. *JAMA* 1995; **274**(14):1152–8.

30. Frantz ID Jr, Dawson EA, Ashman PL, *et al*. Test of effect of lipid lowering by diet on cardiovascular risk. The Minnesota Coronary Survey. *Arteriosclerosis* 1989; **9**:129–35.

31. Miettinen M, Turpeinen O, Karvonen MJ, *et al*. Effect of cholesterol-lowering diet on mortality from coronary heart-disease and other causes. A twelve-year clinical trial in men and women. *Lancet* 1972; **2**(7782):835–8.

32. Dorr AE, Gundersen K, Schneider JC Jr, *et al*. Colestipol hydrochloride in hypercholesterolemic patients — effect on serum cholesterol and mortality. *J Chronic Dis* 1978; **31**(1):5–14.

33. Research Committee of the Scottish Society of Physicians. Ischaemic heart disease: a secondary prevention trial using clofibrate. *Br Med J* 1971; **4**(5790):775–84.

34. Group of Physicians. Trial of clofibrate in the treatment of ischaemic heart disease. Five-year study by a group of physicians of the Newcastle upon Tyne Region. *Br Med J* 1971; **4**:767–75.

35. Hebert PR, Gaziano JM, Chan KS, Hennekens CH. Cholesterol lowering with statin drugs, risk of stroke, and total mortality: An overview of randomized trials. *JAMA* 1999; **278**(4):313–21.

36. National Heart, Lung and Blood Institute. The Lipid Research Clinic's Population Studies' Data Book Vol 1. Bethesda: United States Department of Health and Human Services, National Institutes of Health; 1980.

37. Brown SA, Hutchinson R, Morrisett J, *et al*. Plasma lipid, lipoprotein cholesterol, and apoprotein distributions in selected US communities. The Atherosclerosis Risk in Communities (ARIC) Study. *Arteriosclerosis Thromb* 1993; **13**(8):1139–58.

38. Jenner JL, Ordovas JM, Lamon-Fava S, *et al*. Effects of age, sex, and menopausal status on plasma lipoprotein(a) levels. The Framingham Offspring Study. *Circulation* 1993; **87**(4):1135–41.

39. Gorbach SL, Schaefer EJ, Woods M, *et al*. Plasma lipoprotein cholesterol and endogenous sex hormones in healthy young women. *Metabolism* 1989; **38**(11):1077–81.

40. Crook D, Seed M. Endocrine control of plasma lipoprotein metabolism: Effects of gonadal ste-

riods. *Baillieres Clin Endocrinol Metab* 1990; **4**(4):851–75.

41. Knopp RH. Cardiovascular effects of endogenous and exogenous sex hormones over a woman's lifetime. *Am J Obstet Gynecol* 1988; **158**(6 part 2):1630–43.

42. Pansini F, Bergamini C, Bettocchi S Jr, *et al.* Short-term effect of oophorectomy on lipoprotein metabolism. *Gynecol Obstet Invest* 1984; **18**(3):134–9.

43. Farish E, Fletcher CD, Hart DM, Smith ML. Effects of bilateral oophorectomy on lipoprotein metabolism. *Br J Obstet Gynaecol* 1990; **97**(1):78–82.

44. Bruschi F, Meschia M, Soma M, *et al.* Lipoprotein(a) and other lipids after oophorectomy and estrogen replacement therapy. *Obstet Gynecol* 1996; **88**(6):950–4.

45. Crook D. The metabolic consequences of treating postmenopausal women with non-oral hormone replacement therapy. *Br J Obstet Gynaecol* 1997; **104**(suppl. 16):4–13.

46. Crook D, Cust MP, Gangar KF, *et al.* Comparison of transdermal and oral estrogen-progestin replacement therapy: Effects on serum lipids and lipoproteins. *Am J Obstet Gynecol* 1992; **166**(3):950–5.

47. Meschia M, Bruschi F, Soma M, *et al.* Effects of oral and transdermal hormone replacement therapy on lipoprotein(a) and lipids: A randomized controlled trial. *Menopause* 1998; **5**(3):157–62.

48. Gerhard M, Walsh BW, Tawakol A, *et al.* Estradiol therapy combined with progesterone and endothelium-dependent vasodilation in postmenopausal women. *Circulation* 1998; **98**:1158–63.

49. Kroon UB, Silfverstolpe G, Tengborn L. The effects of transdermal estradiol and oral conjugated estrogens on haemostsis variables. *Thromb Haemost* 1994; **71**(4):420–3.

50. Koh KK, Mincemoyer R, Bui MN, *et al.* Effects of hormone-replacement therapy on fibrinolysis in postmenopausal women. *N Engl J Med* 1997; **336**(10):683–90.

51. Sack MN, Rader DJ, Cannon RO III. Oestrogen and inhibition of oxidation of low-density lipoproteins in postmenopausal women. *Lancet* 1994; **343**:269–70.

52. Scarabin PY, Alhenc-Gelas M, Plu-Bureau G, *et al.* Effects of oral and transdermal estrogen/progesterone regimens on blood coagulation and fibrinolysis in postmenopausal women. A randomized controlled trial. *Arteriosclerosis Thromb Vasc Biol* 1997; **17**(11):3071–8.

53. Castellsague J, Perez GS, Garcia Rodriguez LA. Recent epidemiological studies of the association between hormone replacement therapy and venous thromboembolism. *Drug Safety* 1998; **18**(2):117–23.

54. Campos H, Sacks FM, Walsh BW, *et al.* Differential effects of estrogen on low-density lipoprotein subclasses in healthy postmenopausal women. *Metabolism* 1993; **42**(9):1153–8.

55. Walsh BW, Li H, Sacks FM. Effects of postmenopausal hormone replacement with oral and transdermal estrogen on high density lipoprotein metabolism. *J Lipid Res* 1994; **35**:2083–93.

56. Su W, Campos H, Judge H, *et al.* Metabolism of apo(a) and apob100 of lipoprotein(a) in women: Effect of postmenopausal estrogen replacement. *J Clin Endocrinol Metab* 1998; **83**(9):3267–76.

57. The Writing Group for the PEPI Trial. Effects of estrogen or estrogen/progestin regimens on heart disease risk factors in postmenopausal women. *JAMA* 1995; **273**(3):199–208.

58. Espeland MA, Marcovina SM, Miller V, *et al.* Effect of postmenopausal hormone therapy on lipoprotein(a) concentration. PEPI Investigators. Postmenopausal estrogen/progestin interventions. *Circulation* 1998; **97**(10):979–86.

59. Koh KK, Cardillo C, Bui MN, *et al.* Vascular effects of estrogen and cholesterol-lowering therapies in hypercholesterolemic postmenopausal women. *Circulation* 1999; **99**(3):354–60.

60. Grady D, Sawaya G. Postmenopausal hormone therapy increases risk of deep vein thrombosis and plumonary embolism. *Am J Med* 1998; **105**(1):41–3.

61. Hulley S, Grady D, Bush T, *et al.* Randomized trial of estrogen plus progestin for secondary prevention of coronary heart disease in postmenopausal women. Heart and Estrogen/Progestin Replacement Study (HERS) Research Group. *JAMA* 1998; **280**(7):605–13.

62. Sbarouni E, Kyriakides ZS, Kremastinos DTh. The effect of hormone replacement therapy alone and in combination with simvastatin on plasma lipids of hypercholesterolemic postmenopausal women with coronary artery disease. *J Am Coll Cardiol* 1998; **32**:1244–50.

63. Darling GM, Johns JA, McCloud PI, Davis SR. Estrogen and progestin compared with simvastatin for hypercholesterolemia in postmenopausal women. *N Engl J Med* 1997; **337(9)**:595–601.

64. Rossouw JE. What we still need to learn about hormone replacement therapy. *Menopause* 1999; **10(2)**:189–209.

65. Prentice RL, Rossouw JE, Johnson SR, *et al.* The role of randomized controlled trials in assessing the benefits and risks of long term hormone replacement therapy: Example of the Women's Health Initiative. *Menopause* 1996; **3(2)**:71–6.

66. Walsh BW, Kuller LH, Wild RA, *et al.* Effects of raloxifene on serum lipids and coagulation factors in healthy postmenopausal women. *JAMA* 1998; **279(18)**:1445–51.

67. Clarkson TB, Anthony MS, Jerome CP. Lack of effect of raloxifene on coronary artery atherosclerosis of postmenopausal monkeys. *J Clin Endocrinol Metab* 1998; **83(3)**:721–6.

68. Fisher B, Costantino JP, Wickerham DL, *et al.* Tamoxifen for prevention of breast cancer: Report of the National Surgical Adjuvant Breast and Bowel Project P-1 Study. *J Natl Cancer Inst* 1998; **90(18)**:1371–88.

69. National Center for Health Statistics. Vital Statistics of the United States, Mortality, Part A, Vol II. Washington, DC: Public Health Service; 1992.

70. Lemaitre RN, Furberg CD, Newman AB, *et al.* Time trends in the use of cholesterol-lowering agents in older adults. *Arch Intern Med* 1998; **158**:1761–8.

71. Schrott HG, Bittner V, Vittinghoff E, *et al.* Adherence to national cholesterol education program treatment goals in postmenopausal women with heart disease. The Heart and Estrogen/Progestin Replacement Study (HERS). The HERS Research Group. *JAMA* 1997; **277(16)**:1281–6.

16

An update on the statins
Jean Davignon and Robert Dufour

Introduction

Over the last decade, therapy with HMG-CoA reductase inhibitors (statins) has evolved as much as the context in which these agents are prescribed.[1,2] Advances in atherosclerosis research and cardiology have led to major paradigm shifts, while at the same time results of major clinical trials have provided invaluable lessons for the practice of medicine (see chapter 14). The notion of culprit lesions, the importance of endothelial dysfunction and the contribution of inflammation to atherogenesis have become the focus of attention, raising new questions regarding the beneficial attributes of statins.

Coronary pathologists have shifted the emphasis from high-grade stenotic coronary lesions (which progress slowly, are more stable and allow for a collateral circulation to develop), to the more numerous and infamous ≤50% stenoses.[3,4] It is estimated that 68% of fatal myocardial infarctions are caused by low-grade stenoses.[5] These vulnerable plaques are referred to as culprit lesions because they are more unstable, more likely to erode, hemorrhage or rupture, and more likely to lead to catastrophic luminal obstructions. As they often encroach little, if at all, upon the arterial lumen coronary angiography is not ideal for their investigation. This latter tool is more useful in assessing the progression of high-grade stenoses. New technologies, especially intravascular ultrasound (IVUS) imaging, allow for a better appraisal of vulnerable plaques, which are characterized by a large lipid core, rich in foam cells, with a thin fibrous cap, poor in smooth muscle cells, and rich in activated macrophages and inflammatory cells.[3,6]

More attention is being given to alteration of endothelial function in the presence of cardiovascular risk factors or CAD, resulting in impaired myocardial perfusion.[7] Endothelial dysfunction is characterized by a paradoxical response to arterial infusion with acetylcholine, which induces vasoconstriction rather than vasodilatation. The latter is due to the release of nitric oxide (NO), formerly termed the 'endothelial-derived relaxing factor' or EDRF. The endothelial-mediated vasodilatation is typically inhibited by L-arginine analogues such as L-NMMA (N^{ω}-Nitroso-Mono-Methyl-Arginine), which prevents NO synthesis from L-arginine by constitutive endothelial NO synthase (eNOS). The advent of positron emission tomography (PET) scanning has provided a powerful tool to assess early changes in myocardial perfusion induced by drug therapy.[8]

There has also been a renewed interest in the inflammatory component of atherosclerosis,[9] which is assessed by plasma measurement of inflammatory markers such as C-reactive protein (CRP), IL-6, or serum amyloid-A protein (SAA).[10,11] A sensitive method has been developed to measure local changes in heat produced by the inflammatory reaction over atherosclerotic plaques *in vivo* in coronary arteries.[12] Using this method, a correlation was demonstrated between plasma levels of CRP and increases in heat differences between plaque areas and normal adjacent areas in patients with unstable angina and myocardial infarction.[12]

The use of statins has been greatly influenced by these changes in emphasis and advances in technology. The demonstration that statins may stabilize atherosclerotic plaques, improve endothelial dysfunction and inhibit inflammatory processes has kindled an interest in the multiple actions of these molecules, referred to as pleiotropic effects.[13] Clinical trials and angiographic studies carried out with six different statins have provided complementary information, thus advancing our knowledge of their clinical usefulness. An appreciable beneficial effect on triglyceride-rich lipoproteins, genetic factors modulating their effectiveness, and usefulness in diabetes and stroke have emerged from such studies. The immense experience acquired over 12 years with these widely prescribed drugs has confirmed their overall safety, but has also revealed potentially harmful interactions. Clinical, experimental and cell culture studies have also led to a better appraisal of their pharmacological differences and a better understanding of their mechanisms of action. This chapter will focus on the clinically relevant emergent properties of statins, considering in turn lipid-modulating effects, pleiotropic effects, and the potential for drug interactions.

Lipid-modulating effects

The primary mode of action of statins is a dose-dependent competitive inhibition of HMG-CoA reductase, a key step in cholesterol biosynthesis, resulting in upregulation of the low-density lipoprotein (LDL) receptor and reduction in the plasma concentration of LDL-cholesterol (LDL-C).[1] The magnitude of this effect first overshadowed other lipid-modulating properties such as an increase in high-density lipoprotein cholesterol (HDL-C) concentration and a reduction in plasma triglycerides. With the development of potent synthetic statins of the third generation, for example atorvastatin and cerivastatin, it became evident that the triglyceride-lowering effect could be strong enough to warrant the use of these agents in isolated hypertriglyceridemia as well as in combined hyperlipidemia.[14–16] This effect is a function of baseline triglyceride concentration, increasing in magnitude with the elevation in plasma triglycerides,[16] and it complements the well-known fact that these agents are efficacious in reducing triglyceride-rich remnant lipoproteins in type III hyperlipoproteinemia. Comparative studies with fibrates have indicated that although the latter are more potent in lowering plasma triglyceride levels and increasing HDL-C levels, statins have a stronger effect on the non-HDL-C/HDL-C atherogenic ratio, because they are better at reducing apolipoprotein B (apoB)-containing, cholesterol-rich lipoproteins.[15] Retrospective analyses have revealed that these properties are shared by all statins and were commensurate with their efficacy in lowering LDL-C levels.[16] Simvastatin shares this triglyceride-lowering effect in combined hyperlipidemia,[17] with reductions of 35% at doses of 80 mg/day.[18] The increase in HDL-C concentration associated with statin treatment has also been found to be proportional to baseline plasma triglyceride levels.[19] Plasma apoB, which is readily lowered by statins, reflects the presence of both cholesterol-rich and triglyceride-rich lipoproteins. Furthermore, high apoB levels may indicate the presence of atherogenic small dense LDL particles and an increase in the number of LDL particles. It is remarkable that in the Air Force/Texas Coronary Atherosclerosis Prevention Study (AFCAPS/TexCAPS), a primary prevention trial in low-risk individuals with average plasma LDL-C and low HDL-C levels, plasma apoB concentration, but not LDL-C at 1-year was a good predictor of major coronary events after 5 years.[20] This emphasizes the importance of risk associated with triglyceride-rich lipoproteins and low HDL-C levels, in line with recent epidemiological evidence,[21] giving added value to the non-LDL-related lipid-modulating effects of statins. Small dense LDL particles, which are prone to oxidation, are associated with CAD and predict angiographic changes in response to lipid-lowering therapy. An increase in LDL buoyancy was most strongly associated with regression of coronary lesions in the Familial Atherosclerosis Treatment Study (FATS).[22] This effect of a lovastatin–colestipol combination therapy was associated with a decrease in hepatic lipase activity and a reduced formation of small dense LDL.

Factors that influence the responsiveness of plasma LDL-C to statin therapy have been identified. One of the most studied is the apoE gene, where the ϵ4 allele (apoE4/4 or E4/3 phenotypes) reduces the response.[23,24] In the angiographic Lipoprotein and Coronary Atherosclerosis Study (LCAS), plasma HDL-C determined the magnitude of the effect of statin therapy on coronary lesion progression. Coronary atherosclerosis progressed further in the placebo group, but responded better to fluvastatin therapy (40 mg/day) in patients who had low HDL concentrations (≤35 mg/dl, or ≤0.9 mmol/l) at baseline than in those who had levels ≥35 mg/dl (≥0.9 mmol/l). This was associated with a significant improvement in

the probability of event-free survival over 2.5 years in the subset of patients with low HDL-C levels. Similarly, in the angiographic Regression Growth Evaluation Statin Study (REGRESS), a TaqI-B polymorphism of intron 1 of the cholesteryl ester transfer protein (CETP) gene was found to modulate lesion progression in the placebo group and response to pravastatin in the treatment group.[25] Carriers of the B1B1 allele (frequency 35%) had high CETP activity, high plasma triglyceride and low HDL-C levels. This was associated with a faster rate of progression of coronary atherosclerosis, but a better responsiveness of lesions to statin therapy compared with carriers of the B1B2 (49%) or the B2B2 (16%) alleles. There is a wide range of individual responses to the LDL-C lowering effect of statins that is not fully explained by known sources of variation.[26] A study in familial hypercholesterolemia has indicated that subjects with a high level of cholesterol synthesis, reflected by high plasma concentrations of mevalonic acid, respond better.[27] In this disease, the type of LDL receptor mutation may also influence the response to drug therapy.[28–30]

The magnitude of LDL-C lowering necessary to curb atherosclerosis progression (or lower the rate of major coronary events) has been a matter of debate. An analysis of pooled data from 11 angiographic studies indicates that per cent reduction in LDL-C levels, but not on-trial LDL-C levels, correlates best with per cent change in diameter stenoses.[31] It is estimated that progression of coronary lesions is arrested when a 44% reduction in LDL-C concentration is achieved. There has been some debate about the accuracy of the philosophy 'the lower the LDL-C reduction, the better the outcome', and it has been questioned whether there is a threshold relationship beyond which no further benefit is obtained. However, epidemiological evidence has shown that the relationship between CAD risk and plasma cholesterol level is curvilinear. This implies a diminishing return as the curve flattens in the low cholesterol range.[32] However, in low-risk populations such as that of Shanghai, a linear relationship is observed between risk and plasma concentration in the low cholesterol range.[33] Post-hoc analysis of data from CARE and WOSCOPS introduced the concept of a threshold relationship. No further benefit in risk is achieved below 125 mg/dl (3.23 mmol/l) of LDL-C in CARE in a subset analysis. Re-analysis by quintiles of LDL-C reduction in WOSCOPS showed a plateau in risk reduction after 24% of LDL-C lowering. Similar findings were observed in CARE but not in the Scandinavian Simvastatin Survival Study (4S).[34] However, it has been argued that the confidence limits were high in these analyses and the precise shape of the curve at lower LDL-C values was unclear and did not exclude a curvilinear relationship.[35] Similarly, subset analyses have been criticized as lacking power and being mainly hypothesis-generating exercises. It is also possible that part of the risk reduction in the low concentration range is not entirely reflected in LDL-C changes but could be reflected in total plasma apoB changes, as suggested from further analysis of the AFCAPS/TexCAPS results, as mentioned above.[20] Unfortunately, the relationship between outcome and plasma apoB reduction in CARE, WOSCOPS, LIPID and 4S has not yet been made available. Finally, observations made in clinical trials carried out with pravastatin, but not with simvastatin, may indicate that pravastatin has different properties. This notion was borne out by the fact that pravastatin is hydrophilic compared with the other statins, which are more lipophilic. It implies also that non-LDL mediated pleiotropic effects could be responsible.

An extended analysis of the WOSCOP study[36] has shown that greater cardiovascular benefit is obtained from treatment of patients with pravastatin than would have been anticipated according to the Framingham model (24% predicted, 35% achieved; a 31% underestimation). However, this model predicted with accuracy what was observed in the placebo group. Similarly, post-hoc overlap analysis of WOSCOPS[36] indicated that patients who had achieved similar on-treatment plasma LDL-C levels with pravastatin had lower 4.4-year CAD composite event rates (6.3%) than those who received placebo (9.6%) — a 36% difference. In contrast, two studies comparing mild and aggressive cholesterol-lowering therapy militate in favor of the notion that 'lower is better': the post-coronary artery bypass graft (Post-CABG) study with lovastatin[37] and the Atorvastatin Versus Revascularization Treatment (AVERT) study.[38] The debated issue is not settled, but ongoing clinical trials have been designed to answer this question. The enhanced efficacy of statins at maximum doses has resulted in their application to the treatment of homozygous familial hypercholesterolemia, a disease that is usually poorly responsive to drug therapy.[39,40]

Pleiotropic effects

It is a fundamental attribute of biological molecules to have multiple physiological and biochemical effects. A case in point is clusterin, also known as apoJ, the multiple effects of which explain why it has more than 14 different names, as it was rediscovered many times by different scientists working in widely differing fields.[41] In recent years, it has become evident that part of the cardiovascular benefit associated with statin therapy is probably due to such pleiotropic effects.[13,42] These occur in a wide range of different biological systems, and include vasodilatory, antithrombotic, antioxidant, antiproliferative, anti-inflammatory and plaque-stabilizing effects. They may be related to plasma lipid reduction *per se* but may also be independent. Several observations argue in favor of their existence, in addition to those already mentioned (i.e. overlap analysis and effects beyond the prediction of the Framingham model in WOSCOPS). The early separation of the survival curves in the placebo and treatment groups in 4S, WOSCOPS and AFCAPS/TexCAPS is difficult to explain on the basis of atherosclerosis regression alone, and is in contrast with the late separation of survival curves observed in the Program On the Surgical Control of the Hyperlipidemias (POSCH), in which LDL-C concentration was lowered by partial ileal bypass surgery. The unanticipated beneficial effect on stroke incidence by LDL-C reduction with statins, despite the fact that LDL-C is not highly predictive of stroke,[43] and the remarkable effect of statins on risk reduction in type 2 diabetes in 4S are additional arguments for the existence of pleitropic effects. Similarly, the fact that angiographic changes and LDL-C lowering with statins have not been predictive of cardiovascular event reduction also support their existence. The most compelling evidence is the demonstration by PET scanning that myocardial perfusion can be improved within as little as 90 days in hypercholesterolemic patients, following short-term aggressive lipid lowering with a statin combined with cholestyramine and dietary management.[8]

Even though a large number and wide range of pleiotropic effects have been reported for statins, the difficulty is to determine which have clinical and practical relevance. At present little is known about their relative importance, whether or not they are dose dependent, what part of the molecular structure they can be attributed to, and to what extent they contribute to clinical outcome, independent of reduction in the known CAD risk factors. Regarding the latter, one can speculate that statins might affect the time frame from incipient lesions to first event, reduce the severity of disease, or provide a rationale for the mechanism of action of known risk determinants. A precedent is the recognition that the protective effect of HDL can be explained in a number of ways, from enhancement of reverse cholesterol transport to antioxidant properties, which were not anticipated when the relation was first established between low HDL levels and increased incidence of CAD.

Some pleiotropic effects are specific to a statin type. The inhibitory effect of statins on tissue factor transcription and production by macrophages, demonstrated with fluvastatin and simvastatin but not with pravastatin,[44] is amongst these. Similarly, inhibition of cell proliferation is a property of lipophilic but not of hydrophilic statins.[45] In several cell types, the decreasing order of inhibitory potency is cerivastatin > simvastatin > fluvastatin > lovastatin > atorvastatin >>> pravastatin. Statins have anticarcinogenic properties related to their ability to induce apoptosis[46] and they inhibit cell proliferation, as demonstrated in many cell culture experiments and animal models,[13,47] including melanoma.[48] Lovastatin has been shown to inhibit lung metastasis in the highly metastatic B16F10 melanoma in nude mice.[49] It is tempting to relate these findings to the significant reduction in melanoma frequency observed in the AFCAPS/TexCAPS trial in patients treated with lovastatin.[50] More and more evidence is accumulating to support this antineoplastic effect of statins. In the extended follow-up of the 4S study, curves depicting the cumulative incidence of cancer separate in the long term, suggesting a protective effect of simvastatin (T. Pedersen, personal communication). The recent discovery that lovastatin blocks cell proliferation in the G_1 cell cycle phase through inhibition of the proteasome, independently of its inhibitory effect on HMG-CoA reductase, provides a molecular basis for these effects for the first time.[51] The lactone form (pro-drug) of lovastatin is effective, but neither the open hydroxy-acid form (active) nor pravastatin (also an open acid) show a similar effect. Inhibition of the proteasome results in increased stabilization of p21 and p27 that have tumor suppressor activity. Conversely, some advantageous effects of hydrophilic statins are not shared by lipophilic statins. The limited ability of a hydrophilic statin to penetrate muscle cells, compared with lipophilic statins, is associated with a reduced likelihood of inducing muscle damage, as shown in several experimental animal models.[52–54] These findings, added to an inhibitory effect of statins on platelet aggregation,[55] may account for the remarkable safety profile of statins observed to date.

Early effects of statin therapy on myocardial perfusion can be attributed primarily to improvement of endothelial function, a class effect which is no longer disputed.[56–58] It is in part related to cholesterol reduction, but also ascribed to two other mechanisms: first, a direct effect on nitric oxide (NO) production demonstrated *in vitro*[59,60] and *in vivo*;[61] and second, a reversal of the inhibitory effect of oxidized lipoproteins on endothelial constitutive NO synthase.[62] Experimental evidence in primates indicates that it may occur independently of LDL-C reduction.[63] Acute improvement in myocardial perfusion following treatment with statins can also be attributed to their inhibitory effect on endothelin production,[64] ability to reduce plasma viscosity,[65] and enhancement of erythrocyte deformability which is impaired in hypercholesterolemic subjects.[66] Eventually, such findings may lead

to prescribing statins for their early effect in acute coronary syndromes. Indeed, beneficial effects on endothelial function are reported within 6 weeks in RECIFE (Reduction of Cholesterol in Ischemia and Function of the Endothelium study), when a statin is started shortly after acute myocardial infarction or unstable angina.[67]

Several pleiotropic effects of statins may have a direct impact on atherogenesis. These include their antioxidant properties,[68–71] their ability to promote apoptosis,[46,72,73] their ability to inhibit scavenger receptor activity in macrophages (including SR-A,[74] CD-36,[75] and LOX-1,[76]) and their anti-inflammatory properties. The latter have been postulated from two recent studies. One is a nested case–control study from the CARE trial. Pravastatin was found to be most effective at reducing the relative risk of recurrent events in subjects who manifested signs of inflammation, namely serum amyloid A protein (SAA) and C-reactive protein above the 90th percentile.[10] Compared with the placebo-treated group, those with signs of inflammation had a higher CAD risk but responded better to pravastatin in terms of risk reduction (-54% versus -25%). Interestingly, at baseline these two subsets of patients matched for age and sex had similar levels of LDL-C, HDL-C and triglycerides. The other is a small study which reported that circulating pro-inflammatory cytokines such as IL-6 and TNFα may be lowered by short-term statin therapy.[11]

In the past, it was deduced from the results of regression studies in animals that the mechanism whereby statins slow the progression or induce regression of atherosclerosis was primarily by reducing the cholesterol content of the lipid core of atherosclerotic plaques. Shift in interest to small unstable lesions led to studies aimed at determining whether statins had the ability to stabilize these plaques. Matrix metalloproteinases (MMP), secreted by activated macrophages and other cells in the arterial wall, break down collagen, elastin and other components of the matrix, and thus may contribute to weakening of the fibrous cap which becomes fragile and prone to rupture. *In vitro*, fluvastatin and simvastatin have been shown to inhibit, in a dose-dependent manner, MMP-9 (gelatinase B) activity.[77] Research conducted with the hypercholesterolemic WHHL rabbit has demonstrated that cerivastatin reduces matrix MMP-1 (interstitial collagenase), MMP-3 (stromelysin-1) and MMP-9 in atherosclerotic lesions. A reduced macrophage population, an increased collagen content and a reduction in tissue factor production also accompany statin treatment. The first demonstration that statins might induce plaque stabilization in humans was shown recently by Crisby *et al.*[78] In an open prospective study, patients scheduled for carotid endarterectomy with similar carotid stenoses (>70% diameter reduction) were assigned to receive or not to receive 40 mg of pravastatin for 3 months before surgery. Using immunochemical and histochemical techniques, carotid plaques from treated patients had significantly less lipids and oxidized LDL than controls. Furthermore, there was a significant reduction in the number of macrophages and T-cells and less apoptosis, but no change in smooth muscle cell number. These preliminary findings are encouraging and strongly suggest that plaque stabilization seen in animals occurs in humans and likely applies to small culprit lesions.

Two clinical trials conducted with statins in heart transplant recipients have documented protection from allograft failure during the first year after transplantation. Pravastatin prevented the rise in cholesterol that follows transplantation, markedly decreased the number of rejections with hemodynamic compromise, and significantly improved 1-year survival, in comparison with a control group.[79] A similar benefit was observed over 4 years by maintaining post-transplantation plasma LDL-C concentration at less than 120 mg/dl (3.1 mmol/l) with simvastatin.[80] In this study, a reduction of intimal thickening, assessed by intracoronary ultrasonography, was documented in a subset of patients with LDL-C levels less than 110 mg/dl (2.84 mmol/l). In a head-to-head comparison of pravastatin and simvastatin, 1-year survival after cardiac transplantation was superior with pravastatin and the likelihood of rhabdomyolysis was reduced.[81] Several pleiotropic effects of statins have been considered to account for these observations, including a decrease in natural killer cell cytotoxicity,[79,82,83] inhibition of monocyte chemotaxis,[84] inhibition of smooth muscle cell proliferation,[85] interference with cell cycling,[86] and a putative potentiation of the immunosuppressive effect of cyclosporin A.[80] Data from a pilot study with kidney transplant patients suggest that pravastatin exerts an additional immunosuppressive effect in subjects treated with cyclosporin.[83]

Furthermore, it has been shown recently that lovastatin improves renal blood flow, increases glomerular filtration rate (GFR) and reduces proteinuria in the rat five-sixth nephrectomy model of renal insufficiency.[87] This finding is consistent with the demonstration that lovastatin alone or in combination with enalapril prevents the decline in GFR and glomerular injury in diabetic rats independently of its lipid-lowering effect.[88] Lovastatin and simvastatin are also potent promoters of bone formation in animals by stimulating osteoblast morphogenic protein-2 transcription, another new emergent property.[89] These are promising developments that eventually may lead to prescription of statins for their non-lipid effects.

Pharmacology and drug interactions

Statins have similarities and differences in chemical structure that account for variations in their pharmacokinetic properties.[90,91]

Four of the six commercially available statins are well absorbed in the small intestine (85–99%). The absorption of lovastatin is limited to 30% due to its hydrophobic properties, which prevents complete dissolution in the intestinal fluid. The enterocyte membrane has a low permeability to the hydrophilic pravastatin, which limits its absorption to 35%. Modification of gastric pH by antacids does not alter statin absorption significantly. The cholesterol-lowering effect is not influenced, even though administration of aluminium hydroxide gel (Maalox™) and cimetidine decreases plasma concentration of atorvastatin by 34%.[92] This is also the case when fluvastatin is administered with ranitidine, cimetidine or omeprazole. In spite of an increase in the area under the concentration curve (AUC) of fluvastatin of about 30% and a reduction in plasma clearance of 18–23%,[93] cholesterol lowering is not diminished. Food intake does not affect the lipid-lowering effect, even if in some instances, as with lovastatin, there may be a 50% increase of the active drug plasma concentration when it is given with meals. However, certain food components may substantially affect statin pharmacokinetics. When lovastatin or simvastatin are taken together with modest to large quantities of grapefruit juice (240–600 ml/day), the plasma concentration of these drugs is increased three- to twelvefold, opening the door to potential toxic effects.[94] This interaction is mediated via inhibition of intestinal cytochrome P450 3A4 (CYP3A4) by flavonoids, mostly 6',7'-dihydroxybergamottin which is present in grapefruit.[95,96] Statins that are not metabolized by CYP3A4 (for example, pravastatin), are not affected by this increased bioavailability which is secondary to the decreased intestinal first-pass extraction caused by grapefruit juice.[97] As expected, a clinically significant interaction takes place in the small intestine when bile acid sequestrants (cholestyramine or colestipol) are co-administered with statins. When they are given together, the statin is adsorbed by the resin and its bioavailability, reflected in the AUC, is decreased by 16% to 89%, reducing its lipid-lowering effect.[98] Thus, when prescribing this very effective drug combination (up to 60% LDL-C reduction), instructions should be given to take the resin at least 1 hour before or 4 hours after the statin for maximum efficacy. Caution should be exercised, as combination with a resin, especially useful in the treatment of mixed dyslipidemia, will blunt the triglyceride-reducing effect of the statin.

Statins are absorbed rapidly and the maximum plasma concentration (t_{max}) is reached between 0.5 and 4 hours after oral administration in normal subjects. The plasma half-life is relatively short, at between 1 and 4 hours, except for atorvastatin (14 hours). The longer plasma residence time may have clinical consequences.[99] First, a more stable plasma concentration and persistence of the lipid-lowering effect may be achieved if compliance is erratic. Second, the option is available to take atorvastatin in the morning, while the other statins need to be taken at night, just before maximum circadian cholesterol synthesis takes place, for optimal efficacy. Finally, there might be a prolongation of the period of time before side-effects or biological abnormalities disappear following interruption of treatment. The latter point merits consideration, especially if atorvastatin is given in combination with fibrates or with drugs metabolized by CYP3A4, because of the increased risk of myopathy and rhabdomyolysis. Statins are highly bound to plasma proteins (>95%), mostly albumin, with pravastatin being the only exception (50%). This high affinity of statins for plasma proteins (>99% for cerivastatin) is not affected by other drugs known to be strongly bound to proteins such as warfarin, imipramin or propanolol.[100] Protein binding of these agents is also not affected by statins. Modification of the protein binding of statins by drug interaction is not an issue of clinical importance, since this would result only in a transient increase in plasma free statin concentration which would not increase significantly its lipid-lowering effect or toxicity.

Most statins are lipophilic molecules which need to be rendered more polar by detoxification, primarily through a variety of oxidative transformations. These phase I reactions are catalyzed by the cytochrome P450 isozymes mainly in the liver and small intestine. Lovastatin, simvastatin, atorvastatin and cerivastatin use principally the CYP3A4 system for this purpose. Alternate mechanisms also exist for simvastatin (CYP2D6) and cerivastatin (CYP2C8). Fluvastatin is different since it does not require metabolism by CYP3A4. It is primarily metabolized by CYP2C9 and partly by CYP2D6. The hydrophilic pravastatin is essentially not metabolized by the P450 system.[101] Many of the hydroxylated metabolites of the lipophilic statins retain the pharmacological activity of their parent compound. They may be responsible for a substantial proportion of the observed lipid-lowering effect (approximately 25% for cerivastatin and up to 70% for atorvastatin). The half-life of the active metabolites of atorvastatin is 20–30 hours, further increasing the residence time of active drug. Since the statins are metabolized predominantly in the liver, and since liver enzyme increase is a potential adverse effect of these

drugs, it is important to determine how liver dysfunction affects pharmacokinetic parameters. Unfortunately, information on this subject is sparse: the bioavailability of pravastatin is 34% higher in patients with cirrhosis of the liver, and is increased 11- to 16-fold when atorvastatin is given to patients with moderately severe hepatic impairment.[102,103] Even if metabolites of the lipophilic statins are more polar and water soluble, they are predominantly excreted in the bile. Only pravastatin, cerivastatin, and their metabolites are recovered to a significant extent in the urine. Renal impairment, even when it is severe (creatinine clearance <30 ml/min), does not affect the pharmacokinetic parameters of atorvastatin, pravastatin or cerivastatin, while it doubles the plasma concentration of lovastatin.[104] Hence, it is generally unnecessary to adjust the dosage of statins in patients with mild to moderate renal insufficiency.

The most important clinical consequence of statin metabolism through the cytochrome P450 enzyme system is the risk of interaction with other drugs that are metabolized by or are inhibitors of the same isozymes.[105–108] This is especially important for the statins detoxified by CYP3A4, since many currently prescribed drugs are detoxified by this system. Substrates of CYP3A4 include alprazolam, astemizole, cisapride, felodipine, miconazole, nifedipine, quinidine, terfenadine and triazolam. Inhibitors include azythromycin, clarithromycin, erythromycin, nefazodone, sildenafil and zafirlukast. Diltiazem, cyclosporin, itraconazole and ketoconazole are all both substrates and inhibitors of CYP3A4, the conazoles also being inhibitors of CYP2C9. Although rare, concurrent treatment with one or more of these drugs can dramatically increase the plasma concentration of a statin and induce toxic side-effects such as myopathy, rhabdomyolysis and renal insufficiency. A 20-

fold increase in plasma concentration of lovastatin, with subsequent rhabdomyolysis, has been observed in patients already on itraconazole.[109] CYP3A4 involvement in this toxic interaction is supported by the absence of a similar increase in C_{max} and AUC when itraconazole is given with pravastatin. Other cases of rhabdomyolysis have been reported when lovastatin or simvastatin were given with cyclosporin, erythromycin, clarithromycin, azithromycin, warfarin, nefazodone and mibefradil. Many cases of rhabdomyolysis, 'torsades de points' and early death were observed when simvastatin was combined with mibefradil, a promising selective calcium channel blocker that was withdrawn early.[110,111] A modification of pharmacokinetic parameters has also been observed when fluvastatin was taken with diclofenac, both drugs being metabolized by CYP2C9.

Cases of rhabdomyolysis have been reported in patients treated with a combination of a statin (lovastatin, simvastatin, atorvastatin or cerivastatin) and a fibrate, gemfibrozil being the most frequently involved.[112–115] It was originally believed that an interaction at the level of the cytochrome P450 system was responsible for adverse events, but it seems more likely that a combined toxic effect of both drugs on skeletal muscle is responsible. Increase in the cytosolic free concentration of calcium ions, reduction of chloride conductance and puncture of muscle cells by simvastatin has been demonstrated in rats.[53,116] Combination of a fibrate and a statin may be hazardous, but this is not necessarily so if caution is exercised. Toxic drug interactions are more likely in polymedicated patients at high cardiovascular risk (in other words, those with coexisting hypertension, congestive heart failure, arrhythmia, diabetes, renal insufficiency, etc.). If combination therapy is warranted after careful assessment

of the risk benefit ratio, it is advisable to choose a hydrophilic statin, with a short half-life, small volume of distribution and high liver selectivity. Select a fibrate with a short half-life and give it in the morning, with the statin being taken at night. Begin treatment by using low doses of both drugs, warning patients of potential side-effects, and carefully monitoring for the appearance of muscular symptoms.

The ability of a statin to be detoxified by two or more different cytochrome isozymes does not ensure safety when a drug is administered concurrently. Many different factors influence drug interactions.[108] Some drugs are inhibitors of more than one isozyme (for example, fluvoxamine inhibits the activity of 1A2, 2C9 and 3A4), while others are both substrate and inhibitor of a given isozyme. Genetic polymorphisms of cytochrome P450 isozymes may modulate the interaction (for instance 8% of the American population lack the CYP2D6 gene). Concomitant liver or kidney disease, or hypoalbuminemia enhances the risk of drug interaction, while age, diet, smoking, acute or chronic alcohol consumption can modulate cytochrome activity. It is worth remembering that the magnitude of inhibition tends to be dose related. It is also noteworthy that cases of rhabdomyolysis are usually reported after the drug is released on the market, when large numbers of patients are exposed to numerous drugs, often prescribed by different physicians. Thus, even though rhabdomyolysis is a rare event, it is a trying experience and safety can be ensured only with unrelenting vigilance for potential harmful drug interactions.

Conclusions

In the last decade, advances in cardiology, vascular biology and pharmacology have markedly influenced the use of statins. A large number of well-designed angiographic and clinical trials have clearly demonstrated the efficacy, safety and tolerability of these drugs and provided strong evidence in support of their use in CAD prevention. Their potency and anti-atherogenic lipid-modulating effects on triglyceride-rich lipoproteins, HDL, plasma apoB, and small dense LDL have been fully recognized. Certain statins have had their indications extended to conditions associated with hypertriglyceridemia and even to homozygous familial hypercholesterolemia. A better appraisal of their usefulness followed recognition of factors impacting on their ability to curb atherosclerosis progression, such as low HDL levels and variations in the apoE and CETP genes. A better awareness of their potential dangers has resulted from case reports of drug interactions and careful pharmacokinetic studies. This has led to an improved understanding of differences among the statins and has put into perspective their respective advantages and disadvantages. Recognition of the role of the various cytochrome P450 enzymes in the detoxification process has alerted physicians to potentially dangerous combinations that might lead to myopathy and rhabdomyolysis. This has become especially obvious for concurrent administration of several drugs catabolized via the CYP3A4 pathway.

Studies on the pleiotropic effects of statins have introduced important new notions. They have emphasized the fact that not all statins were created equal (there are class effects and statin-specific effects in the pleiotropic realm). They have strengthened our confidence in their safety (anticarcinogenic and antithrombotic properties). Importantly, they have indicated that statins may have early beneficial effects (improvement in myocardial perfusion) and offered an explanation for reduction in CAD

in the long term (anti-inflammatory and plaque stabilization effects). They have provided new indications for these drugs (use in heart and kidney transplantation). They have also raised the possibility that one day statins might be prescribed for attributes totally unrelated to their lipid effects (anti-osteopenic, improvement of renal function). The ongoing investigation of the emergent properties of statins and their clinical relevance is clearly a worthwhile undertaking.

References

1. Davignon J, Montigny M, Dufour R. HMG-CoA reductase inhibitors: a look back and a look ahead. *Can J Cardiol* 1992; **8**:843–64.

2. Davignon J. Advances in drug treatment of dyslipidemia: Focus on atorvastatin. *Can J Cardiol* 1998; **14**:28B–38B.

3. Lee RT, Libby P. The unstable atheroma. *Arteriosclerosis Thromb Vasc Biol* 1997; **17**: 1859–67.

4. Gutstein DE, Fuster V. Pathophysiology and clinical significance of atherosclerotic plaque rupture. *Cardiovasc Res* 1999; **41**:323–33.

5. Falk E, Shah PK, Fuster V. Coronary plaque disruption. [Review]. *Circulation* 1995; **92**: 657–71.

6. Libby P. Molecular bases of the acute coronary syndromes. [Review]. *Circulation* 1995; **91**:2844–50.

7. Drexler H, Hornig B. Endothelial dysfunction in human disease. *J Mol Cell Cardiol* 1999; **31**:51–60.

8. Gould KL, Martucci JP, Goldberg DI, *et al.* Short-term cholesterol lowering decreases size and severity of perfusion abnormalities by positron emission tomography after dipyridamole in patients with coronary artery disease: A potential noninvasive marker of healing coronary endothelium. *Circulation* 1994; **89**:1530–8.

9. Ross R. Mechanisms of disease — Atherosclerosis — An inflammatory disease. *N Engl J Med* 1999; **340**:115–26.

10. Ridker PM, Rifai N, Pfeffer MA, *et al.* Inflammation, pravastatin, and the risk of

coronary events after myocardial infarction in patients with average cholesterol levels. *Circulation* 1998; **98**:839–44.

11. Rosenson RS, Tangney CC, Casey LC. Inhibition of proinflammatory cytokine production by pravastatin. *Lancet* 1999; **353**:983–4.

12. Stefanadis C, Diamantopoulos L, Vlachopoulos C, *et al.* Thermal heterogeneity within human atherosclerotic coronary arteries detected in vivo — A new method of detection by application of a special thermography catheter. *Circulation* 1999; **99**:1965–71.

13. Davignon J. The pleiotropic effects of drugs affecting lipid metabolism. In: Jacotot B, Mathé D, Fruchart J-C, eds. *Atherosclerosis XI*. Proceedings of the IXth International Symposium on Atherosclerosis. Singapore: Elsevier Science; 1998: 63–77.

14. Bakker-Arkema R, Davidson M, Goldstein M, *et al.* Atorvastatin, a new HMG-CoA reductase inhibitor (HMGRI), is safe and effective in hypertriglyceridemia. *Atherosclerosis* 1994; **109**:313.

15. Ooi TC, Heinonen T, Alaupovic P, *et al.* Efficacy and safety of a new hydroxymethylglutaryl-coenzyme a reductase inhibitor, atorvastatin, in patients with combined hyperlipidemia: Comparison with fenofibrate. *Arteriosclerosis Thromb Vasc Biol* 1997; **17**:1793–9.

16. Stein EA, Lane M, Laskarzewski P. Comparison of statins in hypertriglyceridemia. *Am J Cardiol* 1998; **81**:66B–69B.

17. Bruckert E, de Gennes JL, Malbecq W, Baigts F. Comparison of the efficacy of simvastatin and standard fibrate therapy in the treatment of primary hypercholesterolemia and combined hyperlipidemia. *Clin Cardiol* 1995; **18**:621–9.

18. Hunninghake DB, Plotkin D, Stepanavage M, *et al.* Large, dose dependent effects of simvastatin 40 and 80 mg/day in combined hyperlipidemia. *J Am Coll Cardiol* 1999; **33**:244A.

19. Stein EA, Lane MC, Laskarzewski PM. Comparative effects of statins on plasma lipids and lipoproteins. In: 13th International Symposium on Drugs Affecting Lipid Metabolism [Abstract book] 1998; 18.

20. Gotto AM Jr, Whitney E, Stein EA, *et al.* Predicting risk of first acute major coronary events (AMCEs) in the Air Force/Texas coronary atherosclerosis prevention study (AFCAPS/TexCAPS). *J Am Coll Cardiol* 1999; **33**:263A.

21. Jeppesen J, Hein HO, Suadicani P, Gyntelberg F. Relation of high TG low HDL cholesterol and LDL cholesterol to the incidence of ischemic heart disease — An 8-year follow-up in the Copenhagen Male Study. *Arteriosclerosis Thromb Vasc Biol* 1997; **17**:1114–20.

22. Zambon A, Hokanson JE, Brown BG, Brunzell JD. Evidence for a new pathophysiological mechanism for coronary artery disease regression — Hepatic lipase-mediated changes in LDL density. *Circulation* 1999; **99**:1959–64.

23. Carmena R, Roederer G, Mailloux H, *et al.* The response to lovastatin treatment in patients with heterozygous familial hypercholesterolemia is modulated by apolipoprotein E polymorphism. *Metabolism* 1993; **42**:895–901.

24. Ordovas JM, Lopez-Miranda J, Perez-Jimenez F, *et al.* Effect of apolipoprotein E and A-IV phenotypes on the low density lipoprotein response to HMG CoA reductase inhibitor therapy. *Atherosclerosis* 1995; **113**:157–66.

25. Kuivenhoven JA, Jukema JW, Zwinderman AH, *et al.* The role of a common variant of the cholesterol ester transfer protein gene in the progression of coronary atherosclerosis. *N Engl J Med* 1998; **338**:86–93.

26. Karayan L, Qiu S, Betard C, *et al.* Response to HMG CoA reductase inhibitors in heterozygous familial hypercholesterolemia due to the 10-kb deletion ('French Canadian mutation') of the LDL receptor gene. *Arteriosclerosis Thromb* 1994; **14**:1258–63.

27. Naoumova RP, Marais AD, Mountney J, *et al.* Plasma mevalonic acid, an index of cholesterol synthesis in vivo, and responsiveness to HMG-CoA reductase inhibitors in familial hypercholesterolaemia. *Atherosclerosis* 1996; **119**:203–13.

28. Jeenah M, September W, van Roggen FG, *et al.* Influence of specific mutations at the LDL-receptor gene locus on the response to simvastatin therapy in Afrikaner patients with heterozygous familial hypercholes-

terolaemia. *Atherosclerosis* 1993; **98**:51–8.

29. Leitersdorf E, Eisenberg S, Eliav O, *et al.* Genetic determinants of responsiveness to the HMG-CoA reductase inhibitor fluvastatin in patients with molecularly defined heterozygous familial hypercholesterolemia. *Circulation* 1993; **87**(**suppl. III**):35–44.

30. Leren TP, Hjermann I. Is responsiveness to lovastatin in familial hypercholesterolaemia heterozygotes influenced by the specific mutation in the low-density lipoprotein receptor gene. *Eur J Clin Invest* 1995; **25**:967–73.

31. Thompson GR, Hollyer J, Waters DD. Percentage change rather than plasma level of LDL-cholesterol determines therapeutic response in coronary heart disease. *Curr Opin Lipidol* 1995; **6**:386–8.

32. The International Task Force for Prevention of Coronary Heart Disease. Coronary heart disease: reducing the risk. The scientific background for primary and secondary prevention of coronary heart disease. *Nutr Metab Cardiovasc Dis* 1998; **8**:205–71.

33. Chen Z, Peto R, Collins R, *et al.* Serum cholesterol concentration and coronary heart disease in population with low cholesterol concentrations. *Br Med J* 1991; **303**:276–82.

34. Pedersen TR, Olsson AG, Faergeman O, *et al.* Lipoprotein changes and reduction in the incidence of major coronary heart disease events in the Scandinavian Simvastatin Survival Study. *Circulation* 1998; **97**:1453–60.

35. Grundy SM. Statin trials and goals of cholesterol-lowering therapy. *Circulation* 1998; **97**:1436–9.

36. Packard CJ, Shepherd J, Cobbe SM, *et al.* Influence of pravastatin and plasma lipids on clinical events in the West of Scotland Coronary Prevention Study (WOSCOPS). *Circulation* 1998; **97**:1440–5.

37. Campeau L, Knatterud GLMK, Domanski M, *et al.* The effect of aggressive lowering of low-density lipoprotein cholesterol levels and low-dose anticoagulation on obstructive changes in saphenous-vein coronary-artery bypass grafts. *N Engl J Med* 1997; **336**:153–62.

38. Pitt B, Waters D, Brown WV, *et al.* Atorvastatin versus revascularization treatment investigators. Aggressive lipid-lowering therapy compared with angioplasty in stable coronary artery disease. *N Engl J Med* 1999; **342**:70–6.

39. Raal FJ, Pilcher GJ, Illingworth DR, *et al.* Expanded-dose simvastatin is effective in homozygous familial hypercholesterolaemia. *Atherosclerosis* 1997; **135**:249–56.

40. Marais AD, Naoumova RP, Firth JC, *et al.* Decreased production of low density lipoprotein by atorvastatin after apheresis in homozygous familial hypercholesterolemia. *J Lipid Res* 1997; **38**:2071–8.

41. Rosenberg ME, Silkensen J. Clusterin: Physiologic and pathophysiologic considerations. *Int J Biochem Cell Biol* 1995; **27**:633–45.

42. Davignon J. Methods and endpoint issues in clinical development of lipid-acting agents with pleiotropic effects. *Am J Cardiol* 1998; **81**:17F–23F.

43. Bucher HC, Griffith LE, Guyatt GH. Effect of HMGCoA reductase inhibitors on stroke — A meta-analysis of randomized, controlled trials. *Ann Intern Med* 1998; **128**:89–95.

44. Colli S, Eligini S, Lalli M, *et al.* Vastatins inhibit tissue factor in cultured human macrophages — A novel mechanism of protection against atherothrombosis. *Arteriosclerosis Thromb Vasc Biol* 1997; **17**:265–72.

45. Nègre-Aminou P, van Vliet AK, van Erck M, *et al.* Inhibition of proliferation of human smooth muscle cells by various HMG-CoA reductase inhibitors: Comparison with other human cell types. *Biochim Biophys Acta Lipids Lipid Metab* 1997; **1345**:259–68.

46. Guijarro C, Blanco-Colio LM, Ortego M, *et al.* 3-Hydroxy-3-methylglutaryl coenzyme a reductase and isoprenylation inhibitors induce apoptosis of vascular smooth muscle cells in culture. *Circ Res* 1998; **83**:490–500.

47. Dimitroulakos J, Nohynek D, Backway KL, *et al.* Increased sensitivity of acute myeloid leukemias to lovastatin-induced apoptosis: A potential therapeutic approach. *Blood* 1999; **93**:1308–18.

48. Feleszko W, Zagozdzon R, Golab J, Jakobisiak M. Potentiated antitumour effects of cisplatin and lovastatin against MmB16 melanoma in mice. *Eur J Cancer* [A] 1998; **34**:406–11.

49. Jani JP, Specht S, Stemmler N, *et al.* Metastasis of B16F10 mouse melanoma inhibited by

lovastatin, an inhibitor of cholesterol biosynthesis. *Invasion Metastasis* 1993; **13**:314–24.

50. Downs JR, Clearfield M, Weis S, *et al.* Primary prevention of acute coronary events with lovastatin in men and women with average cholesterol levels — Results of AFCAPS/TexCAPS. *JAMA* 1998; **279**: 1615–22.

51. Rao S, Porter DC, Chen X, *et al.* Lovastatin-mediated G_1 arrest is through inhibition of the proteasome, independent of hydroxymethyl glutaryl-CoA reductase. *Proc Natl Acad Sci USA* 1999; **96**:7797–802.

52. Masters BA, Palmoski MJ, Flint OP, *et al.* In vitro myotoxicity of the 3-hydroxy-3-methylglutaryl coenzyme A reductase inhibitors, pravastatin, lovastatin, and simvastatin, using neonatal rat skeletal myocytes. *Toxicol Appl Pharmacol* 1995; **131**:163–74.

53. Pierno S, De Luca A, Tricarico D, *et al.* Potential risk of myopathy by HMG-CoA reductase inhibitors: A comparison of pravastatin and simvastatin effects on membrane electrical properties of rat skeletal muscle. *J Pharmacol Exp Ther* 1995; **275**:1490–6.

54. Gadbut AP, Caruso AP, Galper JB. Differential sensitivity of C_2–C_{12} striated muscle cells to lovastatin and pravastatin. *J Mol Cell Cardiol* 1995; **27**:2397–402.

55. Rosenson RS, Tangney CC. Antiatherothrombotic properties of statins: implications for cardiovascular event reduction. [Review]. *JAMA* 1998; **279**:1643–50.

56. Egashira K, Hirooka Y, Kai H, *et al.* Reduction in serum cholesterol with pravastatin improves endothelium-dependent coronary vasomotion in patients with hypercholesterolemia. *Circulation* 1994; **89**:2519–24.

57. Anderson TJ, Meredith IT, Yeung AC, *et al.* The effect of cholesterol-lowering and antioxidant therapy on endothelium-dependent coronary vasomotion. *N Engl J Med* 1995; **332**:488–93.

58. O'Driscoll G, Green D, Taylor RR. Simvastatin, an HMG-coenzyme A reductase inhibitor, improves endothelial function within 1 month. *Circulation* 1997; **95**:1126–31.

59. Brandes RP, Behra A, Lebherz C, *et al.* Lovastatin maintains nitric oxide — but not EDHF-mediated endothelium-dependent relaxation in the hypercholesterolemic rabbit carotid artery. *Atherosclerosis* 1999; **142**:97–104.

60. Kaesemeyer WH, Caldwell RB, Huang JZ, Caldwell RW. Pravastatin sodium activates endothelial nitric oxide synthase independent of its cholesterol-lowering actions. *J Am Coll Cardiol* 1999; **33**:234–41.

61. John S, Schlaich M, Langenfeld M, *et al.* Increased bioavailability of nitric oxide after lipid-lowering therapy in hypercholesterolemic patients — A randomized, placebo-controlled, double-blind study. *Circulation* 1998; **98**:211–16.

62. Laufs U, La Fata V, Plutzky J, Liao JK. Upregulation of endothelial nitric oxide synthase by HMG CoA reductase inhibitors. *Circulation* 1998; **97**:1129–35.

63. Williams JK, Sukhova GK, Herrington DM, Libby P. Pravastatin has cholesterol-lowering independent effects on the artery wall of atherosclerotic monkeys. *J Am Coll Cardiol* 1998; **31**:684–91.

64. Hernández-Perera O, Pérez-Sala D, Navarro-Antolín J, *et al.* Effects of the 3-hydroxy-3-methylglutaryl-CoA reductase inhibitors, atorvastatin and simvastatin, on the expression of endothelin-1 and endothelial nitric oxide synthase in vascular endothelial cells. *J Clin Invest* 1998; **101**:2711–19.

65. Tsuda Y, Satoh K, Kitadai M, *et al.* Effects of pravastatin sodium and simvastatin on plasma fibrinogen level and blood rheology in type II hyperlipoproteinemia. *Atherosclerosis* 1996; **122**:225–33.

66. Kohno M, Murakawa K, Yasunari K, *et al.* Improvement of erythrocyte deformability by cholesterol-lowering therapy with pravastatin in hypercholesterolemic patients. *Metabolism* 1997; **46**:287–91.

67. Dupuis J, Tardiff BE, Cernacek P, Théroux P. Cholesterol reduction rapidly improves endothelial function after acute coronary syndromes — the RECIFE (Reduction of cholesterol in ischemia and function of the endothelium) trial. *Circulation* 1999; **99**:3227–33.

68. Aviram M, Dankner G, Cogan U, *et al.* Lovastatin inhibits low-density lipoprotein

oxidation and alters its fluidity and uptake by macrophages: In vitro and in vivo studies. *Metabolism* 1992; 41:229–35.

69. Kleinveld HA, Demacker PN, de Haan AF, Stalenhoef AF. Decreased in vitro oxidizability of low-density lipoprotein in hypercholesterolaemic patients treated with 3-hydroxy-3-methylglutaryl-CoA reductase inhibitors. *Eur J Clin Invest* 1993; 23:289–95.

70. Salonen R, Nyyssönen K, Porkkala-Sarataho E, Salonen JT. The Kuopio Atherosclerosis Prevention Study (KAPS): Effect of pravastatin treatment on lipids, oxidation resistance of lipoproteins, and atherosclerotic progression. *Am J Cardiol* 1995; 76:34C–39C.

71. Aviram M, Rosenblat M, Bisgaier CL, Newton RS. Atorvastatin and gemfibrozil metabolites, but not the parent drugs, are potent antioxidants against lipoprotein oxidation. *Atherosclerosis* 1998; 138:271–80.

72. Jones KD, Couldwell WT, Hinton DR, *et al*. Lovastatin induces growth inhibition and apoptosis in human malignant glioma cells. *Biochem Biophys Res Commun* 1994; 205:1681–7.

73. Buemi M, Allegra A, Senatore M, *et al*. Pro-apoptotic effect of fluvastatin on human smooth muscle cells. *Eur J Pharmacol* 1999; 370:201–3.

74. Umetani N, Kanayama Y, Okamura M, *et al*. Lovastatin inhibits gene expression of type-I scavenger receptor in THP-1 human macrophages. *Biochim Biophys Acta Lipids Lipid Metab* 1996; 1303:199–206.

75. Pietsch A, Erl W, Lorenz RL. Lovastatin reduces expression of the combined adhesion and scavenger receptor CD36 in human monocytic cells. *Biochem Pharmacol* 1996; 52:433–9.

76. Draude G, Hrboticky N, Lorenz RL. The expression of the lectin-like oxidized low-density lipoprotein receptor (LOX-1) on human vascular smooth muscle cells and monocytes and its down-regulation by lovastatin. *Biochem Pharmacol* 1999; 57:383–6.

77. Bellosta S, Via D, Canavesi M, *et al*. HMG-CoA reductase inhibitors reduce MMP-9 secretion by macrophages. *Arteriosclerosis Thromb Vasc Biol* 1998; 18:1671–8.

78. Crisby M, Fredriksson-Norden G, Nilsson J. Pravastatin treatment decreases lipid content, inflammation and cell death in human carotid plaques. The Lancet conference. The challenge of stroke: October 1998.

79. Kobashigawa JA, Katznelson S, Laks H, *et al*. Effect of pravastatin on outcomes after cardiac transplantation. *N Engl J Med* 1995; 333:621–7.

80. Wenke K, Meiser B, Thiery J, *et al*. Simvastatin reduces graft vessel disease and mortality after heart transplantation: a four-year randomized trial. *Circulation* 1997; 96:1398–402.

81. Keogh AM, Macdonald PS, Aboyoun C, *et al*. Pravastatin confers superior survival after cardiac transplantation when compared to simvastatin. *J Am Coll Cardiol* 1999; 33:205A.

82. Cutts JL, Bankhurst AD. Reversal of lovastatin-mediated inhibition of natural killer cell cytotoxicity by interleukin 2. *J Cell Physiol* 1990; 145:244–52.

83. Katznelson S, Wilkinson AH, Kobashigawa JA, *et al*. The effect of pravastatin on acute rejection after kidney transplantation — A pilot study. *Transplantation* 1996; 61:1469–74.

84. Kreuzer J, Bader J, Jahn L, *et al*. Chemotaxis of the monocyte cell line U937: Dependence on cholesterol and early mevalonate pathway products. *Atherosclerosis* 1991; 90:203–9.

85. Corsini A, Raiteri M, Soma MR, *et al*. Simvastatin but not pravastatin has a direct inhibitory effect on rat and human myocyte proliferation. *Clin Biochem* 1992; 25:399–400.

86. Doyle JW, Kandutsch AA. Requirement for mevalonate in cycling cells: quantitative and temporal aspects. *J Cell Physiol* 1988; 137:133–40.

87. Hafez KS, Inman SR, Stowe NT, Novick AC. Renal hemodynamic effects of lovastatin in a renal ablation model. *Urology* 1996; 48:862–7.

88. Inman SR, Stowe NT, Cressman MD, *et al*. Lovastatin preserves renal function in experimental diabetes. *Am J Med Sci* 1999; 317:215–21.

89. Mundy G, Gutierrez G, Garrett R, *et al*. Iden-

tification of a new class of powerful stimulators of new bone formation in vivo, clarification of mechanism of action, and use in animal models of osteoporosis. Second joint meeting of the American Society of Bone Mineral Research & International Bone Mineral Society. San Francisco; 1998.

90. Corsini A, Maggi FM, Catapano AL. Pharmacology of competitive inhibitors of HMG-CoA reductase. *Pharm Res* 1995; **31**:9–29.

91. Lennernäs H, Fager G. Pharmacodynamics and pharmacokinetics of the HMG-CoA reductase inhibitors. Similarities and differences. [Review]. *Clin Pharmacokinetics* 1997; **32**:403–25.

92. Yang B-B, Smithers JA, Abel RB, *et al*. Effects of Maalox TC^R on pharmacokinetics and pharmacodynamics of atorvastatin. *Pharm Res* 1996; **13**(suppl.):S437.

93. Plosker GL, Wagstaff AJ. Fluvastatin — A review of its pharmacology and use in the management of hypercholesterolaemia. *Drugs* 1996; **51**:433–59.

94. Kantola T, Kivistö KT, Neuvonen PJ. Grapefruit juice greatly increases serum concentrations of lovastatin and lovastatin acid. *Clin Pharmacol Ther* 1998; **63**:397–402.

95. Schmiedlin-Ren P, Edwards DJ, Fitzsimmons ME, *et al*. Mechanisms of enhanced oral availability of CYP3A4 substrates by grapefruit constituents. Decreased enterocyte CYP3A4 concentration and mechanism-based inactivation by furanocoumarins. *Drug Metabol Disposition* 1997; **25**:1228–33.

96. Lilja JJ, Kivistö KT, Neuvonen PJ. Grapefruit juice–simvastatin interaction: Effect on serum concentrations of simvastatin, simvastatin acid, and HMG-CoA reductase inhibitors. *Clin Pharmacol Ther* 1998; **64**:477–83.

97. Palmisamo M, Macdonald-Bravo H, Kelley E, Ford NF. A study of the interaction of grapefruit juice with the pharmacokinetics of HMG-CoA reductase. 9th International Symposium on Drugs Affecting Lipid Metabolism; Florence, 1998; 68.

98. Muck W, Ritter W, Frey R, *et al*. Influence of cholestyramine on the pharmacokinetics of cerivastatin. *Int J Clin Pharmacol Ther* 1997; **35**:250–4.

99. Lea AP, McTavish D. Atorvastatin — A review of its pharmacology and therapeutic potential in the management of hyperlipidaemias. *Drugs* 1997; **53**:828–47.

100. Steinke W, Yamashita S, Tabei M. Cerivastatin, a new inhibitor of HMG CoA reductase. Pharmacokinetics in rats and dogs [abstract]. *Jpn Pharmacol Ther* 1996; **24**:1217–37.

101. Jacobsen W, Kirchner G, Hallensleben K, *et al*. Comparison of cytochrome P-450-dependent metabolism and drug interactions of the 3-hydroxy-3-methylglutaryl-CoA reductase inhibitors lovastatin and pravastatin in the liver. *Drug Metab Dispos* 1999; **27**:173–9.

102. Pan HY. Clinical pharmacology of pravastatin, a selective inhibitor of HMG-CoA reductase. *Eur J Clin Pharmacol* 1991; **40**(suppl. 1):S15–S18.

103. Gibson DM, Yang B-B, Abel RB, *et al*. Effects of hepatic and renal impairment on pharmacokinetics (PK) and pharmacodynamics (PD) or atorvastatin. *Pharm Res* 1996; **13**(suppl.):S428.

104. Quérin S, Lambert R, Cusson JR, *et al*. Single-dose pharmacokinetics of ^14C-lovastatin in chronic renal failure. *Clin Pharmacol Ther* 1991; **50**:437–41.

105. Garnett WR. Interactions with hydroxy-methylglutaryl-coenzyme A reductase inhibitors. *Am J Health Syst Pharm* 1995; **52**:1639–45.

106. D'Arcy PF. Drug interactions and drug-metabolising enzymes. In: D'Arcy PF, McElna JC, Welling PG, eds. *Mechanisms of drug interactions*. Berlin, New York: Springer; 1996: 151–71.

107. Bertz RJ, Granneman GR. Use of in vitro and in vivo data to estimate the likelihood of metabolic pharmacokinetic interactions. [Review]. *Clin Pharmacokinet* 1997; **32**:210–58.

108. Hansten PD. Understanding drug–drug interaction. *Sci Med* 1998; **Jan/Feb**:16–25.

109. Neuvonen PJ, Kantola T, Kivistö KT. Simvastatin but not pravastatin is very susceptible to interaction with the CYP3A4 inhibitor itraconazole. *Clin Pharmacol Ther* 1998; **63**:332–41.

110. Schmassmann-Suhijar D, Bullingham R, Gasser R, *et al*. Rhabdomyolysis due to inter-

action of simvastatin with mibefradil. *Lancet* 1998; **351**:1929–30.

111. Wombolt DG, Jackson A, Punn R, *et al.* Case report: Rhabdomyolysis induced by mibefradil in a patient treated with cyclosporine and simvastatin. *J Clin Pharmacol* 1999; **39**:310–12.

112. Pierce LR, Wysowski DK, Gross TP. Myopathy and rhabdomyolysis associated with lovastatin–gemfibrozil combination therapy. *JAMA* 1990; **264**:71–5.

113. Tal A, Rajeshawari M, Isley W. Rhabdomyolysis associated with simvastatin–gemfibrozil therapy. *South Med J* 1997; **90**:546–7.

114. Duell PB, Connor WE, Illingworth DR. Rhabdomyolysis after taking atorvastatin with gemfibrozil. *Am J Cardiol* 1998; **81**:368–9.

115. Pogson GW, Kindred LH, Carper BG. Rhabdomyolysis and renal failure associated with *cerivastatin–gemfibrozil* combination therapy. *Am J Cardiol* 1999; **83**:1146.

116. Nakahara K, Yada T, Kuriyama M, Osame M. Cytosolic Ca^{2+} increase and cell damage in L6 rat myoblasts by HMG-CoA reductase inhibitors. *Biochem Biophys Res Commun* 1994; **202**:1579–85.

17

Is there still a place for the fibrates?

Patrick Duriez and Jean-Charles Fruchart

Introduction

Epidemiological and interventional studies have now confirmed that dyslipidaemias are major risk factors for atherosclerosis and coronary artery disease (CAD). Primary hypercholesterolaemia (increase in LDL-cholesterol levels) is now recognised as highly atherogenic and an important risk factor for CAD. Primary[1] and secondary[2] interventional trials with HMG-CoA reductase inhibitors have undoubtedly proved that a drastic reduction in LDL-cholesterol levels reduces the cardiovascular risk in LDL-hypercholesterolaemic patients and even in patients considered to have normal LDL-cholesterol levels.[3]

Nevertheless other dyslipidaemias, such as hypoalphalipoproteinaemia (low plasma HDL levels) associated or not with concomitant hypertriglyceridaemia, may be the cause of a substantial number of cases of CAD.[4,5] The independent role of triglycerides in CAD has been controversial, but recent evidence suggests that even modest increases in triglycerides increase the risk of coronary events and CAD progression, as well as new lesion formation.[6]

The fasting serum triglyceride level is inversely related to the HDL-cholesterol level. The inclusion of HDL-cholesterol in multiple logistic regression analysis largely excludes or abolishes the effect of serum triglycerides in multiple regression predicting CAD risk.[7] Using this powerful statistical tool to show that serum triglycerides were not an independent coronary risk factor is perhaps not the best approach for an analyte that has a complicated metabolic pathway. Indeed it is recognised that the statistical characteristics of the distribution of triglyceride levels, variability of triglyceride measurements and metabolic relations between triglycerides and other risk factors (in particular HDL-cholesterol) may reduce the ability to detect an association between triglycerides and risk of CAD in standard multivariate analysis.[7]

Nevertheless, in a recent meta-analysis of 17 population-based prospective studies, Hokanson and Austin[8] showed that triglycerides were an independent risk for CAD. On the basis of data from a total of 46 413 men and 10 864 women, they showed that elevated triglyceride levels were associated with a 30% increase in cardiovascular risk in men and a 75% increase in cardiovascular risk in women before adjustment for HDL-cholesterol and other risk factors. Adjustment for these factors attenuated the triglyceride risk factor to 14% in men and 37% in women but did not render it nonsignificant. Recently, Jeppesen *et al.*[9] showed that in middle-aged and elderly white men, a high level of fasting triglycerides is a strong risk factor for CAD independent of other major risk factors, including HDL-cholesterol.

Since the early reports on clofibrate[10] (the first member of the fibrate family to be marketed), fibrates have been used in the treatment of hypertriglyceridaemia with or without hypoalphalipoproteinaemia.[11] Nevertheless, although fibrates have been used in clinical practice for over three decades now, in depth knowledge of the molecular mechanisms of their normolipidaemic effects was lacking until recently. It was known for several years that fibrates induce peroxisome proliferation in rodents and that this process is linked to the induction of the transcription of genes involved in peroxisomal β-oxidation and mediated by specific transcription factors, termed peroxisome proliferator-activated receptors (PPARs).[12] Nevertheless, until recently no direct relationship was evoked between PPAR-activation by fibrates and alteration in lipoprotein metabolism. Furthermore, *in vivo* experiments in animals and *in vitro* studies suggest that in humans fibrates might reduce atherosclerosis development not only through their normolipidaemic properties but also by reducing inflammation at the level of the vascular wall. In this chapter we discuss the recent fundamental and clinical studies of fibrates that suggest that this family of molecules might have a future in clinical practice.

Classification and treatment strategy for raised triglyceride levels

Recent clinical trials documented improvements in coronary mortality and morbidity following the use of drugs (statins) that drastically reduce LDL-cholesterol levels. These have produced a palpable change in the attitude of previously sceptical doctors to the atherogenic role of high LDL-cholesterol plasma levels,[1,2] despite epidemiological arguments that had previously suggested that high LDL-cholesterol strongly increases the risk of CAD. The same type of epidemiological arguments would propose that lowering triglyceride levels would decrease the incidence of CAD in clinical trials. Recently, some clinical trials of therapies that specifically lowered triglyceride levels but did not greatly decrease LDL-cholesterol levels have been reported.

Table 17.1 is adapted from the Adult Treatment Panel (ATP) II guidelines[13] for treatment of patients with elevated triglyceride levels. Those guidelines report 2 mmol/l (175 mg/dl) as the limit of normal fasting serum triglycerides, but data from healthy subjects, case–control studies and epidemiological studies now suggest that there may be benefit in keeping fasting serum triglycerides below 1.5 mmol/l (130 mg/dl). This conclusion is based on the observation that serum triglycerides greater than 1.5 mmol/l (130 mg/dl) are associated with the presence of an LDL subfraction that is small and dense and associated with CAD in some case–control studies.[14] The American Diabetes Association recommends targeting triglycerides to less than 1.70 mmol/l (150 mg/dl) in diabetes while a triglyceride level of less than 2.3 mmol/l (200 mg/dl) has been considered acceptable in CAD and other vascular diseases. However, considering the subgroup analysis in post-MI patients treated with pravastatin in CARE, it may be prudent to target fasting triglycerides to less than 1.70 mmol/l (150 mg/dl).[3]

In mixed lipid disorders, the initial goal is to lower LDL-cholesterol levels. Usually a statin is used but if triglyceride levels remain greater than 2.3 mmol/l (200 mg/dl) or HDL-cholesterol is less than 1.00 mmol/l (38 mg/dl), niacin or alternatively a fibrate may be used as adjunctive therapy.[15,16] This combination increases the possibility of side-effects, in particular, abnormal biochemical liver function

Fasting triglyceride	Clinical status	Target	Recommendations
Normal <200 mg/dl	Healthy	No change	No treatment necessary.
	Diabetes	<150 mg/dl	Weight loss, diet low in fat and simple sugar, control diabetes.
	CAD with low HDL-C	<100–150 mg/dl	Diet, exercise, consider niacin.
Borderline high, 200–400 mg/dl	Healthy	<200 mg/dl	Diet, weight loss, exercise, drug therapy not recommended.
	Diabetes	<150 mg/dl	Treat LDL-C to <100 mg/dl with statin, i.e. atorvastatin or statin with fibrate.
	CAD with low HDL-C	<100–150 mg/dl	Add niacin.
	CAD with low HDL-C and LDL-C >130 mg/dl	<100–150 mg/dl	Niacin, statin with niacin or fibrate, or atorvastatin.
High, 400–1000 mg/dl	Healthy or obese	200–300 mg/dl	Diet low in fat and sugar, weight loss, exercise. After 2–6 weeks add fibrate, niacin or atorvastatin.
	Diabetes	<150 mg/dl	When triglycerides <400 mg/dl calculate LDL-C and treat to <100 mg/dl and add fibrate.
	CAD or PVOD	<200 mg/dl	Obtain LDL-C by beta-quant and treat to <100 mg/dl; add niacin or fibrate if necessary.
Very high, >1000 mg/dl	Healthy or obese	<300 mg/dl	As above.
	Abdominal pain	<300 mg/dl	Clear liquids for 2–3 days and progress dietary fat slowly. Fibrate and add 3-omega PUFAs if necessary.
	Pancreatitis	<300 mg/dl	NPO, IV fluids, begin feeding based on pancreatic enzymes. A liquid diet, very gradual fat restoration. Drugs as above.

CAD = coronary artery disease; HDL-C = high density lipoprotein-C; LDL-C = low density lipoprotein-C; PVOD = peripheral vascular occlusive disease; PNO = nulla per os; IV = intravenous.

Table 17.1
Classification and treatment of high triglyceride levels as modified from ATP II guidelines.[13]

tests and myalgia.[17] The latter is potentially more serious, as myopathy progressing to rhabdomyolysis and renal failure has been reported. The introduction of a new, more powerful statin such as atorvastatin could reduce the need for combination therapy.

In confirmed isolated hypertriglyceridaemia (with exclusion of excess alcohol consumption) and after diagnosis of secondary causes of isolated hypertriglyceridaemia that require treatment (uncontrolled diabetes mellitus, chronic renal failure, etc.), fibrates are among the best options in pharmacological treatment.

Molecular effects of fibrates
Peroxisome proliferator-activated receptors

Peroxisome proliferator-activated receptors (PPARs) are a subfamily of the nuclear receptors.[12] Three distinct PPARs termed α, δ(β) and γ, each encoded by a separate gene and showing a distinct tissue distribution pattern, have already been described. Ligands that induce the transcriptional activity of PPARs have been identified. All PPARs are activated by free fatty acids and derivatives such as leukotriene B4 (LTB4) and prostaglandin J2 (PGJ2). In addition, fibrates bind to and activate PPARα, albeit with low activity and specificity, whereas antidiabetic glitazones are high-affinity ligands for PPARγ. Activated PPARs heterodimerise with another nuclear receptor, the retinoid X receptor (RXR), and alter the transcription of target genes after binding to specific peroxisome proliferator response elements (PPREs), which are a direct repeat of the nuclear receptor hexameric AGGTCA DNA core recognition motif, separated by one or two nucleotides (DR1 and DR2) (Figure 17.1).

Effects of PPARα stimulation by fibrates

Fibrates are first-line drugs in the treatment of primary hypertriglyceridaemia and are very useful in the treatment of combined hyperlipidaemia, type III dyslipoproteinaemia and secondary lipid abnormalities observed in type 2 diabetes and obese individuals.[11,18]

PPARα activation by fibrates leads to the following:

- decreased hypertriglyceridaemia by increasing LPL expression[19] and decreasing apoC-III expression;[20]
- increased HDL-cholesterol, apoA-I and apoA-II levels[21,22] in human plasma, achieved at least partly by increasing apoA-I and apoA-II expression;[21,22]
- reduced LDL-cholesterol levels in combined hyperlipidaemia[23] by decreasing the levels of atherogenic dense LDL, which have poor affinity for the LDL receptor, while increasing buoyant LDL particles which display high affinity for this receptor.

In primary hypercholesterolaemia, fibrates reduce dense LDL, but not light LDL fractions.[24] In hypercholesterolaemic patients, Caslake *et al.*[25] observed that fenofibrate significantly decreased LDL-cholesterol levels (30%) without decreasing LDL-apoB production by shifting LDL from a slowly catabolised pool towards a rapidly catabolised one. Furthermore, the rate of apoB-LDL degradation by the receptor route rose 43% with the drug, whereas the amount cleared by the receptor-independent pathway did not change. It is generally acknowledged that therapeutic concentrations of fibrates do not inhibit HMG-CoA reductase activity.[26]

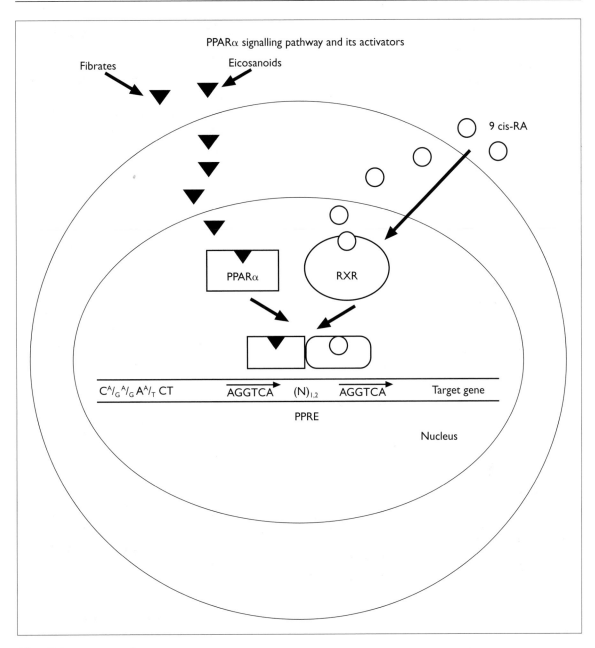

Fig. 17.1
The PPARα signalling pathway and its natural (eicosanoids) and synthetic activators (fibrates). After activation, PPARα heterodimerises with the receptor for 9 cis-retinoic acid (9 cis-RA), RXR, and binds to response elements in the regulatory regions of target genes, termed PPRE, which are composed of two degenerate hexanucleotide repeats (arrows), arranged in tandem as direct repeats and spaced by one or two nucleotides and preceded by an AT-rich region.

Effects of PPARα and fibrates on vascular inflammation and atherosclerosis

Atherosclerosis development is a long-term process which involves the recruitment and activation of different cells such as macrophages, T-lymphocytes, smooth muscle cells and endothelial cells. The accumulation of lipids and of extracellular matrix associated with the activation of the different cells in the arterial intima elicits a local inflammatory response.[27] This inflammatory atheroma may progress silently over decades without inducing acute ischaemic disease but in some cases secretion of matrix metalloproteinases and expression of procoagulant factors, such as tissue factor, will lead ultimately to plaque rupture, inducing thrombus formation and resulting in acute ischaemic disease such as myocardial infarction.

Recent developments in cell biology have shown that PPARs are ubiquitous factors and that, even if they are not continuously expressed during cell life, different biological or chemical events can elicit their expression which will result in profound alterations in cell functioning. PPARs have recently been shown to be expressed in the cells of the vascular wall and to play a role in vascular pathophysiology.

According to Mallat *et al.* (unpublished data), PPARα is expressed in atherosclerotic plaques. These authors showed that PPARα and PPARγ are not found in normal coronary arteries but are expressed in approximately 60% of human coronary or carotid atherosclerotic plaques. Furthermore, they reported that from early atherogenesis until the ultimate stages, PPARα is generally more abundant than PPARγ. Clinical studies in humans and pharmacological assays in animal models have shown that PPARα activators (fibrates) lower the progression of atherosclerosis[16,28–30] in both human and animal models.

PPARα and PPARγ are expressed in primary cultures of endothelial cells,[31] smooth muscle cells[32] and macrophages.[33] Chinetti *et al.*[34] showed that PPARα and PPARγ are expressed in differentiated human monocyte-derived macrophages. PPARα is already present in undifferentiated monocytes but PPARγ expression is induced upon differentiation into macrophages. Chinetti *et al.*[34] showed that ligand activation of PPARγ, but not of PPARα, results in apoptosis induction in unactivated differentiated macrophages. Moreover, both PPARα and PPARγ ligands induce apoptosis of macrophages activated with tumour necrosis factor-α and interferon-γ. The pro-apoptotic activity of PPARs is probably a consequence of their ability to block NF-κB-mediated anti-apoptotic pathways in macrophages. Further, *in vivo* studies are required to determine whether the induction of apoptosis inside atheromatous plaques decreases or increases atherosclerosis development. On the one hand apoptosis might reduce plaque formation but on the other hand, it might weaken the plaque and increase the risk of acute plaque rupture and consequently of CAD.

As early as 1996, Devchand *et al.*[35] reported that leukotriene B4 (LTB4), a pro-inflammatory molecule, is an activating ligand for PPARα which is involved in the regulation of oxidative degradation of fatty acids and their derivatives, amongst which is LTB4 itself. Therefore, the pro-inflammatory effect of LTB4 might be counteracted by the stimulation of its own degradation through its PPARα activation, indicating an anti-inflammatory role for PPARα. Recent data have shown that PPAR agonists inhibit the expression of inducible factors that are implicated in endothelial, macrophage and smooth muscle cell functions, as well as in the promotion of a

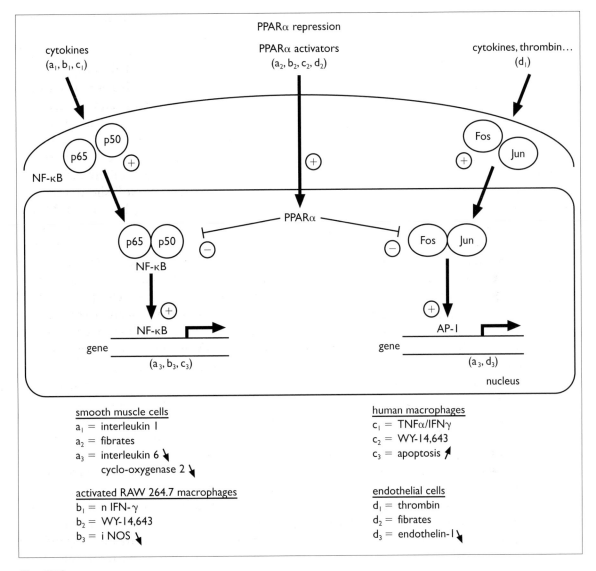

Fig. 17.2
PPARα activators inhibit vascular inflammation, induce apoptosis and decrease endothelin-1 secretion by endothelial cells as a result of PPARα repression of NF-κB and AP-1 signalling.

local inflammatory response within the developing atherosclerotic plaque. Inducible NO synthase (iNOS) in macrophages is a key inflammatory enzyme.[36] A synthetic PPARα agonist (WY-14,643) reduces nitrite accumulation in activated RAW264.7 murine macrophages. Inhibition of nitrite accumulation is associated with a fall in iNOS protein and induction of haeme oxygenase I.

To determine whether PPARα interferes with the response of human aortic smooth muscle cells to inflammatory cytokines, Staels et al.[32] analysed the influence of fibrates on IL-1-mediated activation of IL-6 production, a marker for SMC activation. Fibrates prevented the IL-1-induced secretion of IL-6 in a dose-dependent manner (Figure 17.2). This inhibition occurs at fibrate concentrations required for the induction of positive PPARα response genes and within the range of plasma concentrations found in humans. Incubation of smooth muscle cells with IL-1 increases 6-keto-prostaglandin F1α (6-keto-PGF$_{1\alpha}$) secretion tenfold. Fibrate treatment prevented the formation of 6-keto-PGF$_{1\alpha}$ by preventing COX-2 induction by IL-1 as a result of a negative regulation of COX-2 transcription through NF-κB transcription activity. Recent studies indicate that PPARs negatively interact with different inflammation-activated signalling pathways such as the NF-κB, AP-1 and STAT pathways.

Delerive et al.[37] showed recently that negative interference with AP-1 signalling explains the repression of thrombin-induced endothelin (ET)-1 expression in endothelial cells by PPARα and PPARγ ligands. Using transient co-transfection assays with PPARα and c-Jun and c-Fos expression plasmids, these authors showed that PPARs negatively interfere with the AP-1 signalling pathway, which mediates thrombin activation of ET-1 gene transcription (see Figure 17.2). PPAR activators reduce the thrombin-stimulated binding activity to an AP-1 consensus site and inhibit the transcription of human ET-1. ET-1 is a very strong vasoconstrictor peptide which induces smooth muscle cell proliferation. Therefore, it might promote vasospastic events and atherogenesis. This study shows that PPAR activators might reduce coronary events by reducing vasospasm and atherosclerosis development following fibrate treatment.

Effects of PPARα and fibrates on thrombosis

Acute CAD depends on the activation of the different factors of the pro-thrombotic cascade and/or on the inhibition of the anti-thrombotic factors. Fibrates decrease PAI-1 production in cultured cynomolgus hepatocytes[38] and Kockx et al.[38] showed that there was no correlation between inhibition of PAI-1 production and PPARα transactivation activity, determined by a PPARα-sensitive reporter gene, when cells were stimulated with different fibrates. In humans, gemfibrozil and bezafibrate increased plasma PAI-1 activity[39] but ciprofibrate[40] did not modify its plasma levels.

Furthermore, fibrates influence plasma fibrinogen levels. Gemfibrozil increased plasma fibrinogen levels,[40] while bezafibrate[40] and fenofibrate[41] significantly decreased this concentration and ciprofibrate had no effect.[40] Nevertheless, ciprofibrate undoubtedly decreased the functional fibrinogen activity while the observed effects of gemfibrozil on this parameter depended on the analytic method applied.[40] Recently, Kockx et al.[42] showed that in vivo (in mice) fibrates, but not glitazones, decreased hepatic fibrinogen α-, β- and γ-chain mRNA levels. Nuclear run-on experiments demonstrated that the decrease in fibrinogen expression after fenofibrate treatment occurred at the transcriptional level. Furthermore, plasma fibrinogen concentrations were higher in PPARα-deficient mice compared with the wild type and fibrate treatment decreased plasma fibrinogen levels in wild type but not in PPARα-deficient mice. Therefore, this study established that PPARα plays a role in the regulation of plasma fibrinogen levels by fibrates.

Recent pharmacological trials with fibrates in the treatment of hypertriglyceridaemia and the prevention of CAD

LDL particles constitute a relatively homogeneous family of lipoproteins (although they vary from large buoyant to small, dense particles) and LDL-cholesterol is a reasonable evaluation of the plasma levels of these atherogenic lipoproteins in epidemiological and clinical studies. By contrast, the heterogeneity of triglyceride-rich lipoproteins is an important confounder in determining the relationship between triglyceride plasma levels and CAD risk. Triglyceride-rich particles derived from dietary lipid intake (chylomicrons) are not thought to be associated with increased risk for CHD but chylomicron remnant particles, on the other hand, are thought to be atherogenic. The atherogenicity of large VLDL particles secreted by the liver is uncertain at this time but through the action of lipoprotein lipase, VLDLs are converted to IDLs which are believed to be highly atherogenic.[43]

To focus on the primary targets of fibrates (high triglyceride and low HDL-cholesterol plasma levels) we will present recent clinical data from trials with fibrates that induce a considerable reduction of triglyceride plasma levels but a poor reduction of LDL-cholesterol levels.

Gemfibrozil

In 1997, data from the LOCAT (Lipid Coronary Angiography Trial) study[16] showed that gemfibrozil therapy retarded the progression of coronary atherosclerosis and the formation of bypass graft lesions after coronary bypass surgery in men with low HDL-cholesterol as their main lipid abnormality. Men who had undergone coronary bypass surgery (n = 395) completed a randomised, placebo-controlled study with gemfibrozil (1200 mg/day). They were selected primarily for HDL-cholesterol levels that corresponded to the lowest third for middle-aged men, less than or equal to 1.1 mmol/l (42.5 mg/dl) and had LDL-cholesterol levels less than or equal to 4.5 mmol/l (170 mg/dl). Average baseline lipid and lipoprotein levels were serum triglyceride = 1.60 mmol/l (140 mg/dl), serum cholesterol = 5.17 mmol/l (200 mg/dl), LDL-cholesterol = 3.43 mmol/l (130 mg/dl), HDL2-cholesterol = 0.41 mmol/l (16 mg/dl) and HDL3-cholesterol = 0.61 mmol/l (24 mg/dl). In the gemfibrozil group, these levels were reduced on average by 40%, 9%, and 6% or increased by 5% and 9%, respectively. Coronary angiography was performed at baseline and after an average of 32 months of therapy in patients that had previously undergone coronary bypass surgery. The change in per-patient means of average diameters of native coronary segments was less in the gemfibrozil group (-0.01 ± 0.10 mm) than in the placebo group (-0.04 ± 0.11 mm; $P = 0.009$). The equivalent changes in minimum luminal diameters of stenoses were -0.04 ± 0.15 mm and -0.09 ± 0.18, respectively ($P = 0.002$). In aortocoronary bypass grafts, 23 subjects (14%) assigned to placebo had new lesions in follow-up angiograms, compared with four subjects (2%) assigned to gemfibrozil ($P < 0.001$).

Recently, Syvänne *et al.*[44] studied which lipoproteins, separated by preparative ultracentrifugation, predicted angiographic progression in this population. Analysis of the lipoprotein compositions clearly showed that all lipoprotein classes were significantly depleted of triglycerides by gemfibrozil. VLDL were both decreased in number and depleted of lipid, but there was no suggestion of any reduction of IDL or increase in HDL2 particle numbers. Total serum cholesterol and both triglyceride and cholesterol in the IDL and LDL fractions were positively and significantly associated with the risk of global angiographic progression and HDL-cholesterol concentration was not associated with protection against progression. The components (cholesterol and triglycerides) of all the apoB-containing lipoproteins (VLDL, IDL, LDL), especially IDL, were related to diffuse and focal angiographic progression. Concentrations of esterified cholesterol in the HDL fraction were strongly and inversely related to progression of focal disease but total HDL-cholesterol concentrations were not associated and HDL2-cholesterol levels and even tended to be positively related to the risk of luminal narrowing.

This study adds to the growing evidence of the atherogenicity of triglyceride-rich lipoproteins, especially IDL, and the antiatherogenic influence of HDL3, and suggests that the reductions of triglyceride levels that are commonly considered normal seem to provide protection against progressive CAD.

The goal of the LOCAT study was to test the effects of gemfibrozil on the progression of coronary atherosclerosis and not to evaluate the effects of the drug on CAD death and non-fatal myocardial infarction. The objective the Veterans Affairs-High Density Lipoprotein Cholesterol Intervention Trial (VA-HIT)[45] was to test if gemfibrozil decreased CAD death and non-fatal myocardial infarctions in men with documented CAD (prior myocardial infarctions, prior revascularisation, a history of angina with ischaemia, positive coronary angiogram) and HDL-cholesterol levels less than or equal to 40 mg/dl, LDL-cholesterol levels less than or equal to 140 mg/dl and triglyceride levels less than or equal to 300 mg/dl. Between 1991 and 1993, 2531 patients enrolled into the study and the

median follow-up was 5.1 years. Baseline lipid levels did not differ between the groups: the total cholesterol level was 4.6 mmol/l (175 mg/dl), the HDL-cholesterol level was 0.83 mmol/l (32 mg/dl), the LDL-cholesterol level was 2.90 mmol/l (111 mg/dl) and the triglyceride level was 1.85 mmol/l (161 mg/dl).

Gemfibrozil (1200 mg/day) decreased total cholesterol by 2.8% and triglyceride levels by 24.5%; it had no effect on LDL-cholesterol and increased HDL-cholesterol levels by 7.5%. Drug treatment reduced coronary heart death by 22% ($P = 0.006$) and non-fatal myocardial infarction was reduced by 21.6% (274) and 17.3% (219) in the placebo and gemfibrozil groups, respectively. Furthermore, stroke was less frequent in the gemfibrozil group but there was no difference in the rates of coronary revascularisation, or hospitalisation due to unstable angina between the two groups, as there was no difference in the total mortality between the two groups (210 in the placebo groups versus 197 in the gemfibrozil group) nor in the frequency of new malignancies (173 in the placebo group and 160 in the gemfibrozil group).

Therefore VA-HIT provides direct clinical evidence of the benefit of reducing triglyceride levels and increasing HDL-cholesterol levels without affecting LDL-cholesterol levels as a secondary prevention in patients with low HDL-cholesterol and low LDL-cholesterol levels. It also confirms the beneficial effect of gemfibrozil in terms of reduction of acute vascular events.

Bezafibrate

The Bezafibrate Coronary Atherosclerosis Intervention Trial (BECAIT) was initiated to determine whether bezafibrate retards the progression or facilitates regression of premature coronary atherosclerosis and was the first angiographic study to be conducted with a fibrate.[46-48] Men under the age of 45 years who survived a first myocardial infarction were screened from ten centres in the greater Stockholm area for participation in the study. Patients with a fasting serum cholesterol value of greater than or equal to 5.2 mmol/l (200 mg/dl), a serum triglyceride level of greater than or equal to 1.6 mmol/l (140 mg/dl) and angiographically demonstrable lesions (greater than 20%) in at least one coronary segment were included. Patients with severe angina, severe congestive heart failure, diabetes, hypertension resistant to therapy or very high cholesterol, 10 mmol/l (386.7 mg/dl), or triglyceride, 8 mmol/l (309.36 mg/dl), levels were excluded from entering the study. In total, 47 patients were randomly allocated to treatment with bezafibrate (200 mg twice daily) or placebo and treatment was continued for 5 years, during which angiography was performed again after 2 years and at the end of the study. For the purpose of angiographic analysis, the coronary arterial tree was divided into 15 segments according to the American Heart Association recommendations. The minimum lumen diameter (MLD) was measured in each segment, and the mean of these diameters constituted the basis for comparison between baseline and 2 and 5 years of treatment. The study showed a clear benefit of bezafibrate over placebo in terms of progression of MLD. The angiographic findings over the 5 years of study indicated that the median change in MLD at final assessment was on average 0.13 mm less in the bezafibrate group than in the placebo group ($P < 0.049$). Per cent stenosis was 3.4% less among the bezafibrate treated patients than in the placebo group. Although this difference did not reach statistical significance ($P = 0.069$), the data are consistent with, and thus supportive of, change in MLD.

This study was not designed to detect differences in coronary events, but it is noteworthy that only three patients suffered a coronary event in the bezafibrate group compared with 11 in the placebo group ($P = 0.019$).

The BECAIT data were subjected to subgroup analysis to investigate the effect of treatment in segments with mild-to-moderate lesions causing 20–49% diameter stenosis at baseline compared with segments with lesions causing more than 50% stenosis. The results indicated that, in terms of MLD and per cent stenosis, the entire treatment effect of bezafibrate was directed towards these mild-to-moderate lesions. Furthermore, seven of the ten coronary events that occurred among patients with mild-to-moderate lesions at baseline occurred in those whose lesions progressed to more than the median measurement (>0.052 mm increase in MLD).

In 1998, Ruotolo *et al.*[49] examined the relationship between progression of coronary lesions in the BECAIT study with lipoproteins and lipoprotein subfractions. In addition to the decrease in levels of VLDL-cholesterol (−53%) and triglyceride (−46%), bezafibrate treatment resulted in a significant increase in HDL3-cholesterol level (+9%) and a shift in the LDL subclass distribution towards larger particle species, without any effect on LDL-cholesterol levels. The on-trial HDL3-cholesterol and plasma apoB concentrations were found to be independent predictors of the changes in mean minimum lumen diameter ($r = 0.23$, $P < 0.05$) and per cent stenosis ($r = 0.30$, $P < 0.01$), respectively. Decreases in small dense LDL and/or VLDL lipid concentrations were unrelated to disease progression. These data suggest that the effect of bezafibrate on progression of focal coronary atherosclerosis could be at least partly attributed to a rise in HDL3-cholesterol and a decrease in the total number of apoB-containing lipoproteins.

The goal of the Bezafibrate Infarction Prevention (BIP) was to test the benefit of a therapy that increases serum HDL-cholesterol concentrations and lowers triglyceride concentrations on the incidence of myocardial infarction and mortality among CAD patients.[50] The BIP study randomly allocated men and women with CAD and with total serum cholesterol levels of 4.70–6.50 mmol/l (180–250 mg/dl), LDL-cholesterol levels less than or equal to 4.70 mmol/l (180 mg/dl), HDL-cholesterol levels less than or equal to 1.17 mmol/l (45 mg/dl) and triglyceride levels less than or equal to 3.45 mmol/l (300 mg/dl), to treatment with bezafibrate retard (400 mg/dl) or placebo. By January 1993, 3122 patients were recruited[50] and they were followed up until January 1998, an average of 6.25 years. Baseline serum total cholesterol, HDL-cholesterol, LDL-cholesterol and triglyceride levels were 212 ± 17, 34.6 ± 5.5, 148 ± 17 and 149 ± 52 mg/dl, respectively. Bezafibrate treatment significantly reduced serum triglyceride levels (22%) but not serum total cholesterol (4%) or LDL-cholesterol levels (5%); it significantly increased HDL-cholesterol levels (12%). Bezafibrate decreased coronary atherosclerosis progression (0.13 mm less progression in MLD than in the placebo group),[30] but did not significantly reduce the primary endpoint, fatal or non-fatal myocardial infarction plus sudden death, (-9%, $P = 0.27$) with a median follow-up of 7 years and did not alter total mortality ($P = 0.64$).[51] Nevertheless, subgroup analysis suggested that bezafibrate had only a beneficial effect in patients with serum triglyceride levels above 2.3 mmol/l (200 mg/dl) ($P = 0.03$) where it significantly decreased the primary endpoint ($P = 0.03$).

The Lower Extremity Arterial Disease Event Reduction (LEADER) study[52] is designed to investigate the benefit of lowering fibrinogen in terms of preventing major ischaemic heart disease and stroke in a group of male and female patients less than 75 years of age who had lower extremity arterial disease. The trial has adopted a randomised double-blind design in which bezafibrate (400 mg once daily) was compared with placebo. The results are expected in the year 2000.

Fenofibrate

The incidence of CAD is greatly increased in those with diabetes mellitus. There have been many studies demonstrating that correction of dyslipoproteinaemias will reduce the risk of CAD in non-diabetic populations. Current advice to those with diabetes is based on extrapolations from such studies. However, the justification for this and the treatment targets is unclear as there has been no direct test of the lipid hypothesis in diabetes. The Diabetes Atherosclerosis Intervention Study (DAIS)[53] is the first interventional trial designed to examine directly whether correcting dyslipoproteinaemia in men and women with type 2 diabetes will reduce their CAD. DAIS is a multinational angiographic study using the 200 mg micronised form of fenofibrate in a double-blind, placebo-controlled protocol.

Mixed dyslipoproteinaemia

It has been clearly demonstrated that the most convenient treatments for pure hypercholesterolaemia and pure hypertriglyceridaemia are statins and fibrates, respectively. However, the most appropriate therapy for combined hyperlipidaemia remains to be determined. Zambon et al.[54] used a randomised crossover study to compare the effects of gemfibrozil with lovastatin in familial combined hyperlipidaemia and to measure the additive effects of combination treatment on lipid regulation. Gemfibrozil (1200 mg/day) had no effect on

LDL-cholesterol levels but favourably influenced the triglyceride levels and apoB-containing lipoprotein composition that are related to hypertriglyceridaemia, with a reduction of both the number and size of VLDL particles. Conversely, lovastatin markedly decreased LDL-cholesterol (reduction of the number of LDL particles) but had little effect on triglyceride-rich lipoproteins. Combined treatment was safe and had additive effects on lipids, causing significant reduction in levels of total cholesterol (32%), triglycerides (51%), LDL-cholesterol (34%) and apoB (26%) and an increase in HDL-cholesterol levels (19%). In this condition, target LDL-cholesterol levels of <3.4 mmol/l (130 mg/dl) were achieved in 71% of patients with established CAD. The overall result of the gemfibrozil–lovastatin combination was a return to normal of the lipid profile in 68% of the patients: LDL-cholesterol levels fell to less than 3.9 mmol/l (150 mg/dl) in all cases, triglyceride levels were reduced to less than 2.3 mmol/l (200 mg/dl) in 96% of patients, and HDL-cholesterol levels were greater than 0.9 mmol/l (35 mg/dl) in 68% of patients.

Conclusions

LOCAT, VA-HIT, BECAIT and BIP studies showed that drugs belonging to the fibrate family (gemfibrozil, bezafibrate) and acting through the stimulation of peroxisome proliferator-activated receptors (PPARs) have comparable effects on plasma lipid and lipoprotein profiles and on the inhibition of coronary atherosclerosis progression.

These data suggest that concomitant increases in HDL-cholesterol levels and decreases in triglyceride levels without decreases in LDL-cholesterol levels in patients with intermediate total cholesterol but with low HDL-cholesterol ≤1.17 mmol/l (45 mg/dl), and intermediate triglyceride levels, ≤2.30 mmol/l (200 mg/dl), do not reduce the cardiovascular risk (BIP). Nevertheless, a simultaneous reduction in triglycerides and increase in HDL-cholesterol, without any reduction in LDL-cholesterol, in patients with low LDL- and HDL-cholesterol, intermediate triglycerides (VA-HIT) or intermediate LDL-cholesterol, low HDL-cholesterol and high triglycerides (>2.30 mmol/l (200 mg/dl)) (BIP) decreases cardiac mortality. These studies emphasise the importance of reducing LDL-cholesterol levels when LDL constitutes an apo B-containing lipoprotein risk factor. They also highlight the additional lethal power of triglycerides in hypercholesterolaemic patients, and the lethal power of triglycerides alone in normocholesterolaemic patients with low HDL-cholesterol levels.

Further studies are needed to confirm the beneficial effects of reducing triglyceridaemia and increasing HDL-cholesterol levels in secondary prevention and they are absolutely essential to demonstrate this beneficial effect in primary prevention.

Our knowledge on the physiological role of the PPAR family of transcription factors has evolved enormously over the last 2 years. PPARα regulates lipid metabolism and inhibits the inflammatory response in the vascular wall. PPARα activators such as fibrates inhibit atherosclerosis development through their normolipidaemic activities but it is highly credible that other mechanisms, such as inhibition of vascular inflammation and thrombogenesis, also participate in this beneficial effect. Further studies, with new molecules that are more potent and more specific PPARα activators than the previously available drugs will certainly present new knowledge about the role of PPARα in have also been published in these recommendations. The coronary risk chart is simple to use. An individual's absolute risk of developing a CHD event (angina, non-fatal myocardial infarction, or coronary death) over the next 10 years is found by locating the appropriate box in the coronary risk chart based on the patient's age, gender, smoking habit, systolic blood pressure and total cholesterol level. Those at highest multifactorial risk can be identified and targeted for lifestyle intervention and, where appropriate, drug therapies. Physicians should always use absolute CHD risk when making a clinical judgement about using drugs to treat blood lipids and blood pressure, rather than just considering the level of any one risk factor alone. An absolute CHD risk that exceeds 20% over the next 10 years, or will exceed 20% if projected to age 60 years, and which is sustained despite professional lifestyle intervention, is sufficiently high to justify the selective use of proven drug therapies.

It should be stressed that certain individuals will be at higher risk than is evident from the coronary risk chart. Those with clinically established CHD or other atherosclerotic disease have already declared themselves to be at high risk and this chart is *not* intended for them. Risk is also considerably higher than indicated in the chart for patients with familial hyperlipidaemia and they always require drug therapy. Risk is also higher for those with a family history of premature cardiovascular disease, and those with low HDL-cholesterol or raised triglyceride levels. By substituting the ratio of total cholesterol to HDL-cholesterol for total cholesterol alone, risk prediction can be improved, particularly for women.

The Framingham risk function used to calculate the coronary risk chart has certain limitations. As with other functions, it overestimates risk in young people. Furthermore,

using one coronary risk chart based on a high-risk middle-aged North American population, and applying it to other populations around the world at different levels of CHD risk poses a problem. Whilst the Framingham function predicts absolute risk reasonably well in high-risk populations, it does overpredict absolute risk in low-risk populations. However, estimates of relative risk derived from the chart are likely to be quite robust for all populations.

With these caveats the European coronary risk chart has several functions:

1. An individual's absolute risk of developing a CHD event over the next 10 years can be read from the chart without any calculations.

2. Although young people are generally at lower risk, this will rise steadily as age increases. The chart can be used by following the tables upwards to illustrate the effect of lifetime risk by observing the increased risk with increase in age. In general, risk will rise even further than indicated by the chart since risk factor levels will also tend to increase with age.

3. Relative risk can be estimated readily by comparing the risk in one cell with any other in the same age group. As mentioned, absolute risk may vary considerably from one population to another, but the magnitude of relative risk will usually remain fairly constant.

4. The chart can be used to predict the effect of changing from one risk category to another. Thus, one can readily show an individual the expected reduction in risk associated with stopping smoking, reducing blood cholesterol level or reducing blood pressure.

The coronary risk chart illustrates how the risk of developing CHD can be calculated simply. Ideally, such charts should be constructed from the results of prospective cohort studies undertaken in the population to which the risk chart is to be applied. A coronary risk chart developed by each country is therefore recommended.

Lifestyle and therapeutic goals for patients with CHD, or other atherosclerotic disease, and for healthy high-risk individuals

The new European recommendations have set lifestyle, risk factor and therapeutic goals for secondary and primary prevention of CHD and these are summarised in Table 18.1. As the biology of atherosclerosis does not distinguish those patients with symptomatic CHD,

Patients with CHD or other atherosclerotic disease	**Healthy high-risk individuals** Absolute CHD risk ≥20% over 10 years, or will exceed 20% if projected to age 60 years
Lifestyle Stop smoking, make healthy food choices, be physically active and achieve ideal weight.	
Other risk factors Blood pressure <140/90 mmHg, total cholesterol <190 mg/dl (5.0 mmol/l), LDL-cholesterol <115 mg/dl (3.0 mmol/l) When these risk factors are not achieved by lifestyle changes, blood pressure and cholesterol-lowering drug therapies should be used.	
Other prophylactic drug therapies	
Aspirin (at least 75 mg) for all coronary patients, those with cerebral atherosclerosis and peripheral atherosclerotic disease. β-blockers in patients following myocardial infarction. ACE inhibitors in those with symptoms or signs of heart failure at the time of myocardial infarction, or with LV systolic dysfunction (ejection fraction <40%). Anticoagulants in selected coronary patients.	Aspirin (75 mg) in treated hypertensive patients and in men at particularly high CHD risk.
Screen close relatives	
Screen close relatives of patients with premature (men <55 years, women <65 years) CHD.	Screen close relatives if familial hypercholesterolaemia or other inherited dyslipidaemia is suspected.

Table 18.1
Lifestyle and therapeutic goals for patients with CHD, or other atherosclerotic disease, and for healthy high-risk individuals.

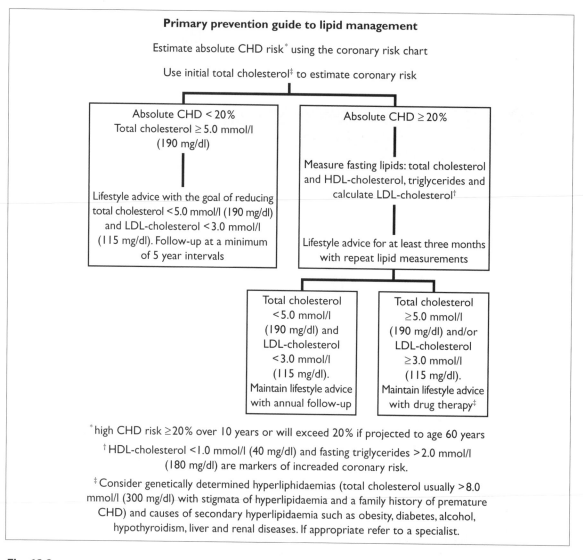

Fig. 18.2
Primary prevention guide to lipid management. Copyright Eur Heart J *1998; **19**:1434–503.*

or other atherosclerotic disease, from high-risk individuals in the population, the European lifestyle and therapeutic goals for secondary and primary CHD prevention are the same. The exception to this rule is the use of prophylactic drug therapies in primary and secondary CHD prevention.

	Europe®	United States®†	IAS Task Force®
Patients with CHD (or other atherosclerotic disease)	TC <5.00 mmol/l (193 mg/dl) LDL-C <3.0 mmol/l (116 mg/dl)	‡Consider drug treatment at LDL-C >130 mg/dl (3.4 mmol/l) Goal LDL <100 mg/dl (2.6 mmol/l)	LDL-C <100 mg/dl (2.6 mmol/l)
Healthy high-risk individuals	Multifactorial* CHD risk ≥20% TC <5.0 mmol/l (193 mg/dl) LDL-C <3.0 mmol/l (116 mg/dl)	Two or more risk factors§ Consider drug treatment at LDL-C >160 mg/dl (4.1 mmol/l) Goal LDL-C <130 mg/dl (3.4 mmol/l)	**High risk¶** LDL-C <100 mg/dl (2.6 mmol/l) **Moderate risk**** LDL-C <135 mg/dl (3.5 mmol/l)
		Fewer than two risk factors‖ Consider drug treatment at LDL-C >190 mg/dl (4.9 mmol/l) Goal LDL-C <160 mg/dl (4.1 mmol/l)	**Small increase in risk††** LDL-C <160 mg/dl (4.0 mmol/l)
			In diabetes mellitus the suggested target lipids levels are <100 mg/dl (2.6 mmol/l) when there is evidence of macrovascular disease, and <130 mg/dl (3.4 mmol/l) with no evidence of macrovascular disease.
General population	TC <5.0 mmol/l (193 mg/dl) LDL-C <3.0 mmol/l (116 mg/dl)	TC <200 mg/dl (5.2 mmol/l)	No goals given for the population.

*Multifactorial CHD risk is calculated from the coronary risk chart (see Figure 18.1) based on age, gender, smoking, systolic blood pressure, total cholesterol and diabetes mellitus. A high-risk individual is defined as >20% probability of developing CHD over 10 years.

†The National Cholesterol Education Program does not define targets for total cholesterol apart from a desirable blood cholesterol for the general population. For dietary therapy the initiation level of LDL-cholesterol and the initiation LDL goals are the same, but for drug treatment the consideration level of LDL is higher than the LDL goal. The LDL goals for diet and drug therapy are the same for all classes of patients.

‡Clinicians are asked to make a judgement about initiating drug treatment below 130 mg/dl (3.4 mmol/l).

§Coronary risk factors are: Age (>45 years in men and >55 years in women), a family history of premature CHD, cigarette smoking, hypertension, low levels of HDL-cholesterol (<35 mg/dl [0.9 mmol/l]) and diabetes mellitus. If a patients' HDL-cholesterol is high (>6.0 mg/dl [1.6 mmol/l]) one risk factor is subtracted from the total number of risk factors for that person.

‖In males <35 years and premenopausal women with LDL-C = 190–219 mg/dl (4.9–5.7 mmol/l) drug therapy should be delayed except in high-risk patients such as those with diabetes.

¶High risk: three or more risk factors OR two risk factors of severe degree OR major genetic hyperlipidaemia OR type 1 or 2 diabetes mellitus with microvascular complications OR absolute CHD risk†† (see below) of about 2.3% per annum (approx. 23% over 10 years) in middle-aged men.

**Moderate risk: one risk factor of severe degree OR two risk factors of moderate degree OR absolute CHD risk of 0.7% per annum (approx. 7% over 10 years) in middle-aged men OR type 1 or 2 diabetes mellitus without microvascular complications.

††Small increase in risk: one risk factor of moderate degree OR plasma cholesterol: HDL-cholesterol ratio 4–5, OR smoking about 10 cigarettes per day but no other risk factor OR absolute CHD risk of 0.3% per annum (approx 3% over 10 years) in middle-aged men.

‡‡PROCAM algorithm for risk (%) of a coronary event (sudden coronary death, definite fatal MI, definite non-fatal MI) over 8 years.

Table 18.2
A comparison of goals for diet and drug management of cholesterol in secondary and primary coronary prevention.

Goals for diet and drug management of cholesterol

Clinical trials of lipid modification by diet and different drugs have convincingly shown that CHD risk associated with rising cholesterol can be substantially reduced in both secondary and primary coronary prevention.[10–14] This risk reduction is likely to be due to the common factor of modifying lipoproteins, principally lowering LDL-cholesterol, rather than any intrinsic property of the lipid-lowering agents used. A decision to treat blood lipids with drugs depends on the absolute CHD risk as well as lipid levels, lipoprotein profile and family history of premature CHD or other atherosclerotic disease. Patients with familial hypercholesterolaemia are at such high risk of premature coronary artery disease that drug treatment is always necessary. Patients with CHD, or other atherosclerotic disease, commonly require drug treatment. Individuals who are at high CHD risk because of a combination of risk factors and whose cholesterol levels are not lowered by diet, also require drug treatment of blood lipids. A comparison of different published goals for diet and drug management of cholesterol in secondary and primary coronary prevention is given in Table 18.2. The European recommendations[5] are compared with those of the United States (National Cholesterol Education Program)[2] and an International Taskforce working in cooperation with the International Atherosclerosis Society.[6]

The European lipid goals are a total cholesterol less than 5 mmol/l (190 mg/dl) and an LDL-cholesterol level less than 3 mmol/l (115 mg/dl). These two values are recommended as goals of dietary and drug therapy for patients with CHD and for patients at high risk of developing CHD. This recommendation differs from that of all earlier guidelines

in which a range of different goals for total and LDL-cholesterol have been given depending on the degree of risk. There are two reasons for this single European recommendation. The first is pathophysiological. There is no reason to think that the atherogenicity of a given concentration of plasma cholesterol, or LDL-cholesterol, depends on whether a myocardial infarction has occurred. The second reason is simplicity. A total cholesterol of less than 5 mmol/l and an LDL-cholesterol less than 3 mmol/l are easy to remember. The accuracy of conversion to mg/dl has also been sacrificed for reasons of simplicity. A cholesterol level of 5 mmol/l equals 193 mg/dl but there is no substantial loss of biological meaning by rounding that number down to 190 mg/dl. Similarly, 3 mmol/l equals 116 mg/dl which can be rounded off to 115 mg/dl. The intensity with which these goals are pursued in primary prevention must be tempered by the calculation of absolute CHD risk. The European recommendations have chosen an absolute CHD risk of 20% as being sufficiently high to justify the use of drug therapies in primary prevention (see Figure 18.2). It is obviously more important to reach these goals in a patient with CHD or in an individual with a 10-year CHD risk greater than or equal to 20%, than it is in an individual whose 10-year risk is less than 20%. In the European recommendations the view was taken that insufficient evidence exists to justify goals for triglyceride and HDL-cholesterol levels. Instead, these measurements should be used to identify individuals at high risk of CHD. An HDL-cholesterol concentration of less than 1 mmol/l (40 mg dl) and triglyceride levels greater than 2 mmol/l (80 mg/dl) identify those at higher risk. A ratio of total cholesterol to HDL-cholesterol greater than 5 is also a marker of higher risk.

The United States (National Cholesterol

Education Program)[2] distinguish lipid levels at which drug treatment should be considered from lipid goals and, with the exception of the cholesterol goal for the whole population (<200 mg/dl or <5.2 mmol/l), only LDL-cholesterol is used. For secondary prevention, the LDL-cholesterol goal of less than 100 mg/dl (2.6 mmol/l) is slightly lower than the European one. The International Task Force (ITF) defines the same goal for secondary prevention as the NCEP.[6] There is genuine uncertainty about the value of cholesterol-modification therapy below an LDL-cholesterol level of about 116 mg/dl (3.0 mmol/l) and this may be resolved with future clinical trial results. The vast majority of coronary patients actually have a total cholesterol level greater than 190 mg/dl (5.0 mmol/l) or LDL-cholesterol level greater than 115 mg/dl (>3.0 mmol/l) and therefore most require drug therapy.[15] Therefore, the issue of whether there is a level of cholesterol below which therapy (other than diet) is not indicated, only affects a small minority of coronary patients.

For primary prevention, the principal of a high-risk approach is advocated in both the NCEP[2] and the ITF[6] but the calculation of absolute risk is more complicated. Whilst the NCEP also uses the Framingham risk function, a dichotomous approach to risk factor evaluation is used by classifying patients into those with two or more risk factors and those with fewer than two risk factors. This LDL-cholesterol goal is less than 130 mg/dl (<3.4 mmol/l) for those at highest risk and less than 160 mg/dl (<4.1 mmol/l) for those with fewer than two risk factors. The dichotomous approach to risk factor classification is disadvantaged by being less precise than estimates of risk derived from using cholesterol, and other continuous risk factors, based on actual levels. The ITF uses a combination of risk factors defined dichotomously but also an estima-tion of absolute CHD risk based on the PRO-CAM function derived from the Munster Heart Study of middle-aged men in Germany.[6] Patients are classified into high risk, moderate risk and a small increase in risk. These three risk levels correspond approximately to an absolute CHD risk of around 23%, 7% and 3%, respectively, over 10 years. The actual published risk estimates are per annum, based on a follow-up study of 8 years. For each level of risk a different LDL-cholesterol goal is defined and these are:

- high <100 mg/dl (<2.6 mmol/l);
- moderate <135 mg/dl (3.5 mmol/l);
- and small <160 mg/dl (4.0 mmol/l).

Patients with diabetes mellitus are singled out as being at particularly high risk and for those with macrovascular disease the LDL goal is less than 100 mg/dl (<2.6 mmol/l), and for those with no macrovascular disease it is less than 130 mg/dl (<3.4 mmol/l).

These international differences in goals for diet and drug management of cholesterol in coronary prevention are a function of several factors, of which scientific evidence is only one. Others include the interpretation of that evidence for clinical practice and the implications for organisation and resourcing of medical care. Unsurprisingly, different groups of experts from different parts of the world, each working in different medical systems, are going to differ to some extent in the goals they define. Importantly, these differences are small for patients with established CHD or other atherosclerotic disease. For the identification and treatment of high-risk individuals there are more differences in defining levels of risk and treatment goals, but the principal of absolute (multifactorial) risk defining intensity of treatment and use of drug therapies is common to all approaches. For sheer simplicity the European recommendations have much to commend them in defining the same simple, practical and achievable lipid goals for coronary patients and high-risk individuals — a total cholesterol level of less than 5.0 mmol/l (190 mg/dl) and an LDL-cholesterol level of less than 3.0 mmol/l (115 mg/dl) — and the coronary risk chart is also the simplest and quickest manual way to estimate coronary risk.

All patients with CHD and high-risk individuals should receive dietary advice. If the total and LDL-cholesterol goals are not achieved with lifestyle changes then drug therapy should be used. It is important to titrate up the dose of lipid-lowering therapy to achieve these goals, and certainly to use a dose no lower than the minimum used in the clinical trials that showed benefit from cholesterol-lowering therapy. There are four classes of lipid-lowering drugs: inhibitors of HMG-CoA reductase (statins), fibrates, bile acid sequestrants (resins), and nicotinic acid and its derivatives. All four classes of drugs, but not all drugs within each class, have been shown in trials to reduce myocardial infarction and sudden death. Nevertheless, the most convincing evidence from angiographic as well as clinical endpoint trials has been obtained using the most potent of the lipid-lowering drugs, namely the statins, which reduce coronary morbidity, mortality and prolong survival.[10–14] This class of drugs also has the best safety record to date and is the easiest to use. Therefore preference should be given to HMG-CoA reductase inhibitors (statins). There is also increasing evidence that statins will reduce the risk of stroke in coronary patients.[11–12] Two other large trials of secondary prevention using fibrates have recently been reported but neither showed benefit in relation to total mortality.[16,17] In addition, earlier clinical trials of fibrates have not yielded results as clear-cut as those from the statin trials.[18,19]

When starting lipid-lowering therapy the drug dose should be titrated up until the cholesterol goal is achieved. It may not be possible for all high-risk individuals to achieve this goal on diet, or with a lipid-lowering drug at the maximum dose, and therefore some will need combination drug therapy.

Clinical opportunities for coronary prevention

Physicians are in an ideal position to encourage healthy lifestyle changes in a large section of the community. The majority of people visit their doctor once a year and research has shown that doctors are considered by society to be a credible and important source of information about the causes of CHD and other atherosclerotic disease, and how these diseases can be prevented. Some doctors view health promotion and disease prevention as an integral part of their role and many patients would like their physicians to advise them on lifestyle change. Starting with patients with established CHD, or other atherosclerotic disease, physicians can facilitate all aspects of secondary prevention and rehabilitation and this will inevitably lead to contact with family members who may themselves be at high risk. Specialists in hypertension, lipids and diabetes have the same opportunity to take a multifactorial approach and address all risk factors. This will ensure that whichever risk factor is identified in a patient, the risk factor intervention will be multifactorial — not just treating blood lipids or blood pressure alone, or only aiming for glucose control in diabetes. Other specialists such as neurologists managing patients with cerebral ischaemia and infarction, or those looking after patients with peripheral arterial disease or renal disease, also have the same opportunity to broaden their assessment and management of these patients to reduce the risk of CHD and its complications. Opportunistic screening of all patients met in connection with ordinary clinical practice, whatever the reason for seeking medical advice, will yield yet more high-risk individuals for primary prevention.

In other words, opportunities for physicians to take preventative action in relation to CHD, or other atherosclerotic disease, in current clinical practice are already considerable and yet this potential is not being realised. Even in patients with established CHD, risk factor recording in medical records is incomplete and the management of risk factors such as obesity, blood pressure or blood lipids is inadequate when compared with the standards set by professional guidelines.[15,20] For many patients with hypertension, dyslipidaemia or diabetes, who are being managed with drug therapies, risk factor goals are not being reached. In their daily clinical practice physicians do not screen routinely for cardiovascular risk factors, other than blood pressure, and even when they do so, appropriate follow-up and action does not always occur.

Preventive cardiology

The organisation of preventive care for coronary patients, high-risk individuals and their families will differ from one country to another, reflecting the wide diversity of medical provision, social, economic and political factors. Therefore, it would not be appropriate to define preventive cardiology as a single model of care, but rather the common principles which differing models of care should embrace. The implementation of current scientific knowledge, as embodied in the guidance of international, continental and national bodies, ultimately depends on the organisation of medical care. Whatever the medical setting, this must be able to deliver effective lifestyle,

risk factor and therapeutic management over the long term.

So much of our scientific knowledge comes from randomised controlled trials, which are themselves models of care. Such care is driven by protocol and patients are usually seen by specialists, and at frequent intervals to ensure continuity of management. Compliance with therapy is carefully monitored, and those who do not attend, for whatever reason, are followed up. This high standard of care is usually maintained over several years in the course of a clinical trial. So the result achieved in the active treatment group is not just a function of the drug used but also the context in which it was prescribed and monitored. When translating a trial result into daily clinical practice, simply prescribing the drug is often not enough. It is also necessary to provide a model of care which emulates the care provided in the clinical trial.

Role of professional and national societies in CHD prevention

Whilst the science base that describes the origins of atherosclerosis and its clinical expression is largely common to every country, there are important differences in political, economic, cultural, social and medical traditions from one part of the world to another. Therefore, whilst there is a need for an international consensus on coronary prevention, reflecting common scientific base, the need to develop *national* guidelines on coronary prevention is essential. These will reflect both scientific evidence and, importantly, address the practicalities of coronary prevention at a population and clinical level for each country. National societies of cardiology, atherosclerosis and hypertension should take the lead in this important professional activity and, wherever appropriate, work in collaboration with members of other specialities such as cardiac rehabilitation, internal medicine and diabetes, as well as primary care physicians, other health professionals and members of heart associations and foundations. When a national society takes responsibility for developing, publishing and disseminating its own guidelines, the members of that society are more likely to read and act on them. This is particularly so if national guidelines are then incorporated into the written guidelines of an institution, department or office.

References

1. Pyörälä K, de Backer G, Graham I, et al. Prevention of coronary heart disease in clinical practice. Recommendations of the Task Force of the European Society of Cardiology, European Atherosclerosis Society and European Society of Hypertension. Eur Heart J 1994; 15:1300–31; Atherosclerosis 1994; 110: 121–61.

2. National Cholesterol Education Program. Second Report of the Expert Panel on Detection, Evaluation, and Treatment of High Blood Cholesterol in Adults (Adult Treatment Panel II). Circulation 1994; 89:1329–445.

3. Fuster V, Pearson TA. 27th Bethesda Conference: Matching the Intensity of Risk Factor Management with the Hazard for Coronary Disease Events. J Am Coll Cardiol 1996; 27:957–1047.

4. Sixth Report of the Joint National Committee on Prevention, Detection, Evaluation and Treatment of High Blood Pressure. National High Blood Pressure Education Program. National Institutes of Health. National Heart, Lung and Blood Institute; 1997. NIH Publication No. 98-4080.

5. Wood DA, de Backer G, Faergeman O, et al., on behalf of the Task Force. Prevention of coronary heart disease in clinical practice. Recommendations of the Second Joint Task Force of the European Society of Cardiology, European Atherosclerosis Society and European Society of Hypertension. Eur Heart J 1998; 19:1434–503. Atherosclerosis 1998;

140:199–270. J Hypertens 1998;16(10): 1407–14.

6. International Task Force. Coronary Heart Disease: Reducing the Risk. The scientific background for primary and secondary prevention of coronary heart disease. A worldwide view. Nutrit Metab Cardiovasc Dis 1998; 8(4):205–71.

7. Murray CJ, Lopez AD. Global mortality, disability, and the contribution of risk factors: Global Burden of Disease Study. Lancet 1997; 349:1436–42.

8. Prevention of coronary heart disease. Report of a WHO Expert Committee. WHO Technical Report Series 678. Geneva: World Health Organisation; 1982.

9. Anderson KM, Wilson PWF, Odell PM, Kanell WB. An updated coronary risk profile: A statement for health professionals. Circulation 1991; 83:356–62.

10. The Scandinavian Simvastatin Survival Study Group. Randomised trial of cholesterol lowering in 4444 patients with coronary heart disease: the Scandinavian Simvastatin Survival Study (4S). Lancet 1994; 344:1383–9.

11. Sacks FM, Pfeffer MA, Moye L, et al. The effect of Pravastatin on coronary events after myocardial infarction in patients with average cholesterol levels. N Engl J Med 1996; 335:1001–9.

12. The Long Term Intervention with Pravastatin in Ischaemic Disease (LIPID) study Group. Prevention of cardiovascular events and death with Pravastatin in patients with coronary heart disease and a broad range of initial cholesterol levels. N Engl J Med 1998; 339: 1349–57.

13. Shepherd J, Cobbe SM, Ford I, et al. Prevention of coronary heart disease with Pravastatin in men with hypercholesterolaemia. N Engl J Med 1995; 333:1301–17.

14. Downs GR, Clearfield M, Weiss S, et al. Primary prevention of acute coronary events with Lovastatin in men and women with average cholesterol levels: results of AFCAPS/TEXCAPS. Air Force/Texas Coronary Atherosclerosis Study. JAMA 1998; 279:1615–22.

15. EUROASPIRE Study Group. A European Society of Cardiology survey of secondary prevention of coronary heart disease: principal

results. European Action on Secondary Prevention through intervention to reduce events. *Eur Heart J* 1997; **18**:1569–92.

16. Rubins HB, Robins SJ, Collins D, *et al*. Gemfibrozil for the secondary prevention of coronary heart disease in men with low levels of high-density lipoprotein cholesterol. Veterans Affairs High-Density Lipoprotein Cholesterol Intervention Trial Study Group. *N Engl J Med* 1999; **341**:410–18.

17. Goldbourt U, Brunner D, Behar S, Reicher-Reiss H. Baseline characteristics of patients participating in the Bezafibrate Infarction Prevention (BIP) Study. *Eur Heart J* 1998; **19(suppl. H)**:H42–H47.

18. Report of the Committee of Principal Investigators. WHO co-operative trial on primary prevention of ischemic heart disease with clofibrate to lower serum cholesterol: Final mortality follow-up. *Lancet* 1984; **2**:600–4.

19. Frick MH, Elo O, Haapa K, *et al*. Helsinki Heart Study: Primary prevention trial with gemfibrozil in middle-aged men with dyslipidaemia; safety of treatment, changes in risk factors, and incidences of coronary heart disease. *N Engl J Med* 1987; **317**:1237–45.

20. Pearson TA, Peters TD, Feury D. The American College of Cardiology Evaluation of Preventive Therapeutics of Cardiology Evaluation of Preventive Therapeutics (ACCEPT) study; attainment of goals for comprehensive risk reduction in patients with coronary disease in the US [abstract]. *J Am Coll Cardiol* 1998; **31(suppl. AS)**:186A.

Index